## DATE DUE

| DATE DUE | |
|---|---|
| OCT 2 1 1994 | |
| JAN 2 9 1995 | |
| APR 1 0 1995 | |
| GUC-346 JUL 21/95 | |
| | |
| FEB 2 3 1996 | |
| MAY - 8 1996 | |
| Metaspina due Nov 26/99 | |
| FEB - 4 2000 | |
| NOV 2 8 2001 | |
| NOV 2 7 2003 | |
| | |
| | |
| | |

# Dual Diagnosis in Substance Abuse

# Dual Diagnosis in Substance Abuse

edited by

## Mark S. Gold
*Fair Oaks Hospital*
*Summit, New Jersey and Delray Beach, Florida*

## Andrew E. Slaby
*Fair Oaks Hospital*
*Summit, New Jersey*

*New York University*
*The Regent Hospital*
*New York, New York*

**Marcel Dekker, Inc.**          **New York • Basel • Hong Kong**

**Library of Congress Cataloging-in-Publication Data**

Dual diagnosis in substance abuse / edited by Mark S. Gold, Andrew E.
   Slaby.
         p.      cm.
      Includes bibliographical references and index.
      ISBN 0-8247-8457-X (alk. paper)
      1. Substance abuse--Diagnosis. 2. Mental illness--Diagnosis.
   3. Substance abuse--Treatment. 4. Mental illness--Treatment.
   I. Gold, Mark S. II. Slaby, Andrew Edmund.
      [DNLM: 1. Mental disorders--complications 2. Substance abuse-
   -complications. WM 270 D8125]
   RC564.D79       1991
   616.86'075--dc20
   DNLM/DLC
   for Library of Congress                                    91-16390
                                                                  CIP

This book is printed on acid-free paper.

MARCEL DEKKER, INC.
270 Madison Avenue, New York, New York 10016

Current printing (last digit):
10  9  8  7  6  5  4  3  2

PRINTED IN THE UNITED STATES OF AMERICA

# Preface

Abusers of alcohol and other substances are as varied as patients with headaches or chest pain. Not all headaches are brain tumors, and not all chest pain signifies a heart attack. The most common cause of headache is stress resulting in muscle tension. Sinus problems, migraines, and eye problems are other common causes. In some instances, headache may be due to a treatable illness that if unrecognized and unattended results in dire consequences and sometimes death. This is the case with meningiomas (tumors of the membranes surrounding the brain), subdural hematomas (blood clots on the brain), and primary tumors of the brain substance itself. In these cases, neglect can lead to severe brain damage and even death.

Lack of clinical acumen and/or economically or politically motivated desire to oversimplify diagnosis and management of substance abuse results in untold pain for patients and their families, as well as in compromised care. The cost is greatest to the young. Undiagnosed and untreated Axis I and II psychiatric disorders in this group, coupled with substance abuse, lead to enduring patterns of maladaptive coping styles: from poor coping to diminished self-esteem, and from low self-esteem, in some instances, to parasuicide and suicide. Repeated and lengthy hospitalizations of young patients due to failure to recognize early, and to treat aggressively, dual-diagnosed patients cost public and private health care systems much money and many man-hours. Dually diagnosed patients rapidly resume substance abuse if their primary psychiatric disorders are not treated. These people do not respond to the best of self-help groups, such as Cocaine Anonymous and Alcoholics Anonymous, and they account for a number of failures in nonmedical treatment centers. Some join the ranks of the homeless. Others resort to suicide.

Dual diagnosis does not simply indicate that alcohol or recreational drugs are abused concomitantly with a psychiatric disorder. Cocaine use may occur in people with preexisting paroxysmal tachycardia. Both cause panic. Both are associated at times with a feeling of impending doom which is, of course, not totally unjustified. Anorexia nervosa may be associated with steroid abuse. Both illnesses impact body-image change. Late-onset alcoholism may be associated with Alzheimer's disease; and sudden excessive use of alcohol and drugs at a younger age, with AIDS. Just because a patient presents with seizures while on amphetamines, cocaine, or meperidine does not mean that he/she does not have epilepsy.

The contributors to this volume, all experts in the topics for which they have been chosen, explore the many facets of the problem of dual diagnosis, with specific information on epidemiology, clinical presentation, and diagnostic-specific management. Specific attention is provided on treatment of dually diagnosed alcoholics, eating-disorder patients, affectively ill patients, anxiety disorder patients, schizophrenics, and neurologically impaired patients. Problems of psychopharmacotherapy and inpatient management of addiction-prone patients are addressed. Genetic trends in psychiatric illness and substance abuse are explored. A special chapter provides a discussion of the problems attendant upon the management of wealthy and famous patients with psychiatric disorders who abuse drugs as a recreational diversion.

This book is unique in its explication of dual diagnosis as a concept and its discussion of management problems peculiar to this population. The material presented here is germane to the practice of all psychiatric clinicians as well as internists, pediatricians, emergency physicians, and family practitioners. Health policymakers, school counselors, employee assistant personnel, and drug addiction researchers and counselors will also find this volume helpful.

Diagnosis is a science. Healing is an amalgam of art and science. The truly successful healer is ever aware that life is never easy but that at times it is more difficult than at others. People are not born thinking that they will be alcoholic or cocaine addicts. Nor do they posit that they will be depressed and want to kill themselves. Loss of control of power to resist drugs or alcohol begets depression. Loss of ability to fight depression, the raging fires of mania, or the hellish torment of racing, disorganized thoughts in schizophrenia can lead to substance abuse. To disentangle the web of human action and reaction in the envelope of social press entails diagnostic sophistication, empathy, sensitivity, and acute awareness that we could someday be like those we treat. We are all human. We all carry genetic and psychological vulnerabilities. This book places the person and the illness in a perspective that facilitates recognition of the role of various contributing factors to patients' problems and provides a framework for humane treatment.

Mark S. Gold
Andrew E. Slaby

# Contributors

**William J. Annitto, M.D.**  Greenbrook Academy, Bound Brook, New Jersey

**Carolyn M. Bell, M.S.W., L.I.C.S.W.**  Harvard Medical School at The Cambridge Hospital, Cambridge, Massachusetts

**Peter M. Bolo, M.D.**  Fair Oaks Hospital, Summit, New Jersey

**Ricardo Castaneda, M.D.**  New York University School of Medicine, New York, New York

**J. Calvin Chatlos, M.D.**  St. Mary Hospital, Hoboken, New Jersey

**Charles Ciolino, M.D.**  Fair Oaks Hospital, Overlook Hospital, and The Summit Medical Group, Summit, New Jersey

**James A. Cocores, M.D.**  Fair Oaks Hospital, Summit, New Jersey

**Gregory B. Collins, M.D.**  The Cleveland Clinic Foundation, Cleveland, Ohio

**William Coryell, M.D.**   University of Iowa, Iowa City, Iowa

**Charles A. Dackis, M.D.**   Hampton Hospital, Rancocas, New Jersey

**Irl L. Extein, M.D.**   Fair Oaks Hospital at Boca/Delray, Delray Beach, Florida

**Marc Galanter, M.D.**   New York University School of Medicine, New York, New York

**A. James Giannini, M.D.**   The Ohio State University, Columbus, Ohio

**Mark S. Gold, M.D.**   Fair Oaks Hospital, Summit, New Jersey and Delray Beach, Florida

**Edward J. Khantzian, M.D.**   Harvard Medical School at The Cambridge Hospital, Cambridge, Massachusetts; and Danvers State Hospital, Danvers, Massachusetts

**Larry Kirstein, M.D.**   The Regent Hospital, New York, New York

**Stuart F. Kushner, M.D.**   Fair Oaks Hospital, Summit, New Jersey

**Norman S. Miller, M.D.**   Cornell University Medical College, White Plains, New York

**Robert Moreines, M.D.**   Fair Oaks Hospital, Summit, New Jersey

**Michael M. Newman, M.D.**   Fair Oaks Hospital, Summit, New Jersey

**Charles R. Norris, Jr., M.D.**   Fair Oaks Hospital at Boca/Delray, Delray Beach, Florida

**Andrew E. Slaby, M.D., Ph.D., M.P.H.**   Fair Oaks Hospital, Summit, New Jersey; New York University and The Regent Hospital, New York, New York

**Judith B. Tufaro, M.A., CAC**   Fair Oaks Hospital, Summit, New Jersey

# Contents

*Preface*                                                                  *iii*
*Contributors*                                                             *vii*

**Introduction**

1.  Dual Diagnosis: Fact or Fiction?                                         3
    *Andrew E. Slaby*

2.  Genetics and Dual Diagnosis                                             29
    *William Coryell*

**Clinical Presentation**

3.  Substance Abuse and Anxiety Disorders                                   45
    *Peter M. Bolo*

4.  Substance Abuse and Thought Disorders                                   57
    *A. James Giannini and Gregory B. Collins*

5.  Substance Abuse and Neurological Disorders                              75
    *Stuart F. Kushner*

6.  Substance Abuse and Mood Disorders                                     105
    *Charles Ciolino*

7.   Substance Abuse and Anorexia Nervosa and Bulimia Nervosa        117
     *Michael M. Newman*

8.   Marijuana and Psychopathology                                   127
     *A. James Giannini*

9.   Studies of Prevalence of Dual Diagnosis in Psychiatric Practice  139
     *Marc Galanter and Ricardo Castaneda*

10.  Diagnosing Dual Diagnosis Patients                              159
     *Charles R. Norris, Jr. and Irl L. Extein*

11.  Drug Use and Addiction as Self-Medication:
     A Psychodynamic Perspective                                     185
     *Carolyn M. Bell and Edward J. Khantzian*

12.  Psychopathology Resulting from Substance Abuse                  205
     *Charles A. Dackis and Mark S. Gold*

**Treatment**

13.  Treatment of the Dually Diagnosed Alcoholic                     223
     *Norman S. Miller and Mark S. Gold*

14.  Treatment of the Dually Diagnosed Adult Drug User               237
     *James A. Cocores*

15.  Treatment of the Dually Diagnosed Adolescent                    253
     *J. Calvin Chatlos and Judith B. Tufaro*

16.  Treating the "High and Mighty" and the "Mighty High"            289
     *William J. Annitto and Mark S. Gold*

17.  Problems with Inpatient Treatment of Substance Abuse
     Patients with Primary Psychiatric Diagnosis                     297
     *Robert Moreines*

18.  Pharmacotherapy and the Dual Diagnosis Patient                  319
     *Larry Kirstein*

*Index*                                                              *337*

# Dual Diagnosis in Substance Abuse

# INTRODUCTION

# 1

## Dual Diagnosis: Fact or Fiction?

**Andrew E. Slaby**

*Fair Oaks Hospital, Summit, New Jersey; New York University, and The Regent Hospital, New York, New York*

Dual diagnosis, simply defined, refers to the concurrence of two separate diagnostic entities in one person. In the area of substance abuse, this means that a substance abuse disorder such as alcoholism occurs together with a psychiatric disorder such as major depression or panic disorder. In most situations, there are actually many concurrent diagnoses. A cocaine user, for example, frequently uses alcohol or heroin to come down. If the same person has a bipolar disorder, he/she would have at least three separate disorders: cocaine abuse, heroin or alcohol abuse, and bipolar disorder. In this chapter, I will discuss how a diagnosis may be confused by the simultaneous occurrence of both a substance abuse disorder and a psychiatric disorder as well as by other substance abuse disorders or medical disorders either induced by substance abuse or occurring independently. Emphasis will be on what is known epidemiologically and clinically of dual diagnosis. Unfortunately, the instability of this patient population over time makes it difficult to follow the group for outcomes of treatment except for those who have a psychiatric disorder that they are self-medicating. The self-medicating group does quite well if the psychiatric disorder is recognized and given diagnostic-specific treatment negating need for further self-medication with recreational drugs. Research into clinical presentation and course of use of recreational drugs is further complicated even in a stable population by the fact that substance abusers often do not know the drug they have taken with any degree of certainty and in most cases do not know the dose or contaminants.

Want of clinical acumen, as well as economically or politically motivated desire to oversimplify diagnosis and management of substance abuse, leads to untold pain for patients and families and to compromised quality of care. Cost is greatest to the young, where concomitant undiagnosed and treated Axis I and II psychiatric disorders, coupled with substance abuse, contribute to the genesis of enduring patterns of maladaptive coping styles and diminished self-esteem. Unrecognized dual-diagnosed patients drain both public and private health care systems by repeated and lengthy hospitalizations. These individuals rapidly resume substance abuse after discharge and fail to comport to treatment plans. These people do not respond to the best of self-help groups such as Alcoholics Anonymous, Narcotics Anonymous, and Cocaine Anonymous. Some join the ranks of the homeless.

As many as 74% of psychiatric inpatients reportedly have abused substances [2]. Thirteen percent consistently abuse drugs other than alcohol. Frank alcoholism occurs in 8.7–17.1% of general medical patients [2]. Psychiatric patients admitted without diagnosed substance abuse problems have been found to differ from medical/surgical controls in quantity and frequency of drug use and problems associated with the drug used [2].

One of the principal clues to differentiating drug users with major psychiatric illness from those whose symptoms are primarily a response to drug abuse is onset of symptoms [3]. Patients with a long history of deterioration prior to hospitalization, as measured by duration of psychotic symptoms, previous psychopharmacotherapy, and poor occupational adjustment, are more likely to be dual-diagnosed. Pattern of drug use and presence or absence of violence does not have as great diagnostic significance [4]. Double depression (i.e., major depressive disorder superimposed on dysthymic disorder) occurs in this population and poses special problems. The double depression group exhibits significantly greater alcohol and amphetamine use [5]. Since both forms of depression are generally antidepressant respondent, identification of this subpopulation can lead to successful treatment of all three disorders: major depression, dysthymia, and substance abuse. Psychic suffering accompanying substance abuse, coupled with psychopathology, results in interpersonal difficulties and impaired social adjustment, contributing to a misimpression of a schizophrenic rather than an affective process [6].

The majority of patients with psychiatric problems are attended by primary care providers rather than mental health professionals, contributing in part to the appalling fact that only about 19% of those affected have been provided help for psychiatric disorders in the previous six months [7]. The impression of many nonpsychiatric health care providers is that substance abuse disorders are different from psychiatric disorders and should receive differential referral. After all, why are there three separate institutes at the National Institute of Health: the National Institute of Mental Health (NIMH), the National Institute of Drug Abuse (NIDA), and the National Institute of Alcoholism and Alcohol Abuse (NIAAA). Specialist, if not subspecialist, care is required to determine the role recreational drugs, concomitant medical and surgical illness, psychosocial variables, and preexistent or precipitated Axis I and Axis II psychiatric disorders play in the development of the clinical picture. Psychiatric disorders, medical disorders, and substance abuse disorders must be independently identified and differentially treated to reduce repeated and lengthy future hospitalizations. Both a differential diagnosis and a differential treatment plan must be elaborated.

## SEXUAL DYSFUNCTION AND OTHER CONCURRENT MEDICAL PROBLEMS

Problems in sexual drive and/or performance frequently precede or correlate with substance abuse. These merit special discussion because, unlike many other medical problems, including the changes in hormonal function with alcoholism that lead to feminization, sexual dysfunction is more frequently due to psychological reasons than organic disease. As the old adage goes, alcohol increases desire but decreases performance. Actually, a small amount of *spiritus fermenti* was once recommended in *The Merck Manual* to overcome inhibitions that entrapped Victorian desire.

There are a number of ways in which drugs and alcohol impact sexual performance:

1. Sexual dysfunction may be a direct side effect of a drug.
2. Stress may lead independently to both sexual dysfunction and substance abuse.
3. Drug abuse may result from anxiety over sexual performance or lack of it.
4. Substance abuse may represent an attempt to self-medicate the primary psychiatric disorder.
5. Poor judgment attendant upon psychiatric disorders such as schizophrenia or medical disorders such as Alzheimer's disease or AIDS dementia may result in substance abuse.
6. Guilt over sexual prowess (e.g., multiple extramarital liaisons) may engender substance abuse.
7. Substance abuse may result from a pattern of socializing required to

meet sexual partners, as in the instance of depressed married men and
women seeking homosexual companionship at gay bars.
8.  Impotence or decreased libido may be entirely independent of drug use
    and due to physical and psychological factors that represent neither a
    drug effect nor a major psychiatric illness.

Drug-associated impotence has been reported to be as high as 25% [8].
Chronic airflow obstruction can occur contemporaneously with psychiatric
problems and drug use, particularly alcoholism and inhalant abuse. Alcohol
abuse is frequently seen in older age groups and in heavy smokers. Emphy-
sema with air hunger is common in both groups. Of 50 consecutive patients
with chronic lung disease in one study assessed both medically and psychiatrically, 58% were found to suffer panic and 34% other anxiety disorders [9].
The role substance abuse and other psychiatric symptoms plays in this
group, as with impotence, is complex. Substance abuse may represent a
response to anxiety associated with the illness. In other instances, a person
may self-medicate the anxiety that is a symptom of air hunger occurring
with chronic lung disease. In both instances, inhalant use or crack smoking
may have contributed to lung problems. Finally, an independent psychiatric
disorder (e.g., panic disorder) may coexist with substance abuse and pulmonary disease. Occurrence of three independent diagnoses, as in the case of
alcoholism, panic disorder *not due to chronic airway obstruction*, and em-
physema, is an example of triple rather than dual diagnosis. The addition of
yet a fourth diagnosis, such as antisocial personality on Axis II, would result
in a quadruple diagnosis [10].
    Substance abuse is associated with a number of medical conditions that
challenge even the most seasoned diagnostician. Historically, various forms
of syphilis and tuberculosis confused all psychiatric pictures. Syphilis
presents as general paresis, cerebrovascular syphilis, meningovascular syphilis, gummas, and tabes dorsalis. Tuberculosis causes tuberculomas, cerebral
abscesses, tubercular meningitis, and the general neurasthenia associated
with pulmonary and other forms of tuberculosis. Today, AIDS complicates
the picture in a myriad of ways, ranging from depression in subclinical
AIDS prior to confirmation by seroassay to AIDS dementia. Hepatitis,
cirrhosis, and other liver diseases are associated with mood change [1].
    Cocaine causes a number of cardiovascular changes, in addition to pul-
monary and upper respiratory problems [1]. Skin and systemic infections are
common sequelae of intravenous drug use. Drug abusers may present with
bilateral pyopneumothoraces and bacteria from jugular vein self-injection
[11]. Factors impacting on the occurrence of medical and dental complications include adulterants present when a drug is taken, nonsterile needles,
overdose tolerance, extant dependence and withdrawal, life-style of drug

user, and age of drug user [12]. Trauma is common with substance use. Unilateral or bilateral subdural hematomas from falls while intoxicated may present solely as depression or may be entirely overlooked because continued intoxication obfuscates recognition on exam in the absence of obvious clinical signs such as a unilateral dilated pupil. As serum alcohol level rises, the risk of any form of accident increases [13]. History of trauma may be a clue to undiagnosed alcohol abuse. Laboratory findings (e.g., elevated GGPT) appear to have a high sensitivity only with more chronic alcoholics and those who have ingested alcohol in the previous 24 hours [1,12].

Psychiatric symptoms reported as complications of AIDS and the AIDS-related complex (ARC) mimic a number of psychiatric disorders and precede seropositivity for HIV. These range from mild chronic dysphoria to acute psychosis. Early symptoms resemble those of advanced cocaine psychosis [14]. Both frequently appear in the same population, confusing the diagnostic picture. Agitation, panic attacks, anorexia, delusions, disorientation, insomnia, hallucinations, depression, impaired memory, and dysattention are reported. Seizures and tachycardia are also seen. Organicity should be suspected in all patients known to be seropositive. Intravenous drug users are the HIV-positive subpopulation that is most rapidly expanding. Heroin and cocaine are the preferred drugs for intravenous use [15]. In the population of IV drug users, acting out behavior due to central nervous system AIDS infection may be seen as sociopathy. In alcoholics, both young and old alike, the fluctuating consciousness of CNS HIV infection may be misconstrued as alcohol withdrawal delirium, and AIDS dementia as alcoholic dementia or Alzheimer's disease, depending on the age of the patient [16].

## DUAL DIAGNOSIS AND ALCOHOL ABUSE

### Alcoholism and Affective Disorders

Uncomplicated alcohol abuse is common only during the initial stages of drinking [1,12]. As desire to drink progresses, so too does frequency of dual or multiple diagnoses, complicating the picture. Therefore, it is rare to see an alcoholic who abuses only alcohol. Multiple drug use is more common [1]. In the final stages, the mental status picture represents the interaction of a number of acute and chronic factors such as delirium and intoxication superimposed on dementia and the other CNS consequences and liver failure.

Depression is usually present. The critical clinical question is not whether a depressed alcoholic suffering the psychosocial consequences of chronic substance abuse is feeling worthless and helpless but rather whether he or she has a treatable affective disorder and whether that affective illness preceded alcoholism. In the later instance, the drinking may represent self-medication of dysthymia.

The relationship between alcoholism and depression has long fomented debate. Schuckit feels this is due to confusing drinking, alcohol problems, and alcoholism on the one hand and sadness, secondary depression, and affective disorders on the other. Of the 80-90% of Americans who drink at some time during their lives, 10-30% develop alcohol-related problems. Only 8-10% of men and 3-5% of women, however, go beyond alcohol problems in their drinking to meet criteria for the diagnosis of alcoholism [17-19]. Many heavy drinkers are remorseful over the social and economic ramifications of their intemperance. Only a fraction of these have significant affective illness requiring more than detoxification and nonmedical rehabilitation. The group with both alcoholism and affective disorders requires greater deployment of medical resources for diagnostic-specific treatment in order to successfully avoid exacerbation of illness and consequences of untreated major affective illness. While one-third of alcoholic patients experience depressive symptoms, only 1-3% of alcoholic men are reported to suffer major depressive disorder [20].

The greater incidence of depressive symptoms as opposed to depressive illness found in actively drinking alcoholics is attributed to the physiological symptoms of withdrawal, the apathy of the alcoholic personality, the state of chronic intoxication, and concomitant drug use [21]. Severity of symptoms independent of affective illness is positively correlated with worse prognosis, suicide, and treatment attrition. For instance, a comparison of nondepressed and depressed alcoholics indicated that the latter have longer histories of problem drinking, more previous treatment for alcoholic misuse, more difficulty controlling alcohol consumption, more mental problems, and more physical symptoms related to alcohol abuse. They have a detached interpersonal style, distracted cognition, alienated self-image, and mixed depressed-anxious emotionality [22].

A number of clues facilitate identification of primary depression (antedating onset of alcoholism) and secondary depression. There is more impairment in patients with primary depression than in those with the secondary or concurrent type [20]. Age of onset and length of illness are two other factors discriminating primary from secondary depression; primary affective illness tends to last longer and have an earlier age of onset. Patients with depression secondary to alcoholism when compared to patients with depression secondary to nonsubstance abuse disorders, excluding schizophrenia, report less severe depression and tend to be predominately male [23].

Family history is important in identifying primary as opposed to secondary depression. Relatives of probands with subtypes of primary affective illness other than bipolar show a greater incidence of alcoholism in addition to affective illness [24]. Data are inconclusive. Other genetic studies indicate that depressives without alcoholism do not transmit alcoholism, while those with both alcoholism and depression transmit both, suggesting that alcoholism and depression are not manifestations of the same disease process [25]. Anxiety disorders are found more frequently in relatives of probands with alcoholism, suggesting self-medication in selected cases [26]. Families with a high incidence of alcoholism exhibit more dysthymic disorder and secondary depression rather than primary major affective illness.

A dose-response relationship between level of depression and alcohol consumption in alcoholic and nonalcoholic women has not been demonstrated. Personality disorder and anxiety level appear more influential. An inverse relationship between depressive symptoms and alcohol consumption exists among healthy women. Nonalcoholic dysthymic women consume significantly more alcohol than major depressive, subclinically depressed, and psychotic nondepressive women and less than the healthy nondepressed population. There is no difference in consumption among major depressive, dysthymic, and other diagnostic groups among alcoholic women. Progression of alcoholism is related to progression of depressive symptoms and correlated with increasing dementia in older age groups [27].

Groups at highest risk for the dual diagnosis of affective illness and alcoholism are females ages 20 through 30, individuals not presently married [28], and patients of low social class [29]. Family history of alcoholism or behavior associated with alcoholism does not differentiate primary alcoholics, alcoholism with secondary affective disorder, and primary affective disorder with secondary alcoholism. The three groups do differ, however, in past personal history and family history of affective disorder and time spent in hospital for both alcoholism and affective disorder. Risk is greater with patients with anxiety disorders and antisocial personality [30,32]. Higher prevalence in the latter group may relate to concomitant factors such as young age and more familial psychopathology, drug use, and subjective anger.

Alcoholics have reason to be depressed. They experience family disintegration, poor social and work role performance, and a myriad of medical problems. Infections, pancreatitis, cirrhosis, and arthritic diseases may themselves contribute to depression [33,34].

In a study of 49 severely depressed alcoholics, 80% with an initial major depression by Research Diagnostic Criteria were no longer depressed two weeks after cessation of drinking, indicating need for at least two weeks of sobriety prior to use of antidepressant therapy [35,36]. Chronic ethanol ingestion may lead to disturbance of the diurnal rhythm of cortisol secretion or stimulation of the adrenocortical activity, raising plasma cortisol levels in chronic alcoholics that is positively correlated with manifest depression [37].

The dexamethasone suppression test (DST) may facilitate rational selection of the subpopulation of alcoholics who will benefit from antidepressant therapy, but false positive results exist with this test [38]. False positives result from hepatic enzyme induction, acute alcoholic withdrawal associated with hypercortisolism and Cushing's disease.

Prognosis of alcoholic patients with affective illness is better if diagnostic-specific treatment is provided for the mood disorder [28]. Incidence of severity of depressive symptoms is greater in alcoholics who relapse than in the general population [39–41]. Debilitating depressive symptoms may first emerge in periods of abstinence. A study of 72 alcoholics abstaining a mean of 64 months revealed a 15% incidence of depressive symptoms beginning after a mean of 35 months of sobriety [42]. Rate for relapse was higher in the symptomatic group. Lithium reduces alcoholic abuse but not depressive symptoms in this group [43]. It is hypothesized that the group that benefits most is cyclothymic, with alcohol abuse exacerbated in the hypomanic rather than depressed phase. Other studies confirm that past psychiatric history is predictive of outcome in both alcoholics and narcotic addicts [44].

Depressive symptoms, as opposed to depressive illness, decrease markedly without treatment as patients progress from active drinking to abstinence [45]. Symptomatic mood changes without affective disorder may relate to major physiologic changes attendant upon alcohol use that abate as drinking ceases, with a concomitant decrease in depressive symptoms. Regardless of what the depressive symptoms relate to, however, depression as measured by the Beck Depression Inventory and Hamilton Psychiatric Rating Scale for Depression in alcoholics directly correlates with self-reports of previous suicide attempts [46,47]. Numerous other studies document the incidence of depression and depressive symptoms among alcoholics [48].

Impact of antidepressants on depression associated with alcoholism is contingent on whether the mood change represents true affective disorder rather than psychological response to a person's feeling out of control with his or her drug use in the absence of genetic predisposition and subsequent manifestation of a DSM-III-R mood disorder. In the absence of diagnostic-specific indications, there is little evidence of efficacy [49].

Psychosocial support mollifies depression associated with perceived consequences of alcoholism [50]. Reordering the social and personal life of the alcoholic and reinforcing valued nondrinking social ties the alcoholic has developed serves to reduce the depression in those without true affective illness. Patients who have a history of drinking primarily to facilitate social aspects of their lives are most likely to have residual depressive symptoms after treatment of alcoholism, indicating need to work aggressively with these patients to develop alternate means of social interaction.

## Alcoholism and Nonaffective Psychiatric Disorders

Less attention has been afforded to concurrence of alcoholism and other psychiatric disorders except for the anxiety disorders already mentioned. Affective illness and anxiety disorders are far more prevalent, and therefore their relationship to alcoholism is easier to study than illnesses with significantly lower prevalence.

Alcoholism is a significant problem for schizophrenic patients [51] but not to the reported degree for mood-disordered patients [52]. Studies of monozygotic and dizygotic twins indicate that alcoholism and schizophrenia are more common in the monozygotic group, suggesting that individuals suffering from both schizophrenia and alcoholism have a genetic predisposition to both disorders of the same nature as that which occurs when alcoholism and schizophrenia appear alone. Schuckit points out that primary alcoholism can mimic almost any psychiatric disorder and that secondary alcoholism can exacerbate any psychiatric symptoms [19].

Diagnoses of character disorders are particularly difficult among alcoholics. This is in part due to the fact that Axis II diagnoses are not as devastating to the integrity of the personality, and therefore may be obfuscated by substance abuse. Alcohol intensifies the moroseness of a depressive and the anxiety of those with anxiety disorders. In a disorder, such as antisocial personality, drinking generally accompanies a behavior pattern that, in the absence of the personality disorder, could be attributed to the drinking alone. Rigorous criteria are required to document the existence of an antisocial personality [19] including, at a minimum, difficulty in at least four life areas, namely, problems with family, peers, school, and police, commencing before age sixteen. By these criteria, approximately 10–20% of male and 5–10% of female alcoholics suffer antisocial personality disorders. These individuals bear a more negative prognosis than those whose difficulty with the law is solely alcohol-related.

Public intoxication, belligerence, driving under the influence, and other alcohol-related crimes generally disappear upon cessation of drinking and are not part of an enduring pattern of antisocial behavior [19]. Because anxiety and insomnia may persist for three to six months following cessation of alcohol use, anxiolytics and hypnotics with any addicting properties should be avoided. This is done to avoid dependency and because anxiolytics and hypnotics seldom maintain effectiveness after two to four weeks, lending to abuse to maintain effect [19]. Nonmedical approaches such as no caffeine after 3 P.M., going to bed and arising at fixed times without any daytime napping regardless of how little sleep was achieved, and use of relaxation techniques such as meditation and self-hypnosis should be prescribed.

The distinction between alcoholic hallucinosis and paranoia and schizophrenia is particularly important. Schizophrenia has a decidedly worse outcome. Alcoholic paranoia and hallucinosis, on the other hand, frequently clears within days or months, regardless of treatment [19]. Embryopathy is greater among offspring of alcoholic than nonalcoholic mothers [53]. Many of the psychiatric disorders seen with alcohol use are the expected depression attendant upon use, which disappears upon cessation of drinking; the occurrence of specific alcohol-related psychiatric disorders such as delirium tremens and paranoia [54]; and what we perceive to be personality disorders [55,56].

Personality disorders may be partially conditioned by the need to secret alcohol as well as to deny alcoholism in order to maintain an amiable relationship at work and with family. Studies of families of alcoholics have failed to demonstrate increased risk for schizophrenia. Family members of schizophrenics are rarely alcoholic [19].

A number of provocative findings reported in the literature merit further investigation. One is that the level of an alcoholic proband's subjective anger is more closely associated with alcoholism than antisocial personality [31]. Another is the finding that while antisocial personality and substance use disorders are common psychopathologics among male alcoholics, major depression and phobias are common among female alcoholics [57–59]. In women, psychiatric disorders often appear to precede alcohol abuse or dependence. In men, however, with the exception of antisocial personality and panic disorder, psychopathology usually occurs subsequent to alcohol use. Other studies [60] indicated that phobias and non-confrontational personality disorders precede abuse of alcohol. Drinking tends to relieve the distress. For both men and women, alcoholism coupled with antisocial personality or drug abuse has a poor prognosis [61–63]. Major depression with alcoholism is associated with a better outcome.

## Alcoholism and Organic Mental Syndromes

Concurrent psychiatric disorders and alcohol abuse are only part of the diagnostic dilemma of dual diagnosis and alcoholism. Chronic and sporadic excess alcohol drinking is associated with more physical problems than other substance abuse. Falls lead to subdural hematomas with organic mental syndromes; sudden cessation of use may result in delirium tremens with seizures. Indiscriminate hetero- and homosexual behavior at times of intoxication leads to AIDs and other sexually transmitted diseases, with their attendant psychiatric syndromes (e.g., AIDS dementia and delirium). Nerve cells die with chronic abuse, leading to alcoholic dementia and peripheral neuropathies mimicking hysterical paralysis. Neglect of diet leads to

Wernicke's encephalopathy and a host of other deficiency diseases associated with changes in mental status.

Chronic alcoholism is a potentially treatable cause of dementia [1,64]. Thiamine deficiency is etiologic in development of Korsakoff's psychosis, the chronic component of the Wernicke–Korsakoff syndrome. Amnesia with relative preservation of other cognitive functions is its most striking feature. Confabulation occurs early. Alcohol dementia, a more global syndrome than Korsakoff's, occurs on autopsy in about two-thirds of patients with alcohol changes in the brain. Cortical atrophy and reduced cerebral blood fluid are found. While end-stage dementia is unremittable, abstinence produces some resolution in less chronic cases if detected early [64]. Neuropsychological impairment appearing upon cessation of drinking becomes less pronounced with continued abstinence [66]. Early remission is attributed to reversal of cerebrospinal fluid acidosis, to other ionic imbalances, and to inhibition of brain protein synthesis. Changes occurring over a longer period include increases in dendritic arborization and glial tissue. As much as two years may be required for reversal of sleep disturbances and electroencephalographic abnormalities. Short-term memory, visual motor performance, and general intellectual functioning all improve [66]. In addition to the Wernicke–Korsakoff syndrome and alcohol dementia, an undetermined number of adult alcoholics suffer the residual form of the attention deficit hyperactivity disorder (ADHD). Some feel that the diagnostic criteria for Wernicke's encephalopathy (confusion, ophthalmoplegia, and ataxia) are too rigid, thereby missing a number who have the disease at necropsy who might have been successfully treated if the disease had been identified early. One of the criteria is absence of any other cause of dementia deemed sufficient for the diagnosis [66].

Seizures are a predictable occurrence with abrupt discontinuation of alcohol intake. Alcohol also lowers the seizure threshold for those with epilepsy. Nearly half of the seizures occur 13 to 24 hours after cessation of use [67]. Therefore, seizures in an alcoholic may be due to cessation of use just as they may be due to excess use of cocaine or amphetamines and *not* represent a separate diagnostic entity.

Alcohol and drug use per se do not lead to AIDS; sharing needles and careless sexual behavior under the influence do. Alcohol and other drugs, however, are known to inhibit the immune system and, therefore, may play a contributing role by impairing initial resistance to the virus. AIDS can present with insomnia, abulia, anhedonia, psychomotor retardation, dysmnesia, anorexia, weight loss, mania, command hallucinations and persecutory delusions mimicking schizophrenia, alcoholic paranoia, and affective illness [68]. The course may be quite prolonged with only subtle changes and may be masked by alcohol use.

Changes in blood pressure and in the heart lead to hypertension and congestive heart failure, both of which can mimic a number of anxiety disorders [69–71]. The Los Angeles Heart Study revealed mean blood pressure of heavy drinkers to be significantly higher than that of light drinkers and nondrinkers. In the Framingham study, rate of hypertension was twice that of nondrinkers [70]. Alcohol-induced blood pressure increase is one of the treatable causes of hypertension [71]. Level of gamma gluytamy/transference (GGPT), an enzyme particularly sensitive to ingestion of alcohol, is related to high blood pressure [72].

Alcohol-induced liver and bone diseases all produce illnesses that may compound the diagnoses of alcohol-induced mental changes [75,76]. Acute and chronic hepatic disease is associated with lethargy and depression.

## DUAL DIAGNOSIS: DRUG USE/AFFECTIVE ILLNESS

Rates of major depressive disorder, scores on depression scales, and rates of self-reported suicide attempts increase progressively with increased use of licit (tobacco, alcohol, and psychotropics without prescription) and illicit substances [77]. A number of depressive scales have been evaluated for relative sensitivity and specificity in detecting depression in substance abusers. On the whole, sensitivity is good (65–94%). Specificity is less impressive (39–61%). Rounsaville et al. [62] have found the 13-item patient self-report the most specific and sensitive test for depression and recommend it for screening for depression in substance abusers. Substance abuse is a particular problem among young patients, particularly young adult chronic patients [78]. Persistent substance abusers have psychiatric hospitalization rates twice as high as patients who are former users or nonusers. Abuse of drugs, in fact, frequently precedes hospitalization. That these patients tend to deny use underscored need for urine and serum screens of all young adult chronic patients to identify and treat substance abuse and minimize readmission. Safer [78] reports that 45% of this subpopulation have been hospitalized three or more times; 60–73% are unemployed. More than 50% receive government assistance; 24–41% have adult criminal records; and 34–50% have documented substance abuse. The young adult chronic population is currently responsible for considerably more community problems than it was in the past. Young handicapped men as a group show more depression and alcohol- and drug-related problems than matched controls, highlighting need for particular care in assessment and treatment of this group [79].

Depression and/or substance abuse are commonly found in eating-disorder patients. Hatsukami and her group [40,41] evaluated 108 women who met DSM-III criteria for bulimia and found that 43.5% had a history of affective illness and 18.5% a history of alcohol or drug abuse. Approximately 56% of the bulimics scored within the moderate-to-severe range of depression on the Beck Depression Inventory. The relationship between affective and eating disorders is a concern of some controversy. On the one hand, it is clear that a significant number of patients with bulimia and/or anorexia respond to antidepressants. On the other hand, people who fear that they cannot achieve a body image to comport with their fantasized ideal may feel that they have reason to be depressed. That greater than one-half of patients with bulimia have been found to have positive dexamethasone suppression tests (DSTs), a rate comparable to that found in patients with major depression, along with the reported high incidence of affective illness in first-degree relatives, suggests a relationship between the two illnesses. Substance abuse in this group is not limited to alcohol and recreational drugs. Marijuana, cathartics, diuretics, and steroids are also abused. The subpopulation of bulimic patients with both substance abuse and affective disorder show a higher incidence of attempted suicide and more social problems [41].

Schizophrenics may have particularly bizarre patterns of substance abuse, given their disorganized thinking. In one study [80], it was found schizophrenics who abused drugs had an earlier age of onset than those who did not. Drugs may have been taken in response to the mounting stress of an incipient psychotic deterioration or may have precipitated it. Low intelligence and academic difficulties are also correlated with early onset and may also contribute to the apparent link between substance abuse and early onset.

Patients with borderline personality are another group at high risk for substance abuse. This group is more pathologic than nonborderline substance abusers, [81] showing more depression, poorer impulse control, impaired reality testing, and antisocial tendencies.

Medical problems compound the picture of any substance abuse disorder. This is particularly true of AIDS which, perforce, is higher in intravenous drug and other substance abusers as well as in patients who experiment with both drugs and sex. The manifestations of AIDS, both medically and psychiatrically, are as legend as those of tuberculosis and syphilis [82]. All organ systems may be impacted by drugs. Even the eyes may be a site of drug absorption or suffer neurologic or vascular damage due to specific drug effects [83–84].

While patients with major psychiatric disorders and substance abuse are in need of more intensive inpatient and outpatient treatment, they more frequently drop out of treatment [85,86]. Outpatient management for the 21–39% of patients with substance abuse disorders who have a concurrent diagnosis usually of a personality disorder, affective illness, or psychosis is particularly problematic [85]. These patients often demand irregular discharges from the hospital, present only partially committed to treatment, and are seen in emergency rooms after failure in standard treatment programs. High symptom level for other disorders is correlated with treatment failure in both outpatient and inpatient settings [85]. These factors have contributed to a therapeutic nihilism that has limited access of dually diagnosed patients to many treatment programs, creating an untested impression that nothing is available to treat this group successfully.

It is true that the patients with more severe psychiatric disorders evince lower levels of improvement [86]. Figures substantiating this fact, however, come from nonmedical programs or treatment centers where limited attention is paid to diagnostic-specific interventions for patients with concurrent DSM-III-R disorders. Traditional nonmedical treatment centers cannot handle such patients. A patient who is accepted and not treated for the concurrent diagnosis frequently fails to improve and is seen as "not committed to treatment." When these patients are included in studies of outcome of inpatient care, it appears that neither inpatient nor outpatient treatment works. Demonstrating differential treatment impact requires a structured medical inpatient program with treatment tailored to individual patient needs. This is especially true for an adolescent population, where patterns of use are less enduring and personality development is in a sufficiently formative stage to allow greater impact. There is, in fact, some evidence to suggest that the severity of psychiatric symptoms and poor treatment outcome is less highly correlated with adolescents than it is with adults.

## DUAL DIAGNOSIS: DRUG USE/SCHIZOPHRENIA

Unusual drug use patterns are seen in schizophrenia. Disorganized and delusional thinking in this group contributes both to bizarre patterns of use as well as to less used routes of administration (e.g., eye, penis, vagina) [1,12]. Certain drugs enhance symptoms of the primary illness or may, in fact, perfectly simulate functional psychosis. Cocaine, amphetamines, and other stimulants create a paranoid psychosis in a clear sensorium that perfectly simulates paranoid disorder and paranoid schizophrenia. Phencyclidine (PCP), in fact, not only creates a paranoid psychosis but is also associated with considerable violence, which may be incorrectly attributed to the schizophrenia, enhancing the stigma associated with the disorder. Fortunately, while there is considerable experimentation among chronic psychiatric patients with stimulants, alcohol, marijuana, and hypnotic sedatives, only a small number actually use PCP [87]. Hallucinogens, on the other hand, do not create psychoses that truly simulate schizophrenia. Drugs like LSD, psilocybin ("mushrooms"), mescaline, and peyote ("cactus buttons") evoke chemical psychoses with characteristic hallucinogenic distortions of perception such as synesthesias (a condensation of two sensations); for instance, a person will "taste" green or "smell" gray. These symptoms suggest concurrent or sole use of a hallucinogenic drug when a patient presents psychotic. The picture in some patients remains sufficiently complex to render a number of LSD psychoses indistinguishable from acute schizophrenia. In one study of 52 LSD psychotics and 29 matched first-break schizophrenics [88], LSD patients did not differ in incidence of psychosis or suicide among the parents. Rate of parental alcoholism, among the parents of those with LSD psychosis, however, far exceeded that of controls and of the general population. While the two groups were distinguishable in some clinical parameters, they were equivalent in premorbid adjustment and by most cognitive measures when initially hospitalized or reassessed three to five years later. Both groups had the same rehospitalization rate.

Many believe that LSD alone does not produce an enduring psychosis but rather precipitates schizophrenia in predisposed personalities. There remains an uncertainty as to the relative role of monoaminergic pathways in schizophrenic illness. LSD is active in serotoninergic systems, and studies indicate serotoninergic aberrations in schizophrenia. Part of the confusion originates in the fact that when an already psychotic patient takes LSD, the preexistent psychosis may be misconstrued as induced. LSD use may have been an attempt either to self-medicate, to help give "insight," or to organize the external world when the internal world is chaotic. It may also simply represent poor judgment or superimposed character disorder, resulting in use of a drug that complicates the clinical picture and can lead to fatal behavior. People on LSD have assumed that they can fly, resulting in a death that may be construed as a suicide when, in fact, it is the result of the distorted thinking symptomatic of hallucinogen use. Incidence of psychiatric illness requiring hospitalization is increased in parents of patients with LSD psychosis [89]. Patients can be singularly inventive in their use of substances that induce psychosis as they seek "insight" or "psychotherapeutic progress." One patient was able to induce a schizophrenic-like psychosis by ingesting isosafrale after he failed to do so with amphetamines and LSD [90].

## DUAL DIAGNOSIS AND COCAINE USE

Cocaine poses special problems in dual diagnosis, given the multiple routes of absorption and the various organ systems on which it impacts. Cocaine is absorbed rapidly from mucous membranes. Commonly taken nasally or via the lungs ("freebasing"), cocaine can also be absorbed through the conjunctiva of the eye, the mucous membranes of the mouth (freezing), the vagina, and the penile urethra. It also can be injected intravenously or subdermally ("skin popping"). This drug is associated with high bioavailability since

there is no hepatic first-pass effect. Cocaine blocks neuronal uptake of norepinephrine and dopamine and reduces the concentration of serotonin. Release
of norepinephrine and dopamine by neurons is facilitated, and tyrosine hydroxylase is activated. Tryptophan hydroxylase activity is inhibited. Net effect: decreased serotonin, dopamine, and norepinephrine turnover [91].

The most common concurrent psychiatric illness with cocaine abuse is
affective illness. Depression is found significantly more often in patients
using cocaine than among opiate and depressant abusers. Remarkably, incidence of affective disorder in first-degree relatives of cocaine abusers is also
increased when compared to the other groups, suggesting that, in the dual-
diagnosis patients, use of cocaine or crack may represent self-medication of
an affective disorder. Early euphorogenic effects are attributed to increased
dopamine and norepinephrine activity due to inhibited reuptake of these
transmitter substances at presynaptic terminals. This effect is similar to that
of some antidepressants and to amphetamines, which cause similar mood
elevation in depressed patients. The effect is not sustained. In most patients,
continued and increased use of cocaine leads to a worsening of depressive
symptoms [92].

The particular psychopharmacologic effects and multiple routes of administration lead to many medical complications that can result in dual,
triple, and more diagnostic problems. Myocardial ischemia [73], myocardial
infarction [93] and cardiomyopathy, myocarditis, and malignant ventricular
arrhythmias are among the most dreaded effects [94]. Risk for myocardial
infarction is greatest among those with preexistent angina. Cocaine is
arrhythmogenic, causing sinus tachycardia, ventricular premature contrac-
tions, ventricular tachycardia and fibrillation, and asystole. Cocaine also
produces hyperpyrexia, leading to seizures and possibly arrthymias. Large
amounts of cocaine can lead to marked increase in systemic arterial pressure
and rupture of the ascending aorta [93].

Pulmonary complications include spontaneous pneumothorax when
"pocket shot" is used by IV drug abusers seeking access to the internal
jugular vein [95]. Freebasing has been reported to cause, or contribute to,
asthma in those predisposed as a nonspecific irritant [96]. Necrosis with
perforation of the nasal septum, atrophy of the nasal mucosa, loss of smell,
lung damage, pulmonary edema, respiratory paralysis, and reduction in the
capacity of the lungs to diffuse carbon monoxide are other respiratory
complications [93].

Cerebrovascular accidents have been found temporally related to cocaine
use. Subarachnoid hemorrhage has been reported within minutes of intranasal administration. Individuals with occult arteriovenous malformations are
at particular risk. Cocaine users with headaches should be apprised of this

risk. A common central nervous system effect is seizures. Cocaine lowers seizure threshold, with the result that a seizure may be caused by as little as a single dose. Cocaine-induced seizures should be considered a possibility in anyone presenting for the first time with epilepsy after age ten [93].

Other complications of cocaine use that may present concurrent use in clude intestinal ischemia with pain or frank gangrene in individuals who take cocaine orally or serve as "mules" or "body packers" by swallowing cocaine to get it through customs; complications of pregnancy (e.g., abruptio placentae, spontaneous abortion, congenital malformations, neurobehavioral impairment, perinatal mortality); severe lactic acidosis, especially in the sprint-trained athlete [97]; precipitation of acute porphyria [98]; spontaneous pneumomediastinum; and pneumopericardium [93]. Aberrations of glucose metabolism can lead to a number of behavioral changes that resemble those of cocaine use itself (e.g., aggressive and depressive behavior) and of other major psychiatric disorders (e.g., major depression). The changes in glucose levels may be due to neglect of diet seen in drug abusers and alcoholics, noncompliance with medication prescribed, and sensitization to epinephrine, which mobilizes blood glucose. Sexual dysfunction may antedate or follow cocaine use. Concerns over lack of sexual responsivity may result in seeking out cocaine as an aphrodisiac to enhance sexual performance. Sparing use can lead to increased sexuality and delayed ejaculation and orgasm-heightening pleasure. Prolonged use is generally correlated with diminished sexual performance and interest. Cocaine becomes the mistress or lover before whom all competitors fail.

## DUAL DIAGNOSIS AND SOLVENT USE

Recreational use of inhalants and solvents for transient highs is correlated with preexistent psychopathology and can induce a number of neuropsychiatric and physical complications, obfuscating the underlying primary pathology. Deliberate inhalation of metallic paints, for instance, leads to hemorrhagic alveolitis [99]. Despite severe and predictable harm to the body from this practice, chronic solvent abusers' response to substance abuse treatment is poor, perhaps because those who abuse solvents over protracted periods of time have behavioral patterns that militate against good social adjustment and positive treatment response. Long-term inhalation of paint thinners, aerosols, gasoline, and cleaning fluids (generally from solvent-soaked rags in plastic bags) leads to some euphoria and disinhibition. Auditory and visual hallucinations occur, coupled with ataxia and tinnitus. The effect wears off in 30–45 minutes as the patient falls asleep with impaired memory of the event [100]. Medical complications include cerebellar toxicity, potentially irreversible encephalopathy, renal dysfunction, cardiac irritability, generalized weakness, and abdominal pain.

Solvent abusers tend to be adolescents. Only a small fraction experiment beyond a few times. Any inhalation of solvents that may lead to permanent damage is distressing. Chronic use entails development of permanent maladapture characteristics in the developing personality in childhood and adolescence. Solvent abusers as a group are more depressed than those who do not abuse solvents [101]. Solvent abusers also more frequently abuse alcohol. Chronic use for some is on the trajectory to heroin addiction. Shoplifting, truancy, and problems in school have been found to coexist with solvent abuse [100]. Lead tetraethyl (the antiknock agent in gasoline) creates a short-term psychosis characterized by hallucinations, mania, fear, and schizophreniform symptoms [102]. These isolated periods of psychosis resemble the micropsychotic episodes of borderline patients and may be misconstrued as such. Obviously, in some instances, the abuse may be symptomatic of a borderline or antisocial personality. One may, in fact, question whether what becomes a borderline personality is, in some cases, the outcome of a multiple substance-abusing episode at a time when the identity is evolving. The adult identity has elements of psychosis that are derived from aberrations of thought and effects of substance abuse.

## DUAL DIAGNOSIS AND BENZODIAZEPINE USE

Benzodiazepines are used by depressed, eating-disordered, and manic patients. Abuse may be intentional to obtain relief or iatry. In the latter instance, anxiotolytics and soporifics have been prescribed for anxiety or panic accompanying a depression or eating disorder or to induce sleep in insomniac depressives and hypomanic and manic patients. With progression of the mood or eating disorder, more is required to achieve the same effect because of either habituation or progressively increasing intensity of symptoms. Eventually, patients are addicted. Any reduction in dosage is fraught with discomfort. Increased doses are required for relief. Intermittent intoxication and withdrawal results in an oneiroid state mimicking schizophrenia. The primary use of benzodiazepines is the management of anxiety and panic with the exception of alprazolam, which also appears to be useful in the management of some depressions.

Despite widespread use of benzodiazepines for anxiety disorders and depression, it is remarkable that many do not become addicted [103]. Dependence occurs at remarkably low doses [104], to the surprise and dismay of patients and physicians alike. Long-term therapeutic use of even small doses can lead to remarkable dependence (so-called low-dose dependence), requiring considerable skill in both management and withdrawal. Symptoms of withdrawal or intoxication are often confused with those of primary anxiety or mood disorder.

## DUAL DIAGNOSIS AND PSYCHOSTIMULANTS

Psychostimulants are commonly abused by psychiatric patients. The most commonly abused, cocaine, has already been discussed. Less commonly used but equally potent in their impact are dextroamphetamine and methylphenidate. These typically cause manic-type highs, the anxiety symptoms of a racing heartbeat, and palpitations. Frank paranoia and profound depression on cessation of use ("crashing") is also seen. Concurrent use of cocaine and amphetamines often occurs. Use of stimulants contributes to relapses in schizophrenia. Short-term use alone of moderately large doses of stimulants without dormant schizophrenia can induce acute paranoid psychosis [105]. These psychoses are usually of brief duration, remitting rapidly upon cessation of stimulant use. There is some question as to whether the facility with which psychoses may be generated relates to the degree psychosis lies dormant in the user.

Stimulant psychoses, more than hallucinogenic psychoses, resemble psychogenic psychoses, particularly paranoid schizophrenia. Paranoia occurs in a clear sensorium with ideas of reference and at times auditory hallucinations. It differs in that delusions tend to be less well developed with stimulant use and stereotopics are more frequent with stimulants. Neuroleptic response is the same for both. Only the fact that the paranoid psychosis passes with cessation of stimulant use is helpful. In addition to causing paranoid psychosis, stimulants intensify or exacerbate symptoms in someone already schizophrenic or manic.

## DUAL DIAGNOSIS AND PSYCHOTROPIC ABUSE

Psychotropic drugs such as thioridazine, doxepin, amitriptyline, and anti-Parkinson drugs, which are sold on the street, to attenuate or qualitatively impact on the character of sensory change with substance abuse. For instance, anti-Parkinson drugs are abused to achieve a euphoric state, for stimulant effect, as hallucinogenics, and for social stimulation [106]. Effect is dose-dependent. Higher doses than that required to manage extrapyramidal side effects are required. Trihexylphidyl has particularly great abuse potential. Termination of anti-Parkinson drugs may lead to premature termination of treatment because of unpleasant symptoms independent of motor problems.

## LABORATORY STUDIES

The dexamethasone suppression test (DST) has been employed to support the diagnosis of depression. Of patients with major depression, 45–50% fail to suppress cortisol after being given a 1-mg oral dose of dexamethasone at 11 P.M. Diagnostic sensitivity varies depending on blood collection times, laboratory accuracy, dexamethasone dosages given, and diagnostic criteria. Numerous medical conditions impact on its validity and reliability, making its use particularly problematic with dually diagnosed patients. Drugs specifically influence the dexamethasone metabolism via liver enzyme alterations. Burch et al. [107] found, in a study of 336 psychotic inpatients, that 60% were taking one or more drugs that changed the DST results in either a false-positive or false-negative manner. Fluctuations in neurotransmitter production affects hypothalamic-pituitary-cortisol feedback mechanisms, altering DST outcome. False-positive results may be found with sedative hypnotics, alcohol, and narcotics. False negatives occur with benzodiazepines and stimulants such as cocaine and amphetamines [107]. Marijuana can cause both false positives and false negatives. Withdrawal phenomena and liver abnormalities altering catabolism of steroids may be responsible for abnormal DSTs during the first two weeks of abstinence. The response with continued abstinence resembles that of normal controls. Nonsuppression of cortisol secretion, coupled with clinical signs of depression, suggests need for a trial of antidepressants or electroshock [108]. Modest hepatic dysfunction does not appear to invalidate DST results [109]. Chronic alcoholism impacts the hypothalamic-pituitary-adrenal axis preventing the cortisol hypersecretion often seen with depression. That this is not always so is indicated by a number of studies showing nonsuppression in a significant number of alcoholics reporting depression [35,36].

The thyrotropin-releasing hormone (TRH) test, which also is abnormal in some patients with depression, is not specific for major depression with cocaine abuse [35,36]. There is evidence that cocaine is associated with blunted results on TRH testing in much the same way that dopamine infusions in humans cause a blunted TRH response. In alcoholics, TRH abnormalities may be due to the fact that chronic alcoholism causes both endocrine abnormalities and hepatic dysfunction.

## PSYCHOTHERAPY WITH DUALLY DIAGNOSED PATIENTS

Group techniques, particularly 12-step programs such as Alcoholics Anonymous and Narcotics Anonymous, are a critical component of substance abuse treatment. For the compliant without a coexistent psychiatric disorder, it may be all that is necessary. When a primary psychiatric illness exists, the attending psychiatrist must be aware of the philosophy of AA, NA, and CA (Cocaine Anonymous) and of the need for concurrent involvement of the patient in these groups. Family members and lovers should be encouraged to attend Nar-Con and Al-Anon. A therapeutic alliance is necessary to assure that patients continue psychopharmacotherapy as prescribed as well as abstinence and involvement in a 12-step program. Therapists should take both an active educational and confrontational role [110]. The clinician's understanding of the pharmacology and pattern of use of substances abused is necessary to achieve continued abstinence and appropriate pharmacotherapy as well as to maintain credibility and respect with users and their families.

## CONCLUSION

In conclusion, it is uncommon today to see any one drug used alone, including alcohol. Polysubstance abuse is more usual. Identification of preexistent or concurrent psychiatric disorders is complicated by the myriad of psychiatric symptoms caused by drug use and by the medical conditions it induces. While a panic attack may be due to the tachycardia and chest pain attendant on cocaine use, the correct identification of true panic disorder leading to substance abuse can lead to diagnostic-specific treatment. Treatment of nonsubstance abuse psychiatric disorder is more effective than treatment of pure substance abuse. In addition, the reported rates of suicide in untreated major depression (15%) and panic disorder (18%) [111] suggest that not only may dually diagnosed patients be self-medicating depression or panic but may also be indulging in a self-destructive behavior that predictably is a consequence of the untreated course of their illness.

## REFERENCES

1. Slaby AE, Lieb J, Tancredi LR. *Handbook of Psychiatric Emergencies* 3rd ed. New York: Medical Examination Publishing, 1986.
2. Davis DI. Differences in the use of substances of abuse by psychiatric patients compared with medical and surgical patients. *J Nerv Ment Dis* 1984; 172:654–657.
3. Perkins KA, Simpson JC, Tsuang MT. Ten-year follow-ups of drug abusers with acute or chronic psychosis. *Hosp Com Psychiat* 1986; 37:481–484.
4. McKelvey MJ, Kane JS, Kellison K. Substance abuse and mental illness: double trouble. *J Psychosoc Nursing* 1987; 25:20–25.
5. Kashani JH, Keller MB, Solomon N et al. Double depression in adolescent substance users. *J Affect Dis* 1985; 8:153–157.
6. Modestin J. Degree of suffering—a neglected variable. *Psychopathology* 1986; 19:317–323.
7. Kamerow DB, Pincus HA, Macdonald DI. Alcohol abuse, other drug abuse,

and mental disorders in medical practice: Prevalence, costs, recognition, and treatment. *JAMA* 1986; 255:2054-2057.

8.  Wein AJ, Van Arsdalen KN. Drug induced male sexual dysfunction. *Urolog Clinics North Amer* 1988; 15:23-31.

9.  Yellowless PM, Alpers JH, Bowder JJ et al. Psychiatric morbidity in patients with chronic airflow obstruction. *Med J Austral* 1987; 146:305-307.

10. Mayou R, Hawton K. Psychiatric disorder in the general hospital. *Brit J Psychiat* 1986; 149:172-190.

11. Zorc TG, O'Donnell AE, Holt RW et al. Bilateral pyopneumothorax secondary to intravenous drug abuse. *Chest* 1988; 93:645-647.

12. Estroff TW, Gold MS. Chronic medical complications of drug abuse. *Psychiat Med* 1985; 3:267-286.

13. Chang G, Astrachan B. Identification and disposition of trauma patients with substance use or psychiatric illness. *Connecticut Med* 1987; 51:4-6.

14. Shaffer HJ, Costikyan NS. Cocaine psychosis and AIDS: A contemporary diagnostic dilemma. *J Substance Abuse Treatment* 1988; 5:9-12.

15. Caputo L. Dual diagnosis: AIDS and addiction. *Soc Work* 1985; 30(4):361-364.

16. Beresford TP, Blow FC, Hall RCW. AIDS encephalitis mimicking alcohol dementia and depression. *Biol Psychiat* 1986; 21:394-397.

17. Schuckit MA. The clinical implications of primary diagnostic groups among alcoholics. *Arch Gen Psychiat* 1985; 42:1043-1049.

18. Schuckit MA. Genetic and clinical implications of alcoholism and affective disorder. *Am J Psychiat* 1986; 143:140-147.

19. Schuckit MA. Alcoholism and other psychiatric disorders. *Hosp Com Psychiat* 1983; 34:1022-1027.

20. Powell BJ, Read MR, Penick EC et al. Primary and secondary depression in alcoholic men: An important distinction? *J Clin Psychiat* 1987; 48:98-101.

21. Clark DC, Gibbons RD, Fawcett J et al. Unbiased criteria for severity of depression in alcoholic inpatients. *J Nerv Ment Dis* 1985; 179:482-487.

22. McMahon RC, Davidson RS. An examination of depressed vs. nondepressed alcoholics in inpatient treatment. *J Clin Psychol* 1986; 42:177-184.

23. Giles DE, Biggs MM, Roffwang HP et al. Secondary depression: a comparison among subtypes. *J Affect Dis* 1987; 12:251-258.

24. Hensel B, Dunner DL, Fieve RR. The relationship of family history of alcoholism to primary affective disorder. *J Affec Dis* 1979; 1:105-113.

25. Merikangas KR, Leebman JF, Prusoff BA et al. Familial transmission of depression and alcoholism. *Arch Gen Psychiat* 1985; 42:367-372.

26. Vaslum S, Vaslum P, Larsen O. Depression and alcohol consumption in nonalcoholic and alcoholic women. *Acta Psychiatrica Scand* 1987; 75:577-584.

27. Curtis JL, Millman EJ, Joseph M et al. Prevalence rates for alcholism, associated depression and dementia on the Harlem Hospital medical and surgery services. *Advances Alcohol Substance Abuse* 1986; 6:45-64.

28. Bedi AR, Halikas JA. Alcoholism and affective disorder. *Alcoholism: Clin Exper Res* 1985; 9:133-134.

29. Goodman AB, Siegel C, Craig TJ et al. The relationship between socioeco-

nomic class and prevalence of schizophrenia, alcoholism, and affective disorder treated by inpatient care in a suburban area. *Am J Psychiat* 1983; 140:166–170.

30. Lewis CE, Rice J, Andreasen N et al. Clinical and familial correlates of alcoholism in men with unipolar major depression. *Alcoholism: Clin Exper Res* 1986; 10:657–662.

31. Lewis CE, Rice J, Andreasen N et al. The antisocial and the nonantisocial alcoholic: clinical distinctions in men with major unipolar depression. *Alcoholism: Clin Exper Res* 1987; 11:176–182.

32. Lindegard B. Physical illness in severe depressives and psychiatric alcoholics in Gothenburg, Sweden. *J Affect Dis* 1982; 4:383–393.

33. Berner P, Lesch OM, Walter H. Alcohol and depressions. *Psychopathol* 1986; 19 Suppl 2:177–183.

34. Nakamura MM, Overall JE, Radcliffe, E. Factors affecting outcome of depressive symptoms in alcoholics. *Alcoholism: Clin Exper Res* 1983; 7:188–193.

35. Dackis CA, Gold MS, Pottash ALC et al. Evaluating depression in alcoholics. *Psychiat Res* 1986; 17:105–109.

36. Dackis CA, Stuckey RF, Gold MS et al. Dexamethasone suppression test testing of depressed alcoholics. *Alcoholism: Clin Exper Res* 1986; 10:59–60.

37. Majumdar SK, Shaw GK, Bridges PK. Relationship between plasma cortisol concentrations and depression in chronic alcoholic patients. *Drug Alcohol Dependence* 1984; 14:45–49.

38. Knoll P, Palmer C, Greden JF. The dexamethasone suppression test in patients with alcoholism. *Biol Psychiat* 1983; 18:441–450.

39. Hatsukami D, Pickens RW. Posttreatment depression in alcohol and drug abuse populations. *Am J Psychiat* 1982; 139:1563–1566.

40. Hatsukami D, Mitchell JE, Eckert EC et al. Characteristics of patients with bulimia only, bulimia with affective disorders, and bulimia with substance abuse problems. *Addict Behaviors* 1986; 11:399–406.

41. Hatsukami D, Eckert E, Mitchell JE et al. Affective disorder and substance abuse in women with bulimia. *Psychol Med* 1984; 14:701–704.

42. Behar D, Winokur G, Berg CJ. Depression in the abstinent alcoholic. *Am J Psychiat* 1984; 141:1105–1107.

43. West AP. Lithium treatment of depressed alcoholics: A hypothesis. *Am J Psychiat* 1983; 140:814.

44. Croughan JL, Miller JP, Matar A et al. Psychiatric diagnosis and prediction of drug and alcohol dependence. *J Clin Psychiat* 1982; 45:353–356.

45. Dorus W, Kennedy J, Gibbons RD et al. Symptoms and diagnosis of depression in alcoholics. *Alcoholism: Clin Exper Res* 1987; 11:150–154.

46. Steer RA, Beck AT, Shaw BF. Depressive symptoms differentiating between heroin addicts and alcoholics. *Drug Alcohol Dependence* 1985; 15:145–150.

47. Steer RA, McElroy MG, Beck AT. Correlates of self-reported and clinically assessed depression in outpatient alcoholics. *J Clin Psychol* 1983; 39:144–149.

48. Lippmann S, Manshadi M. Depression in alcoholics by the NIMH – Diagnostic Interview Schedule and Zung Self-Rating Depression Scale. *Int J Addict* 1987; 22:273–281.

49. Ciraulo DA, Jaffe JH. Tricyclic antidepressants in the treatment of depression associated with alcoholism. *J Clin Psychopharm* 1987; 15:146–150.

50. Bennett LA. Depressive symptoms among hospitalized and post-hospitalized alcoholics in Yugoslavia. *J Nerv Ment Dis* 1986; 174:545–552.

51. Altesman AI, Ayre FR, Williford WO. Diagnostic validation of conjoint schizophrenia and alcoholism. *J Clin Psychiat* 1984; 45:300–303.

52. Bernadt MW, Murray RM. Psychiatric disorder, drinking and alcoholism: What are the links? *Brit J Psychiat* 1986; 148:393–400.

53. Steinhausen HC, Nestler V, Huth H. Psychopathology and mental functions in the offspring of alcoholic and epileptic mothers. *J Amer Acad Child Psychiat* 1982; 21:268–273.

54. Peace K, Mellsop G. Alcoholism and psychiatric disorder. *Austral N Zeal J Psychiat* 1987; 21:94–101.

55. Powell BJ, Penick EC, Othmer E et al. Prevalence of additional psychiatric symptoms among male alcoholics. *J Clin Psychiat* 1982; 43:404–407.

56. Roehrich H, Gold MS. Diagnosis of substance abuse in an adolescent psychiatric population. *Int J Psychiat Med* 1986–87; 16:137–143.

57. Hesselbrock MN, Hesselbrock VM, Tennen H et al. Methodological considerations in the assessment of depression in alcoholics. *J Consult Clin Psychol* 1983; 51:399–405.

58. Hesselbrock MN, Meyer RE, Keener JJ. Psychopathology in hospitalized alcoholics. *Arch Gen Psychiat* 1985; 42:1050–1055.

59. Hesselbrock MN, Tennen H, Hesselbrock VM et al. Assessment of depression in alcoholics: Further considerations—reply to Hagen and Schauer. *J Consul Clin Psychol* 1985; 53:67–69.

60. Shravynski A, Lamantagne Y, Lavalle Y-J. Clinical phobias and avoidant personality disorder among alcoholics admitted to an alcoholism rehabilitation setting. *Can J Psychiat* 1986; 31:714–719.

61. Rounsaville BJ, Weissman MM, Rosenberger PA et al. Detecting depressive disorders in drug abusers. *J Affect Dis* 1979; 1:255–267.

62. Rounsaville BJ, Dolinsky ZS, Babor TF et al. Psychopathology as a predictor of treatment outcome in alcoholics. *Arch Gen Psychiat* 1987; 44:505–513.

63. Rounsaville BJ, Dolinsky ZS, Baber TF et al. Psychopathology as a predictor of treatment outcome in alcoholics. *Arch Gen Psychiat* 1985; 42:1050–1055.

64. Horn GV. Dementia. *Am J Med* 1987; 83:101–110.

65. Goldman MS. Neuropsychological recovery in alcoholics: Endogenous and exogenous processes. *Alcoholism: Clin Exper Res* 1986; 10:136–144.

66. Brew BJ. Diagnosis of Wernicke's encephalopathy. *Austral N Zeal J Med* 1986; 16:676–678.

67. Brennan FN, Lyttle JA. Alcohol and seizures: A review. *J Roy Soc Med* 1987; 80:571–573.

68. Cummings MA, Cummings KL, Rapaport MH. Acquired immunodeficiency syndrome presenting as schizophrenia. *Western J Med* 1987; 146:615–618.

69. Klatsky AL. The cardiovascular effects of alcohol. *Alcohol Alcoholism* 1987; Suppl. 1:117–124.

70. Maheswaran R, Potter JF, Beevers DG. The role of alcoholism in hypertension. *J Clin Hypertension* 1986; 2:172–178.
71. Brecher M, Porjesz B, Begleiter H. Late positive component amplitude in schizophrenics and alcoholics in two different paradigms. *Biol Psychiat* 1987; 22:848–856.
72. Beevers DG, Zezulka AV, Potter JF et al. The clinical relevance of alcohol in the blood pressure clinic. *Europ Heart J* 1987; 8:27–29.
73. Mathias DW. Cocaine-associated myocardial ischemia: Review of clinical and ansiographic findings. *Am J Med* 1986; 81:675–678.
74. McCall D. Alcohol and the cardiovascular system. *Cur Problems Cardiol* 1987; 12:355–414.
75. Bikle DD. Effects of alcohol abuse on bone. *Compr Therapy* 1988; 14:16–20.
76. Zimmerman HJ. Effects of alcohol on other hepatotoxins. *Alcoholism: Clin Exper Res* 1986; 10:3–15.
77. Stefanis CN, Kokkevi A. Depression and drug use. *Psychopathol* 1986; 19 Suppl 2:124–131.
78. Safer DJ. Substance abuse by young adult chronic patients. *Hosp Com Psychiat* 1987; 38:511–514.
79. Motet-Grigoras CN, Schuckit MA. Depression and substance abuse in handicapped young men. *J Clin Psychiat* 1986; 47:234–237.
80. Weller MPI, Ang TC, Zachary A et al. Substance abuse in schizophrenia. *Lancet* 1984; March 10:573.
81. Inman DJ, Bascue LO, Skoloda T. Identification of borderline personality disorders among substance abuse inpatients. *J Substance Abuse Treatment* 1985; 2:229–232.
82. Gabel RH, Barnard N, Norko M et al. AIDS presenting as mania. *Compr Psychiat* 1986; 27:251–254.
83. Mc Lane NJ, Carroll DM. Ocular manifestations of drug abuse. *Survey Ophthal* 1986; 30:298–313.
84. Michelson JB, Friedlaender MH. Endophthalmitis of drug abuse. *Int Ophthal Clinics* 1987; 27:120–126.
85. Kosten TR. Diagnosing depression with the DST and TRH in cocaine and opioid abuses. *J Substance Abuse Treatment* 1986; 3:47–49.
86. Friedman AS, Glickman NW. Effects of psychiatric symptomatology on treatment outcome for adolescent male drug abusers. *J Nerv Ment Dis* 1987; 175:425–430.
87. Ragheb M. Drug abuse among state hospital psychiatric inpatients with particular reference to PCP. *J Clin Psychiat* 1985; 46:339–340.
88. Vardy MM, Kay SR. LSD psychosis or LSD-induced schizophrenia? A multimethod inquiry. *Arch Gen Psychiat* 1983; 40:377–383.
89. Weaver KEC. LSD and schizophrenia. *Arch Gen Psychiat* 1984; 41:631.
90. Keitner GI, Sabaawi M, Haier RJ. Isosafrole and schizophrenia-like psychosis. *Am J Psychiat* 1984; 141:997–998.
91. Annitto WJ, Gold MS. The Fair Oaks Hospital cocaine treatment program. *J Substance Abuse Treatment* 1984; 1:223–226.

92.  Weiss RD, Mirin SM, Michael JL et al. Psychopathology in chronic cocaine abuses. *Am J Drug Alcohol Abuse* 1986; 12:17-29.
93.  Cregler LL, Mark H. Medical complications of cocaine abuse. *NEJ Med* 1986:315:1495-1500.
94.  Lam D, Goldschlager N. Myocardial injury associated with polysubstance abuse. *Am Heart J* 1988; 3:675-680.
95.  Forester D. Pneumothorax in substance abuse. [Letter] *Chest* 1988; 93:670.
96.  Rebhun J. Association of asthma and freebase smoking. *Ann Allergy* 1988; 60:339-342.
97.  Giammarco RA. The athlete, cocaine, and lactic acidosis: A hypothesis. *Am J Med Sci* 1987; 294:412-414.
98.  Dick AD, Prentice MG. Cocaine and acute porphyria. *Lancet* 1987; Nov. 14, p. 1150.
99.  Engstrand DA, England DM, Huntington RW. 3rd Pathology of paint sniffers lung. *Am J Foren Med Path* 1986; 7:232-236.
100.  Dinwiddie SH, Zorumski CF, Rubin EH. Psychiatric correlates of chronic solvent abuse. *J Clin Psychiat* 1987; 48:334-337.
101.  Jacobs AM, Ghodse AH. Depression in solvent abusers. *Soc Sci Med* 1987; 24:863-866.
102.  Daniels AM, Latchman RW. Petrol sniffing and schizophrenia in a Pacific Island paradise. *Lancet* 1984; Feb. 18:389.
103.  Garvey MJ, Tollefson GD. Prevalence of misuse of prescribed benzodiazepines in patients with primary anxiety disorder or major depression. *Am J Psychiat* 1986; 143:1601-1603.
104.  Laux G, Konis W. Long-term use of benzodiazepines in psychiatric inpatients. *Acta Psychiatrica Scand* 1987; 76:64-70.
105.  Rofoed L, Kania J, Walsh T et al. Outpatient treatment of patients with substance abuse and coexisting psychiatric disorders. *Am J Psychiat* 1986; 143:867-872.
106.  Saran AS. Use or abuse of antiparkinsonism drugs by psychiatric patients. *J Clin Psychiat* 1986; 47:130-132.
107.  Burch EA, Goldschmidt TJ, Schwartz BD. Drug intake and the dexamethasone suppression test. *J Clin Psychiat* 1986; 47:144-146.
108.  Kahn A, Ciraulo DA, Nelson WH et al. Dexamethasone suppression test in recently detoxified alcoholics: Clinical implications. *J Clin Psychopharm* 1984; 4:94-97.
109.  Zern MA, Halbreich V, Baron K et al. Relationship between serum cortisol, liver function, and depression in detoxified alcoholics. *Alcoholism: Clin Exper Res* 1986; 10:320-322.
110.  Millman RB. Considerations on the psychotherapy of the substance abuser. *J Substance Abuse Treatment* 1986; 3:103-109.
111.  Slaby AE. Psychopharmacotherapy of suicide. In: Bonger, B ed. *Dangerous Intersections: The Assessment and Management of Suicide in Clinical Practice*. London: Oxford University Press (in press).

# 2

# Genetics and Dual Diagnosis

**William Coryell**

*University of Iowa, Iowa City, Iowa*

Some mental disorders coexist within individuals at far greater than chance rates [1]. Particularly common are combinations of alcoholism with depression, [2] of substance abuse with depression, [3] and of antisocial personality with alcoholism, [4] substance abuse, [3] or depression [5]. These nosological entanglements and the law of parsimony have led to debates over primary and secondary relationships among these disorders. Does one illness, i.e., alcoholism, account entirely for the development of another, i.e., depression? To follow this example, are both alcoholism and an inherent propensity to depression necessary before depression manifests in an alcoholic? Finally, given the high prevalence of depression and alcoholism, does their coexistence represent a predisposition to both illnesses within the same individual? These are not new questions. That they have no widely accepted answers reflects their complexity and the limited power of available research methods.

Standard approaches to delimiting psychiatric illnesses include descriptions of demographic and phenomenological characteristics, follow-up studies, and laboratory studies [6]. If syndrome B follows and is entirely secondary to illness A, then B should differ in important ways from the illness B when it is primary and not preceded by illness A. Important dissimilarities between primary B and secondary B might include symptoms, demographic features (i.e., age of onset and sex), and course. In fact, the literature contains considerable evidence that primary and secondary depressions, for example, do exhibit clinically meaningful differences in demographics, phenomenology, and natural history [7]. Similarly, the course of alcoholism preceded by antisocial personality differs in important ways from alcoholism in non-anti-social individuals [4,8].

Differences in course and outcome have unarguable clinical importance and speak strongly for the practical value of separating chronologically primary and secondary conditions. They do not weigh for or against any of the hypotheses listed above, however. A chronologically secondary illness may occur spontaneously, but its cause may be modified by the persistence of a preexisting illness. On the other hand, the course of the secondary illness may differ because it is etiologically distinct from that same syndrome when it is primary.

This is where genetic studies offer some advantage over other approaches to diagnostic validity. With the possible exception of drug abuse, each of the disorders mentioned so far — alcoholism, depression, and antisocial personality — is strongly familial. This permits investigations into the relative primacy of coexisting disorders. The structure of such investigations then depends on the type of genetic study, and each of the types — twin studies, adoption studies, and family studies — has its own strengths and weaknesses.

Adoption studies are perhaps the most difficult but the most compelling of these methods. The first obstacles to such studies are the confidentiality provisions in place to protect biological parents, adoptive parents, and adoptees. Even with the full cooperation of adoption agencies, the location and evaluation of biological parents may be a very difficult and unevenly successful enterprise. Yet, because they offer a means of separating genetic from environmental factors, these studies are extremely important. They are typically undertaken to show that a given illness has genetic rather than simply familial determinants. Unfortunately, the inherent expense and difficulty of such studies result in numbers rarely large enough to warrant a focus on coexisting illnesses.

Twin studies are likewise intended primarily to separate genetic and environmental influences. The necessary but sometimes questioned assumption is that monozygotic and dizygotic twin pairs both share their environments equally. These studies are, of course, limited to twins, and twin pairs are chosen because at least one twin has the specific disorder of interest. As with adoption studies, coexisting disorders are rarely frequent enough to address questions regarding dual diagnoses.

Family studies are the easiest of these methods and therefore the most commonly undertaken. Unlike adoption and twin studies, they almost always take as probands individuals presenting for treatment at academic facilities. Since patients with multiple diagnoses are probably overrepresented in such settings, there is often ample clinical material for studies relevant to relationships between primary and secondary illnesses. On the other hand, such studies thoroughly confound genetic and environmental factors.

## FAMILY STUDIES: ALCOHOLISM AND DEPRESSION

If, for most patients who exhibit both alcoholism and depression, alcoholism is both a necessary and a sufficient cause of the depression, then their relatives should not be at higher risk for depression than the relatives of alcoholics without depression. If, instead, alcoholism only permits or promotes depression in an otherwise predisposed individual, then depression should appear more often among the relatives of depressed alcoholics than among the relatives of other alcoholics. Finally, if a common familial factor gives rise to both depression and alcoholism, then probands with both conditions should have an excess of relatives with both conditions.

There are almost no data available testing the third hypothesis; data relevant to the other two favor the first. Four of six studies show essentially no difference in familial loading for depression between primary alcoholic probands with depression and primary alcoholic probands without depression (Table 1). In one study, depressed alcoholics had a somewhat higher risk for depression among relatives, but this difference was not statistically significant [9]; in another, siblings but not fathers or mothers of depressed alcoholics had higher rates of depression [10]. However, studies of depression chronologically antecedent to alcoholism (primary depression) have consistently found greater familial loading for depression in comparison to alcoholic probands without primary depression (Table 2). The sequencing of alcoholism and depression is therefore important to the corresponding familial patterns of illnesses.

The importance assumed by the relative timing of syndromes leads to a converse question. Will the proband who exhibits depression and then alcoholism exhibit the same degree of familial alcoholism as the nondepressed proband with alcoholism? This would suggest that, in some cases, depression is a sufficient cause for alcoholism. The data do not support this conjecture (see Table 3). Dual-diagnosis patients with this sequence have a uniformly higher risk for alcoholism among relatives than did depressed patients without alcoholism.

Table 4 displays another strong pattern in the data. In four of four studies, alcoholic probands with depression have more alcoholism among their relatives than do alcoholic probands without depression. Indeed, clinical comparisons of depressed and nondepressed alcoholics have shown the former individuals to have more alcohol-related problems, [9,11] greater general impairment, [12,13] and an earlier onset [12,14,15]. Thus, the earlier

**Table 1** Familial Loading for Depression Among Relatives of Primary Alcoholic Probands with and without Secondary Depression

| Study | Probands | Familial loading for depression | Comments |
|---|---|---|---|
| Cadoret et al. 1974 [27] | *Males* 41 with depression vs. 71 without depression | Depressed probands = nondepressed probands | |
| | *Females* 30 with depression vs. 31 without depression | Depressed probands = nondepressed probands | |
| Schuckit 1983 [11] | *Males* 70 with depression vs. 163 without depression | Depressed probands = nondepressed probands | True of male & female relatives |
| O'Sullivan et al. 1983 [10] | *Males* 72 with depression vs. 194 without depression | Depressed probands > nondepressed probands | True only for siblings |
| Guze et al. 1986 [28] | *Males and Females* 64 with depression vs. 52 without depression | Depressed probands = nondepressed probands | |
| Yates et al. 1988 [9] | *Males* 20 with depression (matched) vs. 20 without depression | Depressed probands = nondepressed probands | Trend toward greater risk in relatives of depressed probands |

**Table 2** Familial Loading for Depression Among Relatives of Alcoholic Probands with and without Primary Affective Disorder

| Study | Probands | Familial loading for depression | Comments |
|---|---|---|---|
| Schuckit et al. 1969 [29] | *Females*<br>19 with depression vs.<br>39 without depression | Depressed probands ><br>nondepressed probands | True only of<br>female relatives |
| Winokur et al. 1971 [30] | *Females*<br>26 with depression vs.<br>63 without depression | Depressed probands ><br>nondepressed probands | True only of<br>female relatives |
| O'Sullivan et al. 1983 [10] | *Males*<br>34 with depression vs.<br>194 without depression | Depressed probands ><br>nondepressed probands | Not true<br>of fathers |
| Schuckit et al. 1979 [31] | *Females*<br>40 with depression vs.<br>154 without depression | Depressed probands ><br>nondepressed probands | |
| Penick et al. 1984 [32] | *Males*<br>71 with mania vs.<br>257 without affective disorder | Manic probands ><br>nonaffective disorder probands | |

**Table 3** Familial Loading for Alcoholism Among Relatives of Primary Depressed Probands with and without Alcoholism

| Study | Probands | Familial loading for alcoholism | Comments |
|---|---|---|---|
| Morrison 1975 [33] | *Males and females* 18 with alcoholism vs. 20 without alcoholism | Alcoholic probands > nonalcoholic probands | All probands had bipolar illness |
| Merikangas et al. 1985 [34] | *Males and females* 19 with alcoholism vs. 114 without alcoholism | Alcoholic probands > nonalcoholic probands | |

**Table 4** Familial Loading for Alcoholism Among Relatives of Alcoholic Probands with and without Depression

| Study | Probands | Familial loading for alcoholism | Comments |
|---|---|---|---|
| Schuckit et al. 1969 [29] | *Females*<br>19 with depression vs. 39 without depression | Depressed probands > nondepressed probands | True only of female relatives |
| Winokur et al. 1971 [30] | *Females*<br>26 with depression vs. 63 without depression | Depressed probands > nondepressed probands | True only of female relatives |
| Woodruff et al. 1973 [13] | *Males*<br>29 with depression vs. 39 without depression | Depressed probands > nondepressed probands | |
| Schuckit 1983 [11] | *Males*<br>70 with depression vs. 163 without depression | Depressed probands = nondepressed probands | Strong trends in fathers and siblings toward more alcoholism among relatives of depressed probands. |

onset and greater overall severity associated with the more familial forms of alcoholism might be expected to result more often in depression.

Is dual diagnosis itself familial? Such a pattern should emerge if a third factor operates to produce both depression and alcoholism. Unfortunately, there are very few data sets appropriate to this question. Table 5 displays results from a large family study of affective disorder [16]. Raters blind to proband diagnosis directly interviewed all available first-degree relatives and applied Research Diagnostic Criteria [17]. Dual diagnoses, depression with alcoholism, was clearly more prevalent among relatives of dual-diagnosis probands.

In summary, depression that precedes alcoholism is clearly associated with familial tendencies to affective disorder while depression that follows alcoholism is not. In contrast, alcoholism following depression is quite familial, and alcoholism with depression may be more familial than the alcoholism not complicated by depression. Finally, the coexistence of these syndromes itself seems familial.

## FAMILY STUDIES: ANTISOCIAL PERSONALITY, ALCOHOLISM, AND DEPRESSION

Antisocial individuals are at increased risk for drug dependence [5,18,19]. This may reflect the recklessness and pervasive disregard for consequences that characterize this disorder. If so, these inherent components of antisocial personality might also predispose to alcoholism. Indeed, alcoholism is a very common though not universal complication of this disorder [20]. Is

**Table 5**  Dual Diagnoses in Probands and Relatives: Primary Depression and Alcoholism

| Diagnosis | No. of interviewed relatives | Percentage with dual diagnosis |
|---|---|---|
| In male probands: | | |
| primary depression with alcoholism | 80 | 12.5[a] |
| primary depression without alcoholism | 316 | 4.4 |
| In female probands: | | |
| primary depression with alcoholism | 117 | 13.7[b] |
| primary depression without alcoholism | 702 | 5.4 |

[a]$\chi^2 = 7.5$, df $= 1$, $p < .01$
[b]$\chi^2 = 11.2$, df $= 1$, $p < .001$

antisocial personality a necessary and sufficient cause of alcoholism when these disorders coexist?

This question is analogous to the one posed earlier regarding alcoholism and depression, as are the means to answer it. If alcoholism is, in these cases, purely the result of antisocial personality, then antisocials with alcoholism should have a familial loading for alcoholism similar to that of antisocials without alcoholism. However, for male probands in one study, [4] antisocial males with alcoholism were much more likely to have a family history positive for alcoholism (61%) than were males without alcoholism (18%), though such family histories were equally common for female sociopaths with and without alcoholism (Table 6). The other relevant study did not separate male and female probands but found a trend toward more alcoholism among the relatives of sociopaths who themselves had alcoholism.

Because antisocial personality by definition has its onset in childhood, it is necessarily antecedent to alcoholism. If alcoholism is caused by antisocial personality, then alcoholics who have antisocial personality should have less familial loading for alcoholism than those who do not have antisocial personality. This is clearly not true (see Table 6). In fact, two studies found a higher familial loading for alcoholism among the dual-diagnosis subjects than among subjects with alcoholism alone. Thus, it appears that alcoholism, when accompanied by another disorder, whether it be depression or antisocial personality, may be a more familial form of alcoholism.

## ADOPTION STUDIES: ANTISOCIAL PERSONALITY AND ALCOHOLISM

As noted earlier, adoption studies bring considerably more power to the question of genetic determinants. They are relatively few, for reasons noted earlier in this chapter, and variations in methodology undermine consensus across studies. Thus, while there is agreement that alcoholism has strong genetic determinants, [21] there is less consensus concerning genetic factors in antisocial personality. Some have found clear evidence for this, [22–24] others have not [25]. Not surprisingly, there are insufficient data available to seek consensus on the genetics of *dual diagnosis*. Several ongoing studies have targeted these issues, and the associated technology for data analysis is evolving rapidly. Cadoret et al., [26] for example, have employed log-linear models to adoption study data in an attempt not only to disentangle genetic and environmental influences, but also to separate determinants of antisocial personality from those of alcoholism (Fig. 1). Results suggest that biologic backgrounds for antisocial personality and alcoholism directly raise risks for the corresponding illnesses in offspring but that either of these illnesses, once present, raises the risk of the other.

**Table 6** Familial Loading for Alcoholism Among Probands with Antisocial Personality (ASP), Alcoholism, or Both

| Study | Dual diagnosis vs. ASP alone | Dual diagnosis vs. Alcoholism alone |
|---|---|---|
| Winokur et al. 1971 [30] | | Males: 28 with dual diagnosis = 112 with alcoholism alone<br>Females: 7 with dual diagnosis = 63 with alcoholism alone |
| Schuckit et al. 1979 [31] | | Females: 40 with dual diagnosis > 154 with alcoholism alone |
| Lewis et al. 1983 [4] | Males: 23 with dual diagnosis > 11 with ASP alone<br>Females: 33 with dual diagnosis = 13 with ASP alone | Males: 23 with dual diagnosis =[a] 25 with alcoholism alone<br>Females: 13 with dual diagnosis = 14 with alcoholism alone |
| Penick et al. 1984 [32] | | Males: 104 with dual diagnosis > 257 with alcoholism alone |
| Lewis et al. 1985 [19] | Males + females: 51 with dual diagnosis[a] = 65 with ASP alone | Males + females: 51 with dual diagnosis = 16 with alcoholism alone |
| Hesselbrock et al. 1985 [35] | | Males: 88 with dual diagnosis = 81 with alcoholism alone |
| Lewis et al. 1987 [36] | | Males: 17 with dual diagnosis = 47 with alcoholism alone |

[a]Strong trend toward greater loading for dual-diagnosis probands.

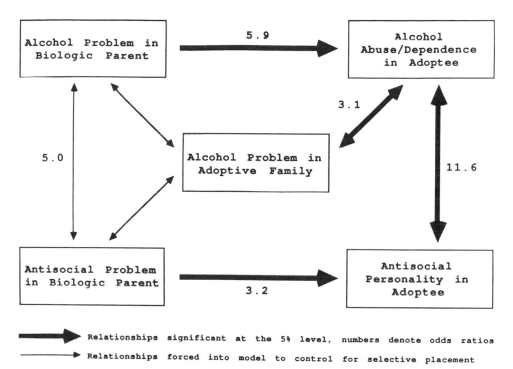

**Figure 1** Log-linear model: 241 male adoptees. (R. Caderet, personal communication.)

## REFERENCES

1. Boyd JH, Burke JD, Gruenberg E, Holzer CE, Rae DS, George LK, Karno M, Stoltzman R, McEvoy L, Nestadt G. Exclusion criteria of DSM-III: A study of co-occurrence of hierarchy-free syndromes. *Arch Gen Psychiat* 1984; 41:983–989.
2. Weissman MM, Myers JK. Clinical depression and alcoholism. *Am J Psychiat* 1980; 137:372–373.
3. Rounsaville BJ, Weissman MN, Kleber H, Wilbur C. Heterogeneity of psychiatric diagnosis in treated opiate addicts. *Arch Gen Psychiat* 1982; 39:161–166.
4. Lewis C, Rice J, Helzer J. Diagnostic interactions: Alcoholism and antisocial personality. *J Nerv Ment Dis* 1983; 171:105–113.
5. Woodruff RA, Guze SB, Clayton PJ. The medical and psychiatric implications of antisocial personality. *Dis Nerv System* 1971; 10:712.
6. Robins E, Guze SB. Establishment of diagnostic validity in psychiatric illness: Its application to schizophrenia. *Am J Psychiat* 1970; 126:107–111.
7. Coryell W. Secondary Depression. In: Michels R, Cavenar J, Cooper A, Guze SB, Judd LL, Klerman G, Solnit A (eds.) *Psychiatry*. Philadelphia, J.B. Lippincott Company, 1988, pp. 1–9.

8.  Schuckit MA. The clinical implications of primary diagnostic groups among alcoholics. *Arch Gen Psychiat* 1985; 42:1043–1049.
9.  Yates W, Petty F, Brown K. Factors associated with depression among primary alcoholics. *Compr Psychiat* 1988; 29:28–33.
10. O'Sullivan K, Whillans P, Daly M, Carroll B, Clare A, Cooney J. A comparison of alcoholics with and without coexisting affective disorder. *Br J Psychiatry* 1983; 143:133–138.
11. Schuckit M. Alcoholic patients with secondary depression. *Am J Psychiat* 1983; 140:711–714.
12. Alterman A. Patterns of familial alcoholism, alcoholism severity, and psychopathology. *J Nerv Ment Dis* 1988; 176:167–175.
13. Woodruff RA, Guze SB, Clayton PJ, Carr D. Alcoholism and depression. *Arch Gen Psychiatry* 1973; 28:97–100.
14. Buydens-Branchey L, Branchey M, Noumair D. Age of alcoholism onset I. Relationship to psychopathology. *Arch Gen Psychiat* 1989; 46:225–230.
15. Penick EC, Read MR, Crowley PA, et al. Differentiation of alcoholics by family history. *J Stud Alcohol* 1978; 39:1944–1948.
16. Andreasen NC, Rich J, Endicott J, Coryell W, Grove WM, Reich T. Familial rates of affective disorders. *Arch Gen Psychiat* 1987; 44:461–469.
17. Spitzer RL, Endicott J, Robins E. *Research Diagnostic Criteria* 3rd ed. New York: Biometrics Research, New York State Department of Mental Hygiene, 1978.
18. Guze SB, Goodwin DW, Crane JB. Criminality and psychiatric disorder. *Arch Gen Psychiat* 1969; 20:583–591.
19. Lewis C, Robins L, Rice J. Association of alcoholism with antisocial personality in urban men. *J Nerv Ment Dis* 1985; 173:166–174.
20. Lewis C. Alcoholism, antisocial personality, narcotic addition: An integrative approach. *Psychiatr Devel* 1984; 3:223–235.
21. Cloninger C, Reigh T. Genetic heterogeneity in alcoholism and sociopathy. In: *Genetics of Neurological and Psychiatric Disorders*, ed. Kety SS, Rowland LP, Sidman RL, Matthysse SW, eds. New York: Raven Press, 1983:145–166.
22. Crowe RR. An adoption study of antisocial personality. *Arch Gen Psychiat* 1974; 31:785–791.
23. Hutchings B, Mednick A. Registered criminality in the adoptive and biological parents of registered male criminal adoptees. In: *Biosocial Basis of Criminal Behavior*. Mednick SA and Christiansen KO, eds. New York: Gardner Press, 1977:127–141.
24. Cadoret RF, O'Gormann T, Heywood E, Troughton E. Genetic and environmental factors in major depression. *J Affect Dis* 1985; 9:155–164.
25. Bohman M. Some genetic aspects of alcoholism and criminality. *Arch Gen Psychiat* 1978; 35:3.
26. Cadoret RJ, Troughton E, O'Gorman TW. Genetic and environmental factors in alcohol abuse and antisocial personality. *J Stud Alcohol* 1987; 48:1–8.
27. Cadoret R, Winokur G. Depression in Alcoholism. *Annals of the New York Academy of Sciences* 1974; 233:34–39.

28. Guze SB, Cloninger CR, Martin R, Clayton PJ. Alcoholism as a medical disorder. *Compr Psychiatry* 1986; 27:501–510.

29. Schuckit M, Pitts FN, Reich T, King LJ, Winokur G. Alcoholism I. Two types of alcoholism in women. *Arch Gen Psychiat* 1969; 20:301–306.

30. Winokur G, Rimmer J, Reich T. Alcoholism IV: Is there more than one type of alcoholism? *Br J Psychiat* 1971; 118:525–531.

31. Schuckit MA, Morrissey ER. Psychiatric problems in women admitted to an alcoholic detoxification center. *Am J Psychiatry* 1979; 136:4B, 611–617.

32. Penick ED, Powell BJ, Othmer E, Bingham SF, Rice AS, Liese BS. Subtyping alcoholics by coexisting psychiatric syndromes: course, family history, outcome. In: Goodwin DW, VanDusen KT, Mednick SA (eds.). *Longitudinal Research in Alcoholism.* Boston, Kluwer-Nijhoff Publishings, 1984. pp. 167–196.

33. Morrison JR. The family histories of manic-depressive patients with and without alcoholism. *J Nerv Ment Disease* 1975; 160:227–229.

34. Merikangas KR, Leckman JF, Prusoff BA, Pauls DL, Weissman NM. Familial transmission of depression and alcoholism. *Arch Gen Psychiatry* 1985; 42:367–372.

35. Hesselbrock MN, Meyer RE, Kener JJ. Psychopathology in hospitalized alcoholics. *Arch Gen Psychiatry* 1985; 42:1050–1055.

36. Lewis C, Rice J, Andreasen N, Endicott J, Roschberg N. The antisocial and the non-antisocial alcoholic: clinical distinctions in men with major unipolar depression. *Alcoholism: Clinical and Experimental Research* 1987; 11:176–182.

# CLINICAL PRESENTATION

# 3

## Substance Abuse and Anxiety Disorders

**Peter M. Bolo**

*Fair Oaks Hospital, Summit, New Jersey*

## INTRODUCTION

In the last several years, there has been a growing interest in the coexistence of drug and alcohol abuse and the various anxiety disorders. Panic disorder, agoraphobia, and post-traumatic stress disorder (PTSD) are especially elaborated upon in the literature. Generalized anxiety disorder, social phobia, simple phobia, and obsessive-compulsive disorder (OCD) are less thoroughly explored.

Most work focuses on alcohol rather than other substances of abuse. Some authors suggest that what has been learned from alcohol abuse may be generalizable to other drugs.

The problem is a common one. A number of epidemiologic studies exist on the co-occurrence of substance abuse disorders and anxiety disorders. Most involve surveys of inpatients in alcohol treatment units. In one of the only outpatient community samples of alcoholics surveyed, Weissman et al. [1] found a 9% lifetime prevalence of generalized anxiety disorder and a 3% lifetime prevalence of phobia (type unspecified).

Surveying for rates of all anxiety disorders in alcoholic inpatients, Halikas et al. [2] estimated 10% (in an exclusively female sample). Weiss and Rosenberg [3] 23%, and Bowen et al. [4] 44%.

Rates of various phobias have been estimated, again, in samples of alcoholic inpatients. In a classic early paper, Mullaney and Trippet [5] found agoraphobia in 17%, social phobia in 24%, and phobic symptoms in 37% of their hospitalized alcoholics. Bowen et al. [4] discovered agoraphobia and/or social phobia in 24% of their alcoholics, and Smail et al. [6] estimated a doubly high rate: 53%. Weiss and Rosenberg [3] found 12% of their inpatient alcoholics had phobic disorder, 10% panic disorder, and 6% generalized anxiety states.

Peace and Mellsop [7] posit that the presence of a coexistent anxiety disorder increases the likelihood of an alcoholic seeking treatment, explaining the higher rates of anxiety disorders found in inpatient alcoholics versus community samples.

The Epidemiologic Catchment Area (ECA) study found the risk of alcoholism 2.5 times higher for individuals with any type of phobia. The risk for those with panic disorder is four times that of the general population [8].

Family studies demonstrate that first-degree relatives of individuals with anxiety disorders are at a higher risk of alcoholism, suggesting a relationship between the two illnesses. Dramatically, Noyes et al. [9] estimated 30.8% of male relatives of agoraphobics were alcoholics. Munjack and Moss [10] found that 26.5% of relatives of agoraphobics abused alcohol.

Most of these epidemiologic studies have ignored obsessive compulsive disorder (OCD). In a recent survey of inpatient alcoholics, however, Eisen and Rasmussen [11] found that 6% met DSM-III-R criteria for OCD, three times the lifetime prevalence in the general population.

Weissman [8] remarks on the absence of long-term studies following subjects from the onset of alcoholism or an anxiety disorder; such studies could elucidate the order of development of the two illnesses in the dual-diagnosis patient. Only retrospective accounts from patients are available, and their validity is questionable. Many researchers postulate that alcoholism develops from an attempt at self-medicating anxiety symptoms. Others note the similarity of alcohol withdrawal symptoms and panic symptoms and suggest that anxiety disorders result from alcohol effects in susceptible individuals. Or perhaps alcoholism and anxiety disorders are part of a spectrum of related disorders. Interestingly, cocaine and certain other drugs can directly precipitate panic attacks.

Kranzler and Liebowitz [12] propose a clinically useful concept: a bidirectional interaction between psychopathology and substance abuse. They also argue the importance of drawing a distinction in these dual-diagnosis patients based on persistence of anxiety symptoms. For instance, anxiety symptoms persisting beyond several weeks of abstinence from alcohol suggest an independent anxiety disorder deserving specific treatment.

## PANIC DISORDER AND AGORAPHOBIA

### Alcohol

That panic disorder/agoraphobia and alcoholism frequently co-occur in individuals is demonstrated by two studies examining the alcohol histories of individuals in outpatient treatment for their anxiety disorder. Breier et al. [13] found that 17% had a history of alcoholism, and Reich and Chaudry [14] estimated 28% in their sample, with a higher rate among males.

Quitkin et al. [15] pioneered the concept that a subset of alcoholics are treatable by medicating their underlying phobic-anxiety syndrome (equivalent to agoraphobia with panic attacks). This inspired further work in the area, which has led to today's growing focus on the simultaneous treatment of both the substance abuse disorder and the anxiety disorder in the dual-diagnosis patient.

However, panic states remain commonly overlooked in the treatment of alcoholics. Among inpatients at a Veterans Administration alcoholism unit, Johannessen et al. [16] found that only two of twenty patients with clear-cut spontaneous panic attacks were diagnosed, and neither had been treated.

In the Quitkin et al. [15] formulation of the phobic-anxiety syndrome with alcoholism, spontaneous panic attacks occur first. Anticipation of these panics results in a prolonged feeling of tension and dread. It is this anticipatory anxiety that leads to substance abuse. Alcohol and other sedatives are somewhat useful in the management of anticipatory anxiety but do not treat the panic attacks themselves. This caveat leads to an escalating pattern of alcohol use and eventually to the development of a true dual-diagnosis condition. Quitkin and co-workers encourage a careful assessment of any alcohol or sedative abuser with complaints of anxiety attacks or phobias, searching for this syndrome. They recommend the use of imipramine for these patients, suggesting that the alcoholism will remit with definitive treatment of the underlying panic/agoraphobic disorder.

Blankfield [17] formulates a different relationship between alcoholism and panic disorder/agoraphobia. She attributes anxiety disorder symptoms to alcohol withdrawal. Withdrawal symptoms appear following cessation of alcohol consumption in physically dependent persons but also in between drinks as the blood alcohol level falls. These symptoms are physical—tremor, palpitations, sweating, lightheadedness—as well as psychological—nervousness, irritability, and even agoraphobia. For this reason, she recommends allowing a two- to four-week period of abstinence before making an anxiety disorder diagnosis in an actively alcoholic individual complaining of anxiety symptoms.

To see whether alcoholics with panic disorder could discriminate with-drawal symptoms from panic attacks, George et al. [18] asked alcoholics with panic disorder to describe both phenomena, using a list of 29 physical and cognitive symptoms. The only symptom that discriminated alcohol withdrawal from panic attack was tremor, being associated with withdrawal. Otherwise, the descriptions were indistinguishable. George et al. speculate that this common symptomatology suggests a similar or overlapping neuro-chemical perturbation, specifically alterations in the noradrenergic system. They go on to speculate that experiencing the hyperadrenergic alcohol with-drawal state may sensitize the individual to overinterpret stimuli with a panic response.

In a similar vein, Stockwell et al. [19] surveyed alcoholic inpatients with panic agoraphobia. Most recognized a clear relationship between their drinking and anxiety symptoms. For the majority, symptoms of social phobia and agoraphobia predated drinking. Fears were estimated to be at their worst, however, following the development of full-blown alcoholism, and a bout of heavy drinking tended to heighten anxiety. The severity of phobias diminished substantially with large reductions in alcohol consump-tion. This group, too, was unable to discern panic attacks from alcohol withdrawal "dry shakes." In some patients, agoraphobia followed a bereave-ment in which alcohol was consciously used to manage panic symptoms; all believed their alcohol consumption worsened or prolonged their anxiety and phobias. The authors conclude that alcohol abuse fuels agoraphobia or severe social anxiety and that it is futile to treat anxiety symptoms while alcohol consumption continues. They do, however, believe that treating an underlying anxiety disorder during periods of abstinence decreases the likeli-hood of alcoholic relapse.

That a difference exists between panic disorder patients with or without history of alcoholism is born out by a differential response to intravenous lactate infusion. George et al. [20] found that those with a history of alco-holism tend not to panic with lactate infusion, in contrast to those without a history of alcoholism in whom lactate does induce panic attacks. The few with alcoholism history who did panic with lactate were distinct in that their panic disorder had clearly predated the onset of alcohol abuse. The authors postulate several explanations for this phenomenon. Perhaps alcoholics, because of repeated alcohol withdrawal experiences, are desensitized to the peripheral symptoms, such as tachycardia or tremor, that may elicit a panic attack. Or perhaps alcoholics are desensitized to lactate because they have elevated baseline plasma lactate concentrations. George and co-workers also posit that alcoholism may lead to a pathophysiologically different but symp-tomatically similar syndrome in predisposed individuals. Perhaps alcohol withdrawal kindles limbic structures to a heightened state of excitability that could promote panic attacks through increases in norepinephrine and cortisol release.

Reich and Chaudry [14] noted that their panic disorder patients with a history of alcoholism were less independent and less aware of social cues on personality trait assessments than those without a history of alcoholism. The patients with alcoholic histories benefited less from supportive psychotherapy and required the addition of medication to achieve significant improvement on anxiety scales.

## Cocaine

The ECA study demonstrates substantial comorbidity of panic attacks and cocaine abuse, with the highest relative risk — 13.0 — in the group of cocaine users who reported no marijuana use during the study interval [21]. Washton and Gold [22] estimate the prevalence of panic attacks among chronic cocaine abusers to be as high as 64%.

Aronson and Craig [23] were first to describe several patients whose panic disorder began during chronic cocaine abuse and continued autonomously for up to three years following abstinence from cocaine. The lengthy period of sustained symptoms following cessation of cocaine makes a prolonged cocaine abstinence syndrome an implausible explanation. Rather, the authors propose, by depleting biogenic amines, chronic cocaine use causes increased noradrenergic activity centrally.

Louie et al. [24] described ten patients who developed panic attacks after one to six years of cocaine use. Only one of these patients had a first-degree relative with panic disorder, suggesting that this was an acquired, rather than a primary, panic disorder. Their patients, too, had persistent panic attacks following cocaine abstinence for up to seven years. Of note, these patients worsened with tricyclic antidepressant treatment, responded partially to alprazolam, and improved substantially with carbamazepine or clonazepam. Louie and co-workers suggest that cocaine induces panic disorder through increased limbic excitability. Post et al. [25] propose that cocaine use produces acquired panic disorder by kindling of the limbic area.

"Crack" cocaine has also been associated with panic attacks [26]. Other drugs known to precipitate or induce panic attacks include phencyclidine and marijuana [27].

In a sample of cocaine-dependent outpatients, Nunes et al. [28] found 9 of 29 to have a coexisting anxiety disorder: 4 with social phobia, 4 with generalized anxiety disorder, 2 with panic disorder, and 1 with OCD. Those with social phobia reported that cocaine boosted their self-confidence in social situations. The authors suggest that socially anxious individuals may be particularly prone to self-medicating with cocaine.

## POST-TRAUMATIC STRESS DISORDER

Substance abuse and post-traumatic stress disorder (PTSD) frequently coexist, and much appears in the literature, both epidemiologically and therapeutically, on this topic. Most of what we know has been learned from the approximately 1 million Vietnam veterans who saw active combat, placing them at risk for developing PTSD. To some extent, what has been gained from studying this large available population may be generalizable to those with PTSD following trauma of other sorts, such as victims of violent crimes and natural disaster survivors.

Substance abuse disorders are the most commonly occurring psychiatric problems with PTSD, according to a number of epidemiologic studies of both inpatients and outpatients [29]. Rates of alcohol abuse among veterans with PTSD range from a low of 41% in Davidson et al. [30] to an astounding high of 80% in Escobar et al. [31] Between these estimates, Behar [32] found 45%, Faustman and White [33] 54%, and Sierles et al. [34] 64%.

The rates for drug abuse (all substances other than alcohol combined) are likewise impressive in PTSD patients. Davidson et al. estimate 16%, Sierles et al. 20%, Behar 23%, Faustman and White 36%, and, again estimating the highest rate, Escobar et al. 50%.

La Coursiere et al. [35] propose a self-medication model to explain alcohol abuse among individuals with PTSD. They point out that alcohol relieves many of the PTSD symptoms, at least initially. Alcohol suppresses anxiety; eases muscle tension, irritability, and sometimes depression; and induces sleep. Alcohol also suppresses REM sleep, during which most frightening post-traumatic dreams occur. Over time, however, alcohol tolerance builds, PTSD symptoms break through, and alcohol consumption needs to increase: alcoholism develops. In addition, alcohol withdrawal symptoms further reinforce the vicious circle of escalating alcohol consumption by overlapping with and heightening the PTSD symptoms.

McCormack [36] points out a potential treatment pitfall of the self-medication model. There is a danger in focusing less on the substance abuse disorder, assuming it will remit with treatment of the underlying PTSD. He warns that there is little evidence to support this assumption and stresses the need to treat specifically the coexisting substance abuse disorder. Bartucci and Stewart [37] recommend treatment of the substance abuse disorder prior to the PTSD, given their complex interactions.

But Wedding [38] argues that treatment focused solely on substance abuse is unlikely to return a functionally impaired veteran with PTSD to a more functional state. He recommends that treatment be tailored for this dual-diagnosis patient.

Drawing on extensive clinical experience with Vietnam veterans, Jelinek and Williams [39] tailor their treatment by dividing their patients into three categories: those who are free of substance abuse; those whose alcohol use began in Vietnam to relieve stress and who continue to self-medicate their PTSD symptoms; and those with substance abuse predating their Vietnam experience and PTSD symptoms and who frequently also have a family history of alcoholism. Jelinek and Williams do not intermingle these patients in therapy groups as their primary issues, and goals differ substantially. For the group who began abusing alcohol in Vietnam for self-medication of stress, they conceive of PTSD as primary and alcoholism as secondary. They recommend treatment in a therapy group where PTSD is the main focus and alcohol abuse is viewed as inhibiting the progress of treatment. In their experience, as PTSD symptoms lessen, veterans reduce or discontinue their alcohol consumption. For the group whose alcohol abuse predates their Vietnam experience, Jelinek and Williams suggest referral to a formal detoxification program first. The primary goal for these veterans is detoxification and abstinence; PTSD therapy is secondary. They report that "detoxing" veterans often experience rebound PTSD symptoms. Post-traumatic stress disorder therapy becomes the focus after abstinence from alcohol is achieved. Jelinek and Williams caution that veterans are generally very resistant to relinquishing alcohol — a cheap, available, and temporarily effective tool for managing disturbing PTSD symptoms. They suggest that a variety of alternate tools be offered: breathing exercises, progressive muscle relaxation, visual imagery, and peer support systems.

Nace [40] offers another perspective on the treatment of this population. He believes that the first priority is treatment of the substance abuse disorder because unchecked abuse will inhibit therapy aimed at other issues. He warns clinicians to avoid assuming that substance abuse is driven by PTSD symptoms and that treatment of PTSD will lead to spontaneous remission of substance abuse. He believes that the euphoria of intoxication can serve as a reward and reinforcement for PTSD symptoms. By the time these individuals present for treatment, Nace feels that their drinking or drugging has already led to dependence and has taken on a life of its own — even if it began with self-medication — and deserves a specific focus in treatment. He adds that abstinence often heightens PTSD symptoms and renders the patient more amenable to psychotherapeutic intervention. Interestingly, Nace modifies his confrontation of the pathological defenses — denial and rationalization — in the treatment of substance abuse in the setting of PTSD. In the presence of PTSD, even more care is needed in nurturing the treatment alliance to keep the patient in treatment than while confronting the uncomplicated substance abuser. Nace stresses how important it is for the therapist to convey respect for the patient — recognizing the validity of the patient's viewpoint without necessarily reinforcing it — and to communicate warmth and genuineness.

## THE BENZODIAZEPINE CONTROVERSY

With the widespread use of benzodiazepines for the treatment of anxiety disorders has come a concern about the abuse potential of these medications. Are physicians introducing patients to a substance abuse disorder? The use of benzodiazepines in the dual-diagnosis patient is especially controversial.

Authors like Ellis and Carney, [41] worried about a potential epidemic of benzodiazepine abuse/dependence, warn that medications are largely inappropriate for the management of generalized anxiety by general medical practitioners. Instead, they suggest the use of supportive psychotherapeutic intervention, behavior modification, physical activity, and relaxation techniques.

Garvey and Tollefson [42] examined benzodiazepine use in a group of patients with major depression, panic disorder, or agoraphobia with panic attacks, who had no history of substance abuse. Only 7% (all with major depression) misused the prescribed benzodiazepines, and each reported this misuse directly to their physician. Furthermore, most of the misusers also admitted to past alcohol abuse during depressive episodes. They conclude that benzodiazepines can be used safely in individuals free of history of substance abuse. They caution that those with history of substance abuse, even highly circumscribed histories, need close supervision if any benzodiazepine is to be used.

Ciraulo et al. [43] recently reviewed the literature on benzodiazepine use in alcoholics. They argue that, although there is a risk in prescribing a potentially abusable medication to an addict, there is likewise a danger in unconditionally withholding a potentially helpful medication from an individual with a serious anxiety disorder. They do find support for the notion that alcoholics are more susceptible to benzodiazepine abuse. However, this does not apply across the board to all, or even most, alcoholics, particularly if benzodiazepines are prescribed in a rational manner. Paramount in this rational use is a clear understanding of what one is treating. For instance, it should be clear that one is treating symptoms of a primary, independent anxiety disorder rather than alcohol withdrawal–related or alcohol-induced anxiety symptoms. Ciraulo and co-workers also encourage trials of alternative treatments prior to the use of benzodiazepines: psychotherapy, behavior therapy, nonaddictive medications. If benzodiazepines are used, they suggest close follow-up,prescribing limited amounts of medication, and urine toxicologies to exclude surreptitious abuse of other substances.

Malka [44] agrees that benzodiazepines may be helpful when anxiety states accompany alcoholism. He recognizes the risk of developing benzodiazepine dependence but believes that this risk is often less than the risk of relapse into excessive alcohol intake at times of heightened anxiety.

Those involved in traditional substance abuse treatment object to views like those of Ciraulo and Malka above. Annitto [45] believes it is impossible for a physician to choose rationally those alcoholics who can safely use benzodiazepines.

Naidoo [46] relates his experience with the development of troublesome benzodiazepine dependence in patients treated for panic disorder. They frequently become tolerant to the benzodiazepine, have breakthrough panic symptoms, and effectively become dual-diagnosis patients. He warns that these patients are difficult to manage since they are frequently hypersensitive to even low-dose tricyclic antidepressants, experiencing sudden increases in anxiety symptoms, complicating their compliance.

Clearly, the jury is still out on this benzodiazepine controversy.

## CONCLUSION

Substance abuse commonly coexists with the various anxiety disorders. The nature of the relationship between the two is somewhat controversial.

With panic disorder, some believe alcoholism develops from an individual's attempt to self-medicate anticipatory anxiety; this model suggests that medical treatment of the underlying panic disorder is the most important intervention. Others point out the similarity between panic symptoms and alcohol withdrawal—even minor withdrawal symptoms between drinks— and how increasing alcohol use exacerbates panic symptoms; this model stresses the need for a period of alcohol abstinence before a valid diagnosis of panic disorder can be made. Cocaine abuse is highly associated with panic attacks and may actually cause panic disorder, which may last years beyond cocaine abstinence.

Among those with post-traumatic stress disorder, especially in the Vietnam veteran population, substance abuse is astoundingly common. A self-medication model exists here, too, although alcohol abuse predates the war experience in many veterans. Most recommend a treatment that focuses on both disorders. The substance abuse interventions should be informed by an understanding of post-traumatic symptoms, and the need for abstinence should be underscored while the anxiety disorder is addressed psychotherapeutically.

# REFERENCES

1.  Weissman MM, Myers JK, Harding PS. Prevalence and psychiatric heterogeneity of alcoholism in a United States urban community. *J Stud Alc* 1980; 41:672–681.
2.  Halikas J, Herzog M, Mirassou M, Lyttle M. Psychiatric diagnosis among female alcoholics. In: M. Galanter, ed., *Currents in Alcoholism*. Vol. 8. New York: Grune and Stratton, 1982.
3.  Weiss KJ, Rosenberg DJ. Prevalence of anxiety disorder among alcoholics. *J Clin Psychiat* 1985; 46:3–5.
4.  Bowen RC, Cipywnyk MD, D'Arcy C, Keegan D. Alcoholism anxiety disorders, and agoraphobia. *Alc: Clin Exp Res* 1984; 8:48–50.
5.  Mullaney JA, Trippett CJ. Alcohol dependence and phobias: clinical description and relevance. *Brit J Psychiat* 1979; 135:565–573.
6.  Smail P, Stockwell T, Canter S, Hodgson R. Alcohol dependence and phobic anxiety states I. A prevalence study. *Brit J Psychiat* 1984; 144:53–57.
7.  Peace K, Mellsop G. Alcoholism and psychiatric disorder. *Aust N Zeal J Psychiat* 1987; 21:94–101.
8.  Weissman MM. Anxiety and alcoholism. *J Clin Psychiat* 1988; 49:17–19.
9.  Noyes R, Crowe RR, Harris EL, Hamra BJ, McChesney CM, Chaudhry DR. Relationship between panic disorder and agoraphobia: A family study. *Arch Gen Psychiat* 1986; 43:227–232.
10. Munjack DJ, Moss HB. Affective disorder and alcoholism in families of agoraphobics. *Arch Gen Psychiat* 1981; 38:869–871.
11. Eisen JL, Rasmussen SA. Coexisting obsessive compulsive disorder and alcoholism. *J Clin Psychiat* 1989; 50:96–98.
12. Kranzler HR, Liebowitz NR. Anxiety and depression in substance abuse: clinical implications. *Med Clin N Amer* 1988; 72:867–885.
13. Breier A, Charney DS, Heninger GR. Agoraphobia with panic attacks: Development, diagnostic stability, and course of illness. *Arch Gen Psychiat* 1986; 43:1029–1036.
14. Reich J, Chaudry D. Personality of panic disorder alcohol abusers. *J Nerv Ment Dis* 1987; 175:224–227.
15. Quitkin FM, Rifkin A, Kaplan J, Klein DF. Phobic anxiety syndrome complicated by drug dependence and addiction: a treatable form of drug abuse. *Arch Gen Psychiat* 1972; 27:157–162.
16. Johannessen DJ, Cowley DS, Walker RD, Jensen CF, Parker L. Prevalence, onset, and clinical recognition of panic states in hospitalized male alcoholics. *Am J Psychiat* 1989; 146:1201–1203.
17. Blankfield A. Psychiatric symptoms in alcohol dependence: diagnostic and treatment implications. *J Subst Abuse Treat* 1986; 3:275–278.
18. George DT, Zerby A, Noble S, Nutt DJ. Panic attacks and alcohol withdrawal: can subjects differentiate the symptoms? *Biol Psychiat* 1988; 24:240–243.
19. Stockwell T, Smail P, Hodgson R, Canter S. Alcohol dependence and phobic anxiety states II. A retrospective study. *Brit J Psychiat* 1984; 144:58–63.
20. George DT, Nutt DJ, Waxman RP, Linnoila M. Panic response to lactate

administration in alcoholic and nonalcoholic patients with panic disorder. *Am J Psychiat* 1989; 146:1161 1165.

21. Anthony JC, Tien AY, Petronis KR. Epidemiologic evidence on cocaine use and panic attacks. *Am J Epidem* 1989; 129:543–549.
22. Washton AM, Gold MS. Chronic cocaine abuse: Evidence for adverse effects on health and functioning. *Psychiat Ann* 1984; 14:733–743.
23. Aronson TA, Craig TJ. Cocaine precipitation of panic disorder. *Am J Psychiat* 1986; 143:643–645.
24. Louie AK, Lannon RA, Ketter TA. Treatment of cocaine-induced panic disorder. *Am J Psychiat* 1989; 146:40–44.
25. Post RM, Uhde TW, Joffe RT, Bierer L. Psychiatric manifestations and implications of seizure disorders. In Extein I, Gold MS, ed., *Medical Mimics of Psychiatric Disorders*. Washington, D.C.: American Psychiatric Press, 1986.
26. Price WA, Giannini AJ. Phencyclidine and "crack" — precipitated panic disorder. *Am J Psychiat* 1987; 144:686–687.
27. Roy-Byrne PP, Uhde TW. Exogenous factors in panic disorder: clinical and research implications. *J Clin Psychiat* 1988; 49:56–61.
28. Nunes EV, Quitkin FM, Klein DE. Psychiatric diagnosis in cocaine abuse. *Psychiat Res* 1989; 28:105–114.
29. Rundell JR, Ursano RJ, Holloway HC, Silberman EK. Psychiatric responses to trauma. *Hosp Comm Psychiat* 1989; 40:68–74.
30. Davidson J, Swartz M, Storck M, Krishman RR, Hammett E. A diagnostic and family study of post traumatic stress disorder. *Am J Psychiat* 1985; 142:90–93.
31. Escobar JI, Randolph ET, Puente G, Spiwak F, Asamen JK, Hill M, Hough RL. Post-traumatic stress disorder in Hispanic Vietnam veterans. *J Nerv Ment Dis* 1983; 171:585–596.
32. Behar D. Confirmation of concurrent illnesses in post-traumatic stress disorder. *Am J Psychiat* 1984; 141:1310.
33. Faustman WO, White PA. Diagnostic and psychopharmacological treatment characteristics of 536 inpatients with posttraumatic stress disorder. *J Nerv Ment Dis* 1989; 177:154–159.
34. Sierles FS, Chen JJ, McFarland RE, Taylor MA. Posttraumatic stress disorder and concurrent psychiatric illness: A preliminary report. *Am J Psychiat* 1983; 140:1177–1179.
35. LaCoursiere RB, Godfrey KE, Ruby LM. Traumatic neurosis in the etiology of alcoholism: Vietnam combat and other trauma. *Am J Psychiat* 1979; 137:966–968.
36. McCormack NA. Substance abuse among Vietnam veterans: a view from the CAP control perspective. *Int J Addict* 1988; 23:1311–1316.
37. Bartucci RJ, Stewart JT. Doctors Bartucci and Stewart reply. *Am J Psychiat* 1986; 143:1203.
38. Wedding D. Substance abuse in the Vietnam veteran. *AAOHN J* 1987; 35:74–76.
39. Jelinek JM, Williams T. Post-traumatic stress disorder and substance abuse in Vietnam combat veterans: treatment problems, strategies and recommendations. *J Subst Abuse Treat* 1984; 1:87–97.

40. Nace EP. Posttraumatic stress disorder and substance abuse: clinical issues. In: M. Galanter, ed., *Recent Developments in Alcoholism*. Vol. 6. New York: Plenum Press, 1988.
41. Ellis P, Carney MWP. Benzodiazepine abuse and management of anxiety in the community. *Int J Addict* 1988; 23:1083–1090.
42. Garvey MJ, Tollefson GD. Prevalence of misuse of prescribed benzodiazepines in patients with primary anxiety disorder or major depression. *Am J Psychiat* 1986; 143:1601–1603.
43. Ciraulo DA, Sands BF, Shader RI. Critical review of liability for benzodiazepine abuse among alcoholics. *Am J Psychiat* 1988; 145:1501–1506.
44. Malka R. Role of drug therapies in the treatment of alcoholism: alcohol and anxiety — alcohol and depression. *Clin Neuropharm* 1988; 11:S69–S73.
45. Annitto WJ. Alcoholics' use of benzodiazepines. *Am J Psychiat* 1989; 146:683.
46. Naidoo P. Benzodiazepine addiction. *N Zeal Med J* 1988; 101:88–89.

# 4

# Substance Abuse and Thought Disorders

**A. James Giannini**

*The Ohio State University, Columbus, Ohio*

**Gregory B. Collins**

*The Cleveland Clinic Foundation, Cleveland, Ohio*

The treatment of dual-diagnosis psychotic patients has, traditionally and unfortunately, been one of extremes rather than means. There has been a clinical tendency to separate the psychosis from the drug abuse. While traditional psychiatrists have usually limited their focus to the underlying motivation, internists and psychiatrists specializing in drug abuse have isolated the overdose or withdrawal state, and a bevy of drug counselors have emphasized the addictive behavior. Historically, these professional groups have tended to operate in either less than splendid isolation or in a lockstep, assembly-line procedure. Fortunately, a more recent trend has tended to combine these approaches into a holistic, mutually supportive, unified treatment model. This comprehensive strategy involves the extension of the "disease model" to the dual treatment of the diagnosis psychotic patient.

Approximately 10% of addicts have a coexisting major psychiatric disorder [1]. Anticholinergic effects are often sought by schizophrenics, while manics rely on alcohol to "bring them down." In addition, some drugs such as phencyclidine and lysergic acid produce acute psychoses in over three-fourths of the abusing population [2]. Detoxification from cocaine, barbiturates, and ethchlorvynol can produce psychotic withdrawal symptoms. Amphetamine, taken chronically and acutely, can produce a paranoid psychosis. Alcohol can produce a variety of acute and chronic psychotic states, including the acute agitation of intoxication, the acute paranoid psychoses, and the agitated confusion of delirium tremens. Alcohol also causes many nutrition-related psychotic states, most notably the Wernicke–Korsakov dementia.

Ideally, psychiatric illness in a substance abuser should be coordinated with a drug-rehabilitation program. Neither detoxification nor psychotherapy is independently an effective treatment for the addictive behavior. Similarly, the psychiatrist must take caution not to sabotage the rehabilitation process by prescribing addictive medications. Definitive and psychotic pharmacological therapy, however, remains the same in both abusing and nonabusing psychotic patients.

The psychedelic drugs are well known for their ability to provoke psychotic reactions. They produce sensory distortion by their actions on central serotonin. The major concentration of serotonergic neurons is found in the five pairs of pontine raphe nuclei in the brainstem. These fibers then project to the other parts of the brainstem, to the forebrain, and to the spinal cord.

The psychedelics apparently act at both inhibitory presynaptic and excitatory postsynaptic sites. The major clinical effect, however, appears to be excitatory. Most psychedelics bind in the auditory and visual areas, the limbic system (especially the amygdala, hippocampus, and striate bodies), and the cerebral cortex. In this manner, these drugs are able to alter the perception and integration of sensory stimuli [3].

The peculiar dreamlike quality produced by the psychedelics may also be due to serotonergic action. Most serotonergic neurons fire in a slow, rhythmic action. This activity naturally ceases only during the REM phase of sleep. Lysergic acid diethylamide (LSD) and possibly other related drugs also inhibit this activity, possibly inducing a dreamlike state. Supporting this finding is the observation that REM suppression can be overridden by serotonergic antagonists [4].

Most psychedelics are alkaloids. Prehistoric man may have discovered these effects in the mushroom fly agaric (*Amanita muscaria*). Recorded history reveals a succession of culturally bound psychedelic episodes. In the West, the minted ceremonial drink *kykyion*, which contained LSD derived from infested grain, was used in the Eleusinian rites in Athens 3,500 years ago [5].

In modern times, Albert Hoffman synthesized LSD in 1943. He inadvertently absorbed some through his skin and experienced a psychotic reaction. Aldous Huxley experimented with mescaline in the early 1950s and published his results in *Doors of Perception*. In the 1980s, carboxylated amphetamine derivative, "ecstasy" (methylenedioxyamphetamine), was used briefly in psychoanalysis because of its "bonding" effects. Because of its psychedelic abuse potential, however, the U.S. Food and Drug Administration reclassified methylenedioxyamphetamine as an "experimental" drug. All psychedelics produce vivid visual and auditory imagery, accompanied by depersonalization, derealization, hallucinations, disorientation, and dissociation. Physical changes are not clinically significant. They include mydriasis, diaphoresis, and resting and intention tremor. In addition to this general presentation, many of these drugs have their own distinctive sign or symptom [6].

Absorption of most psychedelics occurs through the gastrointestinal tract and nasal mucosa. Metabolism is oxidative and via hepatic pathways. Primary distribution is in the kidney, liver, and lungs [7]. Treatment is basically psychologically supportive.

Reassurance and reality-oriented therapy are sufficient in a low-intensity environment to treat most psychedelic states. When this fails, lorazepam 1–2 mg IM may be given to soothe agitation. (Be aware, however, that benzodiazepines decrease the rate of psychedelic metabolism.) If the psychosis persists, neuroleptics are generally effective. Haloperidol is recommended since the psychedelic may be adulterated with phencyclidine [8].

Lysergic acid diethylamide (LSD) is a substance that is usually vended as a synthetic derivative. It naturally occurs in morning glory seeds and, to a lesser extent, in wheat fungus and nutmeg. It produces a unique cross-sensory distortion, or "synesthesia." In a synesthetic experience, the abuser can "hear" color, or "see" sounds [8–10].

Mescaline causes an illusory "flattening" and "geometricization" of three-dimensional objects in the visual field. The result is that humans and animals can be seen as cubist images. Dimethyltryptamine, dioxymethylamphetamine, and dioxymethylmethamphetamine produce powerful illusions of emotional bonding and physical merging. This property has made those drugs extremely popular as sexual aids [8,10,11].

Psilocybin use causes an intensification of perceived color. Because of this, abusers are able to "see" thousands of variations on the primary colors and their derivatives [12].

Nutmeg and its rind, mace, are the sources of many psychedelics, including myristicin, borneol, eugenol, and LSD. These spices also are powerful emetics. Doses necessary to produce psychosis also can produce ipecaclike effects. The abuser typically presents with psychosis and severe emesis [13].

## DISSOCIATIVES

The dissociatives are a class of drugs with effects on most major neurotransmitter systems. They include phencyclidine (PCP), the prototypical member, as well as ketamine, which is still used in anesthesiology. The primary source of their psychotic changes appears to be increased activity at the presynaptic (DA-2) dopamine receptors [14]. This provides excitation, paranoia, delusions, and hallucinations. It may also account for much of the postingestion amnesia. Dopaminergic binding occurs in the nucleus accumbens and nigrostriatal areas. Dopaminergic activity is paramount in doses of 10–20 mg of phencyclidine [15].

At lower doses of 5–10 mg, anticholinergic effects seem to predominate [15]. Phencyclidine has the cationic head, bulky phenyl group, and large hydroxyl group typical of atropinic and muscarinic agents. PCP competes directly with acetylcholine for binding sites. It also disrupts the linkage between the acetylcholine receptor and the associated potassium channel [16]. Clinical effects include confusion, dissociation, disorientation, hyperreactivity of deep tendon reflexia, pupillary dilatation, decreased corneal reflex, horizontal nystagmus, flushed dry skin, and elevated body temperature [15,17].

At all doses, phencyclidine agonizes $\beta$-opioid receptors in the thalamus, the periaqueductal gray area, and the substantia gelatinosa [15]. This opioid receptor agonism may cause the indifference to pain reported in abusers. It also may cause miosis and respiratory depression, and it may exacerbate anticholinergic confusion and dopaminergic delusions. Finally, antagonistic actions at the NMDA (N-methyl-D-aspartate) receptor (primarily in the cerebral cortex and hippocampus) may result in amnestic episodes, seizures, and anoxic effects [18].

The overall clinical presentation of PCP psychosis typically involves agitation, disorientation, and confusion. The skin is hot and dry. Eye examination is remarkable for mydriasis, mild exophthalmos, and decreased corneal reflex; nystagmus in horizontal, vertical and, occasionally, rotatory planes may be seen. There may be paranoid suspicious trends with great potential for violence. Typically, the abuser is amnestic for most of the episode. Tolerance for pain is much increased. As a result, the patient may tear muscle tissue without being aware of it. Myoglobinuria is a sometimes fatal result of this [19,20].

Phencyclidine, like the other dissociatives is an arylcyclohexylamine. It is a weak base that is soluble in both water and lipid. It produces a dopamine-dependent psychosis. Detoxification treatment is based on these two characteristics and utilizes dopamine blockade plus ion trapping. A dopamine receptor blocker such as haloperidol 5 mg IM or PO q. 20–30 min will usually block the psychotic symptoms. Since phencyclidine is a specific DA-2 receptor agonist, haloperidol's DA-2 antagonism provides specific antipsychotic effects. Additionally, unlike many neuroleptics, haloperidol has no anticholinergic actions to synergize those of phencyclidine [21].

Ion trapping involves the rapid neutralization and elimination of phencyclidine. Ingested PCP is first neutralized in the gastrointestinal tract with magnesium sulfate. It is also neutralized in the serum via intramuscular injections of 1 g ascorbic acid. (In addition to its ion-trapping effects, ascorbic acid also directly augments haloperidol's dopaminergic effect.) Once "trapped," phencyclidine can be eliminated renally with furosemide 40 mg IM [22].

Withdrawal dysphoria, depersonalization, and derealization can occur after cessation of prolonged use of PCP [23,24]. To decrease these symptoms, high doses of the noradrenergic tricyclic antidepressant desipramine can be given for a two- to eight-week period [24]. Usually, the maximum dose ranges from 200–300 mg/day. Daily dosage begins at 50 mg hs and is raised by 50-mg increments until the maximum tolerated dosage in the 200–300-mg range is achieved. Psychotherapy should focus on dealing with residual aggressive impulses, dissociation, and amnestic gaps. Psychotic relapses have reportedly occurred in the context of psychoanalytic therapy. PCP is a nonreinforcing drug with no stimulus triggers [23,25].

In part because of its low price, PCP abuse is a blue collar phenomenon. Because of its multiple effects and multiple forms of abuse, it is an adulterant of many other drugs of abuse. It has been estimated that fully two-thirds of all PCP sold is vended as another drug. It can be inhaled, snorted, injected, smoked, ingested, and even used as a douche or enema. Because of its dopaminergic activity, it is often sold as amphetamine. Its combined dopaminergic and noradrenergic stimulating effects allow it often to be vended as cocaine. Its sedating effects make it an ideal mimic for the GABAergic drugs such as barbiturates, ethchlorvynol, and meprobamate. Its action on the opiod receptor makes it a credible substitute for heroin and morphine. Dusted on low-grade marijuana, or even oregano, it can be smoked in a simulation of high-grade "Colombian" marijuana [23].

## ANTICHOLINERGICS

Abuse of anticholinergics is rare, but the anticholinergics are the drugs most commonly abused by schizophrenics. These patients are first exposed to members of this class when being treated for neuroleptic-induced parkinsonism. Benzotropine (Cogentin), biperiden (Akineton), and diphenhydramine (Benadryl) are the most commonly prescribed and subsequently abused drugs for this purpose. Typically, the patients discontinue the neuroleptic but continue to use the anticholinergic [26].

Anticholinergics produce their psychotic states by blocking potassium channels in central neurons [27]. The gross anatomical sites of action include the nucleus basalis of Meynert and the nigrostriatal bodies. By way of comparison, primary degenerative loss of cholinergic activity in these areas produces, respectively, Huntington's chorea and primary Parkinson's disease. In addition, anticholinergics block activity in the reticular activating substance (RAS) [26]. These actions are caused by three essential structural features of the molecule: there must always be a cationic head, a bulky phenyl group, and a hydroxy group [28]. Anticholinergics also block electrical polarization throughout the periphery. As a result, high doses or overdoses produce paralytic ileus and atonic bladder [29].

More significantly, anticholinergics can affect the electrical conductivity of the heart itself. T-wave flattening, or inversion, QRS prolongation, circus rhythms, and asystole have all been reported. The cardiac effects make anticholinergic psychosis the most dangerous of the drug-induced psychotic states. Activity can be measured by cardiac monitor. When the QRS widens to 10, administer physostigmine salicylate 2 mg IM. Since physostigmine, a semireversible cholinesterase inhibitor, passes the blood-brain barrier, it can also be used to treat psychosis. Allow 20 min between each injection. If bronchial oversecretion results, suction immediately. The patient may be at risk for up to 72 h, and so cardiac monitoring should be maintained for that time period [30].

In addition to aggravating the underlying psychosis of schizophrenia, anticholinergics also produce a classical "signature." These features, as enunciated by Sir William Osler, result in a patient who is "mad as a hatter, red as a beet, and dry as a bone." Other distinctive psychotic features include Lilliputian hallucinations, visual hallucinations of dark flying shapes, photophobia, grandiose delusions, and illusions of flying [8].

Anticholinergic medication, especially tripelennamine, can be used to boost the effectiveness of opiates. The enhancement is a result of the interrelationship between the opioid receptors and potassium channels. Decreased potassium activity results in magnification of opiate action. As a result, relatively weak opiates such as pentazocine (Talwin) can, when combined with tripelennamine, give the equivalent opiate action of heroin. This combination is known as "T's and blues." This interactive effect operates between all anticholinergics and opiates: not surprisingly, the methadone analog propoxyphene (Darvon) has recently been reported to have been abused with diphenhydramine (Benadryl) [31,32].

## OPIATES

Although not considered producers of psychosis, opiates in high dosages can produce intense visual hallucinations. These were described in Thomas De Quincey's *Confessions of an English Opium-Eater* nearly two centuries ago. The opiate-induced dreamlike states can become intensely vivid if the dosage strength is sufficiently high.

Opiates evidently produce these psychotic effects by secondary actions on norepinephrine [33]. In addition to their pleasure-producing actions at the nucleus accumbens, they also block noradrenergic release at the locus ceruleus in ventral floor of the pons [34]. The psychosis is produced when high levels of opiates are consumed. Since the necessary psychotogenic doses are often fatal if produced by intravenous administrations, most delusional/hallucinatory experiences occur when heroin or morphine is smoked. This was the attraction of nineteenth-century "opium dens." Also, similar effects can be produced by dissolving opium or morphine in alcoholic beverages and then drinking the potent cocktail. This combination was first made by the Renaissance physician Paracelsus in the early sixteenth century.

The psychotic state can be easily blocked with injections of naloxone. If addiction is present, detoxification can be effected using clonidine 17 $\mu$/kg/day in divided dosages, titrating downward over a seven-day period. Neuroleptics are not indicated for these relatively brief psychotic states [35].

Detoxification must be done on an inpatient unit since opiate cravings are strongly environment-dependent. Abstinence systems may be classically conditioned responses, since chills, cramping, and nausea can emerge long after detoxification in an environment with "stimulus triggers," such as friends from the opiate subculture or exposure to needles and spoons. In controlled studies, former addicts were found to get "high" when injected with placebo under triggered conditions [36].

For this reason, therapy should be geared to major changes in the addict's life-style. An alternative peer structure drawn from recovery groups such as Narcotics Anonymous is often the best starting point. Behavior therapy aimed at stimulus decrement is also important. To assist in maintenance of an opiate-free life-style, the inert opiate blocker naltrexone 25–50 mg qd may be prescribed [8].

## SYMPATHOMIMETICS

Another drug that may activate the pleasure centers in the nucleus accumbens is cocaine [37]. This derivative of the leaves of the coca plant has been used in the Americas probably since the tenth century. Employed by the armies of the Inca, it could ward off hunger and fatigue as well as precipitate a "berserk" state in warriors. Psychotic features were achieved by chewing leaves mixed with ashes. This latter practice produced an early primitive form of "crack." [8]

Chronic cocaine use produces many tactile hallucinations of "cocaine bugs" as well as of terrifying figures [38,39]. Thinking can be distorted by paranoid trends. The patient's sleep is frequently troubled by multiple checks under the bed, in the closets, and at the doors for whatever phantoms might occupy the crevices of the dark [37].

The cause of cocaine addition and psychosis may be central dopamine depletion. In addition to causing a massive release of dopamine into the synaptic cleft, cocaine blocks reuptake. Consequently, dopamine cannot be recycled, and a progressively declining supply is the result [37]. Therefore, neuroleptics that produce antipsychotic actions by blocking dopamine should be used with great caution [38]. Also, they are often not particularly effective. Agitation can be treated with intramuscular lorazepam (Ativan) 1–2 mg on an acute basis. Bromocriptine (Parlodel) 1.25–2.5 mg q. 6 h on a gradually declining basis can decrease psychotic perceptions as well as block symptoms of cocaine withdrawal [40,41]. At present, cocaine use is prevalent in all strata of society.

In therapy, patients must be educated to recognize and identify their sympathomimetic cravings so that they can avoid those decisions that predispose toward relapse. Urges are tied to visual and emotional stimuli and need to be modulated or eliminated. Assertiveness training, peer-group therapy, family therapy, relaxation training, and goal-oriented individual therapy are stressed. The goal is the development of an alternative, drug-free life-style. Commercial treatment programs, Narcotics Anonymous, and Cocaine Anonymous generally follow these cognitive-behavioral guidelines. When cocaine and other sympathomimetics are used for their anorectic effects, weight/feeding intake programs such as TOPS, Overeaters Anonymous, and Weight Watchers can be useful. The treatment professional can also give the patient the toll-free number of BASH (Bulimia Anorexia Self-Help Foundation, St. Louis, Missouri), which is (800) 227-4785 [42].

Amphetamine and similar sympathomimetics produce psychotic reactions similar to cocaine, but these psychoses are quantitatively and qualitatively less severe [43]. Amphetamine is abused by long-distance truck drivers seeking endurance as well as by overweight (and self-perceived overweight) individuals in search of a svelte silhouette courtesy of amphetamine's anorectic affects [8]. Its paranoid tendencies are a bit greater than cocaine, while the incidence of visual hallucinations is much less. The treatment with benzodiazepines and bromocriptine is identical to that of cocaine [42].

Phenylpropanolamine (PPA) and cinnamedryl are over-the-counter sympathomimetics with abusive and psychosis-inducing potential. The former is sold as an anorectic and cold preparation, while the latter is advertised for treatment of menstrual cramps. Abusers of both are generally adolescent females. Anorexia, anxiety, irritability, and visual hallucinations have been noted after chronic abuse. Paranoia is not common. Usually, bromocriptine and neuroleptics are not necessary. Reality-oriented psychotherapy, combined with anxiolytics such as hydroxyzine (Vistaril) 25–50 mg IM or PO, usually suffice to reduce psychotic symptoms. Acute psychosis seen in overdoses respond to propranolol 10–40 mg qid PO [44,45].

A more exotic sympathomimetic source is the botanical "khat" ("qat") (*Cutha edulis Forsk*). This plant was originally cultivated in Yemen and now is in widespread use throughout the Mideast. Its use has also been reported in Europe and the United States. The leaves of this plant contain phenylpropanolamine, cathine, cathinone, and an analog of ephedrine. When chewed, they produce an intense "rush," which may result in manic or paranoid psychoses. Haloperidol 5 mg IM, carbamazepine 100 mg PO, or reserpine 0.1 mg IM have all been reported to block these short-lived psychoses [46,47].

## STEROIDS

Anabolic steroid psychosis has been, until now, a relatively rare occurrence. However, it is estimated that 20% of all male and 10% of all female high school athletes abuse anabolic steroids to enhance muscular development and athletic performance [48]. Irritability, accompanied by mixed paranoid delusions of grandeur and persecution, makes these testosterone derivates and analogs important, albeit atypical drugs of abuse. Visual hallucinations are generally limited to yellow, or more often, white chromatopsia. Virilization in women and persistent erections with hypogonadism in men are often seen. Stretch marks across the pectorales major, rectus femoris, and biceps-triceps are typical signatures marking a particular psychosis as steroid-induced [49].

The retention of nitrogen to build up muscular protoplasm also affects functioning of neural tissue. This results in changes in central catecholamine metabolism. The resultant psychosis can be treated with any neuroleptic. In many cases, maintenance lithium therapy will protect the individual against residual grandiosity, irritability, and aggressivity [50].

Psychotherapy should focus on body image and self-image. Frequently, a strong need for achievement-dependent acceptance is key. Outpatient drug-rehabilitation programs and Narcotics Anonymous have not proved particularly useful. Therapists need to work closely with the individual's coach or athletic trainer. It is essential to involve the patient's designated "authority figure" to remove perceived stressors predisposing toward relapse.

## ALCOHOL

Alcoholism is a disease of chronic abuse of, and dependence on, ethanol. It may be that pathological Picket–Spengler condensation of acetaldehyde and biogenic amines to form tetrohydroisoquinolone (THIQ) predisposes one to alcohol cravings and addictions [8,51]. There are many direct and indirect manifestations of alcoholic psychosis. Directly, acute and chronic alcohol intoxication may produce alcoholic paranoia, "pathological intoxication" with agitation and violence, acute alcoholic psychosis, and delirium tremens. Indirectly, alcoholism may cause nutrition-related psychoses, including Wernicke–Korsakov psychosis, pellagra, hypomagnesemia, and vitamin B-12 deficiency [52].

Alcohol is often favored by manics to bring relief from uncontrollable mood swings [1]. This may account for the high incidence of alcoholism in this subgroup. (Since mania is a disease of upward mobility that allows for rapid informational processing, many of its sufferers are propelled into the boardrooms and higher-status professions. This may account for the use of alcohol at a higher strata of society.) Alcohol has traditionally been abused at the bottom of the social scale to ward off effects of hunger, deprivation, boredom, and failure. William Hogarth's "Gin Lane" gave graphic evidence of this.

The effects of simple ingestion of alcoholic beverages can be magnified by dissolving metronidazole (Flagyl) in the glass. Metronidazole decreases alcoholic absorption in the gastrointestinal tract and slows metabolism in the liver. The result is an excited state that may proceed to psychosis. There is hypersexuality, with delusions of grandeur. Confusion and disorientation are not uncommon [53].

Chronic alcohol abuse decreases the amount of available central glucose. This, in turn, causes a compensatory shunting of gamma-aminobutyric acid (GABA) to succinate pathways to create a reserve energy supply. GABA inhibition over biogenic and amino acid amines is thereby decreased. Acting on GABA coreceptor, it increases neuronal membrane fluidity by cephalin methylation. This, in turn, counteracts the antifluidizing effects of ethanol-induced increase in the cholesterol-phospholipid ratio. Membrane excitability is also altered by suppression of Na/K ATPase and consequent sodium-potassium transport. There is also some evidence that alcohol operates in inhibition coupling of adenylate cyclase [51,54,55].

Although GABA inhibition is decreased by chronic alcoholism, there is still a minor direct inhibitory effect. When alcohol is withdrawn, all inhibition is removed. This then results in the manifestations of delirium tremens. There is a massive release of biogenic amines and amino acid neurotransmitters. As a result, gross tremors are seen. Visual hallucinations and delusions are thought to be due to diminished dopaminergic inhibition. Hyperpyrexia is caused by hypothalamic effect. Nystagmus is also due to indirect dopaminergic effects originating in the occiput. While many mechanisms may be operative during withdrawal, treatment is organized about reintroducing GABAergic control. Benzodiazepines are always indicated; neuroleptics are not. Librium 10–50 mg qid or lorazepam 1–2 mg qid will usually reassert neurotransmitter control [8,54,56,57].

When delirium tremens is under control, the psychosis may still remain. This may be due to nutritional deficiencies, not uncommonly from inadequate intake of vitamin B-12 and folic acid. Typically, these patients have group visual hallucinations and well-organized paranoid delusions. There are also other associated nonpsychiatric signs that help to reveal the diagnosis. Peripheral blood smears demonstrate macrocytic anemia. Physical examination can show spasticity, diminished vibratory sense, and a "beef-red" tongue. These patients also complain of paresthesias, numbness, tinnitus, and dim vision [56].

When alcoholics reach this stage, they are usually in need of serious therapy. The Alcoholics Anonymous 12-step program seems historically to have been the most successful. In addition, the family should be strongly encouraged to participate through such ancillary programs as Al-Anon and Ala-Teen. Outpatient rehabilitation, as initially developed by such pilot programs as Chemical Abuse Centers, Inc., in Ohio, provides a useful four-point program that enlists the support network of the patient, including the employer. In such a protocol, patients are able to live with their families and continue working while participating in the 12-point process.

Vitamin B-12 (cyanocobalamin) is essential for synthesis and maintenance of the myelin sheath throughout the central and peripheral nervous system. Damage to this myelin sheath results in the large number of symptoms. Replacement of vitamin B-12 is essential. Vitamin B-12, given 2 cc IM, is usually sufficient when combined with sound nutritional support. A supplementary treatment of folic acid 1 mg qd PO will protect from hematological damage. Complete recovery occurs in 30%, and incomplete recovery in about 60%, of severe cases [8,56].

A second deficiency state with psychotic symptoms is the well-known Wernicke–Korsakov psychosis. This is due to a vitamin B-1 (thiamine) deficiency and is similar to beriberi. The classic presentation of Wernicke–Korsakov psychosis is amnestic episodes accompanied by confabulation. There can also be delirium, ophthalmoplegia, ataxia, nystagmus, misrecognition of others, and misperception of situations. These symptoms are associated with hemorrhagic necrosis of the mammillary bodies. These interrupt the Papez circuit, which coordinates information between the neocortex and hypothalamus. Other lesions in the periaqueductal region disrupt the ascending fibers of the RAS and the median forebrain bundle. Yet another focal degeneration is in the dorsomedial thalamic nucleus [58,59].

Thiamine is needed for several steps in carbohydrate metabolism, including decarboxylation of pyruvic acid, decarboxylation of $\alpha$-ketoglutaric acid, and pentose utilization in the hexose monophosphate shunt [43]. Treatment consists of an initial dose of thiamine 200 mg IM, followed by daily doses of 200 mg PO for 8–12 months. About 55% show partial recovery after five years and 25% show no significant improvement [58,59].

Niacin deficiency (pellagra) is marked by the "four D's": diarrhea, dermatitis, and dementia, followed by death. Other symptoms include confusion and mood-congruent delusions. Niacin acts as an enzyme in the synthetic and metabolic pathways of many neurotransmitters. Consequently, in niacin deficiency, there is neuronal degeneration throughout the neocortex, pyramidal, and extrapyramidal tracts as well as the cerebellum. Demyelination of the lateral column of the spinal cord may also occur. Rapid treatment is essential. Nicotinic acid 50 mg should be given 10 times qd or 25 mg IV bid or tid. Delirium usually improves within two days [60].

Magnesium is essential to neuronal catecholamine uptakes. It also helps regulate calcium intracellular/extracellular balance. Alcohol-induced hypomagnesemia causes irritability and suspiciousness, which may assume the proportions of paranoid delusions. Degenerations in the cerebellum and basal ganglia cause coarse irregular resting tremors and intention tremors. Treatment is relatively straightforward, and 1.0–4.0 g $MgSO_4$ IM may be given in divided doses of 0.5–1.0 g in alternating buttocks on successive days while titrating for serum magnesium levels daily [52,61].

A number of relatively rare psychoses can also occur with alcohol abuse. Marchiafava–Bignami disease, paranoid delusional states with apraxia, aphasia, and mixed manic and depressive features are seen. These changes have, reportedly, been due to a symmetrical bilateral degeneration of the myelin sheath in the corpus callosum and, less consistently, to accompanying degeneration of the anterior commissure and midcerebellar peduncles. Though the exact pathogenesis is unknown, there seems to be an association with cheap homemade red wine. The course is invariably fatal after a few years of progressive deterioration. There is no known treatment [8].

Alcoholic paranoia has been theorized to occur by precipitation of latent paranoid schizophrenia by chronic alcoholic disinhibition of the exact cause is unknown. It is marked by morbid jealousy, ideas of reference and outside influence, sexual delusions that one's lover is promiscuous, rage reactions, and distrust of nearly everyone. Chlorpromazine in doses adequate to relieve agitation or violence, over several months, may be indicated. Treatment on a psychiatric unit is recommended, with the focus on paranoid trends [62].

A related presentation occurs in acute alcoholic psychosis. This occurs in chronic alcoholism when a latent schizophrenia is precipitated by a period of abstinence. Symptoms include auditory command hallucinations, persecutory delusions, auditory and olfactory hallucinations, and panic. It is distinguished from delirium tremens by the fineness of the resting tremor, absence of hyperpyrexia and visual hallucinations, presence of auditory hallucinations, and well-organized delusions. Treat, initially, with chlordiazepoxide 50 mg PO. If no improvement occurs, give haloperidol 5–10 mg bid-qid IM or PO. Stress reality-oriented psychotherapy as well as alcohol counseling [63].

Paradoxical intoxication occurs acutely after ingestion of small amounts of alcoholic beverages. Delusions, impulsivity, and visual hallucinations are typical. Lesions of the uncinate and other areas contribute to the presentation. The disinhibitory effects of alcohol seem to magnify underlying pathology in the cortical area. Since the presentation is short-lived, sedation with any benzodiazepine is usually effective. This type of intoxication is seen predominantly in schizophrenics and epileptics [64].

The thought disorders occurring in substance abuse may arise from the drug abused or from the underlying psychopathology of the abuser. Some psychotic reactions may reflect severe or borderline-integrated psychopathology, which is easily decompensated into psychosis by drug or alcohol abuse. Other psychoses, such as those induced by PCP, reflect the dangers and profound psychiatric risk inherent in these profoundly mind-altering drugs, even to well-integrated individuals. While some of the drugs of abuse produce characteristic psychotic symptomatology, most often the pattern is a nonspecific one characterized by agitation, confusion, paranoia, or loss of mental acuity, making a definitive clinical diagnosis of a specific substance very difficult. Where confronted with an acute psychosis, the clinician is strongly advised to maintain a high index of suspicion for substance abuse as a coincident or causative factor and to search for a drug-induced etiology. Such a search must include serum and urine toxicology screening for any potentially mind-altering or therapeutic substance. Ruling out the presence of mind-altering substances should occur before the aggressive use of neuroleptics to manage agitation or violent behaviors. Precipitous therapy with neuroleptics in the face of a psychosis caused by an unknown drug ingestion may worsen the psychotic process, as is the case with anticholinergics. While the laboratory results are pending, the physician might be well advised to medicate cautiously, using neuroleptics judiciously, if at all, and preferring benzodiazapines for their safety as a short-term measure.

The substance abuser with the frank psychosis presents a problem that is challenging indeed for the diagnostic and treatment skills of the physician. While the physician may realize that the psychosis could be drug-induced and is cautious in the prescription of neuroleptics or sedatives to control the symptoms, he or she may also be under pressure to respond to the manifestation of bizarre or potentially destructive thinking or behavior. Such situations often constitute a psychiatric emergency that is generally best met in an inpatient setting, with adequate nursing care to provide close supervision, and the necessary means to provide controls for extreme agitation, violence, or suicidal behavior. A multidisciplinary approach is clearly called for, with intensive intervention by psychiatrists knowledgeable about drugs, chemical-dependency professionals, nurses, and clinical laboratory specialists. Such a team can effectively diagnose the nature of the chemical psychosis, can protect the patient from harm to self or others, and can detoxify or medicate as needed to resolve the acute psychosis. The next phase of treatment, abstinence-oriented psychotherapy, must be initiated promptly to prevent the patient's return to the offending substances or others. To this end, long-term follow-up with abstinence-oriented counseling, community self-help groups (such as Alcoholics Anonymous, Cocaine Anonymous, and Narcotics Anonymous), combined with periodic urine monitoring, should provide a foundation for sustained recovery.

## REFERENCES

1. Sternberg DE. Dual diagnosis. In: Giannini AJ, Slaby AE. *Drugs of Abuse*. Oradell, N.J.: Medical Economics, 1989.
2. Giannini AJ. Phencyclidine. In: Miller NS ed. *A Handbook of Drug and Alcohol Addiction*. New York: Marcel Dekker (in press).
3. Aghajanian GK, Sprouse JS, Rasmussin K. Physiology of the midbrain serotonin system. In: Meltzer H ed. *Psychopharmacology, The Third Generation of Progress*. New York: Raven Press, 1987.
4. Aghajanian GK. LSD and serotonergic dorsal raphe neurons. In: Jacobs B ed. *Hallucinogens: Neurochemical, Behavioral and Clinical Perspectives*. New York: Raven Press, 1984.
5. Seigel R. The natural history of hallucinogens. In: Jacobs B ed. *Hallucinogens: Neurochemical, Behavioral and Clinical Perspectives*. New York: Raven Press, 1984.
6. Shulgin AT. The background and chemistry of MDMA. *J Psychoactive Drugs* 1986; 18:291–304.
7. Siva-Sankar DV. *LSD: A Total Study*. New York: PJD Publications, 1975.
8. Giannini AJ, Slaby AE, Giannini MC. *Handbook of Overdose and Detoxification Emergencies*. New York: Medical Examination/Excerpta Medica, 1983.
9. Bowers MS, Friedman DX. Psychedelic experiences in acute psychosis. *Arch Gen Psychiat* 1966; 120:13–19.
10. Valette G, LeClaire M. Effects of mescaline and lysergide. *C R Acad Sci (Paris)* 1978; 287:1055–1059.
11. Climko RP, Roehrich H, Sweeney DR. Esctasy: A review of MDMA and MDA. *Int J Psychiat Med* 1986–87; 16:359–372.
12. Freedman DX. The psychopharmacology of hallucinogenic agents. *Ann Rev Med* 1964; 20:409, 214.
13. Painter JC, Shanor SP, Winck CL. Nutmeg poisoning. *J Toxicol: Clin Toxicol* 1971; 4(1):1–8.

14. Giannini AJ, Eighan MI, Giannini MC, Loiselle RH. Comparison of haloperidol and chlorpromazine in the treatment of phencyclidine psychosis. Role of the DA-2 receptor. *J Clin Pharmacol* 1984; 24:202–205.

15. Giannini AJ, Giannini MC, Sangdahl C. Antidotal strategies in phencyclidine intoxication. *Int J Psychiat Med* 1984; 14:315–321.

16. Albuquerque EX, Aguago LG, Warnick JE. Interactions of phencyclidine with ion channels of nerve and muscle. *Fed Proc* 1983; 42:2854–2859.

17. Castellani S, Adams PM, Giannini AJ. Physostigmine treatment of acute phencyclidine intoxication. *J Clin Psychiat* 1982; 43:10–11.

18. Compton RP, Contreras PC, O'Donohue TL. The NMDA antagonist, 2-amino-7-phosphoheptanoate produces phencyclidine like behavioral effects in rats. *Eur J Pharmacol* (in press).

19. Giannini AJ. PCP: Detecting the abuser. *Med Aspects Human Sexuality* 1987; 21(1):100–112.

20. Dandarino R, Friborg J, Bendry C. Un cas d'intoxication aigue a la phencyclidine avec atteinte muscarlaire importante et insuffisance renale aigue. *L'Union Med Can* 1975; 104:57–60.

21. Giannini AJ, Nageotte C, Loiselle RH, Malone DA. Comparison of chlorpromazine, haloperidol and primozide in the treatment of phencyclidine psychosis. Role of the DA-2 receptor. *J Toxicol: Clin Toxicol* 1985; 22:573–578.

22. Giannini AJ, Loiselle RH, Giannini MC, DiMarzio LR. Augmentation of haloperidol with ascorbic acid in phencyclidine intoxication. *Am J Psychiat* 1987; 144:1207–1210.

23. Giannini AJ, Loiselle RH, Giannini MC, Price WA. Phencyclidine and the dissociatives. *Med Psychiat* 1987; 3(3):197–214.

24. Giannini AJ, Malone DA, Giannini MC, Price WA, Loiselle RH. Treatment of chronic cocaine and phencyclidine abuse with desipramine. *J Clin Pharmacol* 1986; 26:211–215.

25. Fauman B, Aldinger G, Fauman M. Psychiatric sequelae of phencyclidine abuse. *J Toxicol: Clin Toxicol* 1976; 9:529–538.

26. Borison RL, Evans DR, Elia HW, Evans DD, Diamone BI. Anticholinergics. In: Giannini AJ, Slaby AE, eds. *Drugs of Abuse.* Oradell, N.J.: Medical Economics, 1989.

27. Albuquerque EX, Aguayo LG, Warnick JE. Interactions of phencyclidine with ion channels of nerve and muscle: Behavioral implications. *Fed Proc* 1983; 42:2854–2859.

28. Lien EJ, Ariens EJ, Beld AJ. Quantitative correlations between chemical structure and affinity for acetylcholine receptors. *Eur J Pharmacol* 1976; 35:245–251.

29. Ketchun JS, Sidell FR, Crowell EB, Aghajanian GK, Hayes AH. Atropine, scopolamine and ditran: Comparative pharmacology and antagonists in man. *Psychopharmacologia* 1973; 28:121–145.

30. Davchut P, Gravenstein JS. Effects of atropine on the electrocardiogram in different age groups. *Clin Pharmacol Ther* 1971; 12:274–280.

31. Giannini AJ, Gregg LO, Andriano J. P's and blues. *J Toxicol: Clin Toxicol* 1984; 22:397–402.

32.  Butch AJ. Abuse and pulmonary complications of injecting pentazocine and tripelennamine tablets. *J Toxicol: Clin Toxicol* 1979; 14:301–304.
33.  Kline NS. Beta endorphin induced changes in schizophrenia and depressed patients. *Arch Gen Psychiat* 1977; 34:1111–1115.
34.  Gold MS, Byck R, Sweeney DR. Endorphin locus coeruleus connection mediates opiates action and withdrawal. *Biomedicine* 1974; 30:1–3.
35.  Gold MS, Pottash ALC, Sweeney DR, Kleber HD. Clonidine detoxification. *AM J Psychiat* 1979; 136:982–984.
36.  Miller NS, Giannini AJ, Gold MS, Philomena JA. Drug abuse and drug testing: Medical, legal and ethical issues in drug abuse. *J Substance Abuse Treatment* 1990; 3:231–239.
37.  Gold MS, Giannini AJ. Cocaine. In: Giannini AJ, Slaby AE eds. *Drugs of Abuse.* Oradell, N.J.: Medical Economics, 1989.
38.  Giannini AJ, Gold MS. Cocaine Abuse: Demons within. *Emergency Dec/Primary Care* 1988; 4(9):34–39.
39.  Magnan MM, Saary T. Trois cas de cocainiame chronique. *C R Heb Mem, Societe de Biologies. Paris* 1889; 60–63.
40.  Dackis CA, Gold MS. Bromocriptine as a treatment of cocaine abuse. *Lancet* 1985; 1:1151–1152.
41.  Giannini AJ, Baumgartel P, DiMarzio LR. Bromocriptine therapy in cocaine withdrawal. *J Clin Pharmacol* 1987; 27:267–270.
42.  Giannini AJ, Gold MS. Anorexia Nervosa and Bulimia Nervosa. In: Taylor DB, ed. *Difficult Medical Management.* Philadelphia: WB Saunders, 1989.
43.  Cameron JS, Specht PG, Wedf GR. Effects of amphetamines on moods, emotions and motivation. *J Psychol* 1965; 61:93–95.
44.  Norvemius G, Widerlov E, Lonnerhulm G. Phenylpropanolamine and mental disturbances. *Lancet* 1979; 2:1367.
45.  Fellows KW, Giannini AJ. Cinnamedryl: Potential for abuse. *J Toxicol: Clin Toxicol* 1983; 20:93–96.
46.  Giannini AJ, Burge H, Shaheen JD. Khat: Another drug of abuse. *J Psychoact Drugs* 1986; 18:155–164.
47.  Giannini AJ, Castellani S. A manic-like psychosis due to Khat. *J Toxicol: Clin Toxicol* 1982; 19:455–559.
48.  Steroid abuse. *U.S. News & World Report* 1989; 106:12.
49.  *Physician's Desk Reference.* Oradell, N.J.: Medical Economics, 1989.
50.  Kochakian CD, Morlin JR. The role of hydrolytic enzymes in some of the metabolic activities of steroid hormones. *Rec Prog Hormonal Res* 1947; 1:177–214.
51.  Blum K, Hamilton MG. Potative role of isoquinolone alkaloids in alcoholism. *Alc Clin Exp Res* 1978; 2(2):113–116.
52.  Hill R, Hoffman, Beresford T. Hypomagnesia in eating disorders. *Psychosomatics* 1988; 29:264–267.
53.  Giannini AJ, DeFrance DT. Metronidazole and alcohol   Potential for combinative abuse. *J Toxicol: Clin Toxicol* 1984; 20:509–515.
54.  Tran VT, Snyder SH, Magor L, Hawley RF. GABA receptors are increased in brains of alcoholics. *Ann Neurol* 1982; 9:289–292.

55. Gilman AG. Receptor regulated G-protein. *Trends Neurosci* 1986; 10:460–463.
56. Thompson WL. Management of alcohol withdrawal syndromes. *Arch Int Med* 1978; 138:278–283.
57. Miller NS, Giannini AJ. The disease model of addiction. *J Psychoactive Drugs* 1990; 22:83–85.
58. Parsons GA, Leher WR. The relationship between cognitive dysfunction and brain damage in alcoholics. *Alcoholism: Clin Exp Res* 1981;5:326–343.
59. Miller NS, Dackis CA, Gold MS. The relationship of addiction and tolerance. *J Subst Abuse Treatment* 1987; 4:197–207.
60. Spies TD, Bean WB, Ashe WF. Recent advances in treatment of pellagra and associated deficiencies. *Ann Int Med* 1969; 12:1830–1844.
61. Traviesa DC. Magnesium deficiency. *J Neurol, Neurosurg Psychiat* 1974; 37:959–961.
62. Wacker WEC, Parisi AF. Magnesium metabolism. *NEJM* 1968; 278:658–660.
63. Marinacci AA, Von Hagen KO. Alcohol and temporal lobe dysfunction. *Behav Neuropsych* 1972; 3:2–5.
64. Giannini AJ, Black. *Psychiatric, Psychogenic and Somatopsychic Disorders*. Garden City: Medical Examination/Excerpta Medica, 1978.

# 5

## Substance Abuse and Neurological Disorders

**Stuart F. Kushner**

*Fair Oaks Hospital, Summit, New Jersey*

## INTRODUCTION

The area of dual diagnosis of substance abuse disorders and neurological disorders actually encompasses a wide range of patient populations but will be divided for purposes of this chapter into two broad categories: (1) neurologic complications of substance abuse disorders, and (2) substance abuse as a complication of neurologic disorders. Much more is known about the first of these two categories which, of course, includes the familiar neurologic sequelae of alcohol abuse, such as Wernicke–Korsakoff syndrome, alcoholic dementia, cerebellar degeneration, peripheral neuropathy, and other less common disorders. Since all these have been written about extensively and are familiar to most medical students and neuropsychiatric specialists, they will not be included in this chapter (with the exception of alcoholism and epilepsy, which will be discussed briefly). Comparable to that group of disorders, however, there has emerged a relatively new cluster of neurological complications that is secondary to other substance abuse disorders. Included here are the complications of cocaine, amphetamines, narcotics, hallucinogens, and even a group of organic solvents. These disorders, newer and generally less familiar to the medical community at large, will be reviewed in more detail, with particular emphasis on cocaine since it has emerged as the drug of the eighties.

The second broad category, namely, substance abuse developing as a complication of primary neurological disorders, is poorly defined and certainly less well understood than the first group. Primarily included here are the various neurologic pain syndromes — headaches, migraines, neuralgias — which, not surprisingly, by their very nature could lead to secondary substance abuse disorders. Aside from these, considering the variety of neurological illnesses both common and uncommon, relatively little research seems to have been undertaken to explore the question of whether other diseases such as demyelinating diseases, extrapyramidal disorders, and seizure disorders have any association with, or causal connection to, substance abuse. One interesting exception to this observation is the diagnostic category of attention deficit hyperactivity disorder (ADHD) for which, although it cannot be considered in the exclusive domain of the neurologist (and in fact may more typically be treated by the child psychiatrist), few will argue against an underlying neurologic basis. There is, as we shall see, some preliminary suggestive evidence for an association between this disorder and the occurrence later in life of cocaine abuse. Some possible explanations for this association will be discussed.

## NEUROLOGICAL DISORDERS COMPLICATING SUBSTANCE ABUSE

## Cocaine

It has been estimated that as many as 30 million Americans have used cocaine, with up to 5 million abusing it on a regular basis, [1] making this clearly a problem of epidemic proportions with overwhelmingly important medical and social implications. Most of the literature on the neurologic complications of cocaine has appeared within the past five years, consistent with the patterns of increasing use during this period. The major categories of neurologic disorders that have been identified include seizures, neurovascular disorders (both ischemic and hemorrhagic), and headaches. In addition, a number of other disorders have been described, often as single-case reports or small study samples. Included among them are the postpartum and perinatal neurological complications, as well as transient focal signs, syncope, neuroleptic malignant syndrome, hyperthermia, and a few others that will be briefly mentioned.

### Seizures and Cocaine

This complication of cocaine abuse is among the most significant clinically because of its potential lethality. Cocaine alone can, of course, cause seizures in any individual, although the patient with a preexisting seizure disorder is, not surprisingly, at higher risk (just as the individual with a preexisting aneurysm or AVM is at increased risk for vascular complications, as will be discussed subsequently). Seizures are well known to occur in cases of cocaine overdose or poisoning due to the drug's CNS-stimulant and local anesthetic effects; however, interestingly, other cases have occurred in chronic users at lower than expected doses that were previously well tolerated by the same individual. Post et al. [2] have hypothesized a mechanism of pharmacologic kindling to explain this phenomenon based on animal studies in which the repetitive administration of high doses of cocaine lead to the emergence of seizures at a dose that was previously subconvulsant. (They enlist the same mechanism to explain the occurrence of cocaine-induced panic attacks that initially occur in conjunction with use but later become spontaneous.) In spite of this phenomenon, seizures are generally found to be dose-related, associated with high blood levels of cocaine [3] and, because of this, during periods of seizures, arrhythmias and hypertension may coexist. In fact, in cocaine poisoning, seizures are a major determinant of lethality since they lead to lactic acidosis and hyperthermia, with resultant impairment of myocardial contractility [4]. The importance and high incidence of seizures as a complication of cocaine has been confirmed in a number of recent reviews [5,3]. Although seizures have usually been found to be generalized, isolated, and self-limited, some earlier animal studies have shown that seizure activity induced by cocaine begins in the temporal lobe and then generalizes [6]. Lowenstein et al., [5] in a large retrospective study, observed the development of status epilepticus in two patients, both of whom went on to have chronic encephalopathies, emphasizing the need for prompt early treatment of seizure activity when it does occur. In another interesting and related case report, Merriam et al. [7] describe a 20-year-old chronic cocaine user with a two-week history of "disturbed behavior," who developed what at first appeared to be a cocaine psychosis, with symptoms of agitation, incoherence, and paranoid thinking. Subsequently, she was found to have a clouded sensorium and motor automatisms on examination. Her EEG revealed right-hemisphere seizure activity and interictal bursts of right-sided slow waves and was interpreted as partial complex status epilepticus. In this case, Merriam and co-workers felt that it was the presence of a clouded sensorium that tipped them off to a seizure disorder rather than just a cocaine-induced psychosis. They again emphasize the importance of arriving at a correct diagnosis and administering anticonvulsants since, if left untreated, partial complex status (and other seizure types as well) may lead to residual cognitive impairment. In this case, the etiology of the seizure may have been the direct epileptogenic effect of cocaine or possibly a new cocaine-related cerebrovascular event or even a preexisting structural lesion that served as a focus.

In terms of the management of the patient with suspected cocaine-induced seizures, Rowbotham [3] has set forth some particular guidelines for the practitioner, but foremost is the importance of ruling out all other potentially treatable causes. Brain-imaging studies (CT or MRI scans), lumbar puncture, and EEG may be necessary to exclude stroke, subarachnoid hemorrhage, or infection (discussed below). If status develops, most recommend phenobarbital loading and/or pentobarbital anesthesia. Long-term anticonvulsant treatment is probably *not* necessary in most cases unless there is focal brain injury or a persistently abnormal EEG [3].

In light of the fact that elevation of body temperature and reduction of blood pH *both lower* seizure threshold, as well as cause cardiac complications, the importance of preventing hyperthermia and minimizing acidosis are obvious. For a similar reason, the use of neuroleptics such as haloperidol or chlorpromazine to calm the excited hyperkinetic cocaine-intoxicated patient would probably be contraindicated in most cases since they also may *lower* seizure threshold as well as aggravate cardiac arrhythmias [4]. Probably a benzodiazepine would be preferable to use in such a situation. Calcium-channel blockers are also gaining increasingly in popularity and may be effective antidotes for cocaine toxicity, antagonizing both cardiac effects such as hypertension and tachycardia as well as *central* effects such as motor tremors and seizures. Another well-known anticonvulsant, carbamazepine, may also prove useful in cocaine-induced seizures in that it has been found experimentally that chronic pretreatment with it can inhibit the occurrence of high-dose cocaine seizures. The mechanism is uncertain but has been proposed to be related to the drug's interacting with local anesthetic mechanisms at the level of the sodium channel [8].

*Neurovascular Complications of Cocaine*

Both ischemic and hemorrhagic infarctions are now well documented and frightening complications of cocaine abuse just as, in the earlier literature of the 1960s, they were reported as complications of amphetamines and LSD, the recreational drugs most prevalent in that era. The first case of cerebral infarct related to cocaine was reported in 1977 in a 43-year-old man with mild hypertension, who sustained a left middle cerebral artery infarct 1–2 h after injecting cocaine [9]. Since that original description, a number of case reports and review articles have appeared describing intracranial hemorrhages and cerebral infarctions in cocaine-abusing patients. In 1986, Cregler and Mark summarized five cases since the original, four with subarachnoid hemorrhage and one with middle cerebral artery occlusion [10]. In the four cases of hemorrhage, the event occurred within minutes of intranasal use, and they all were found to have underlying aneurysms or arteriovenous malformations. The authors propose that although the incidence of subarachnoid hemorrhage from intranasal cocaine is probably low, individuals harboring an occult aneurysm or AVM may be at special risk; therefore, physicians treating patients with headaches following cocaine use should be aware of the possibility in their differential diagnoses. In a more recent review, Rowbotham summarizes 15 more articles describing a wide variety of stroke types (in all vascular territories) in a total of 41 patients including subarachnoid hemorrhage, intracerebral hemorrhage, and ischemic stroke [3]. In nine of these cases, angiography documented either an aneurysm or AVM and, in several of them, there were middle cerebral artery branch occlusions in association with 'crack' smoking. Similarly, in another earlier report, six cases of neurovascular complications are reviewed and, again, most were found to have underlying vascular lesions [11]. In one of these cases, the hemorrhage occurred into an occult astrocytoma, presumably as the cocaine-induced elevation of blood pressure caused a rupture of already weakened vessels in the tumor bed.

Another recent extensive review of neurovascular complications was completed by Jacobs and co-workers as a retrospective review of the medical records of close to 4000 drug abusers admitted to Detroit Receiving Hospital from 1984 to 1987 and found 13 cases with neurologic deficits attributable to use of cocaine [12]. Ischemic manifestations were the most frequent, followed by an equal distribution of subarachnoid and intracerebral hemorrhage. Once again, systemic hypertension associated with an underlying cerebral abnormality appeared to be the mechanism in most cases of subarachnoid hemorrhage and in some cases of intracerebral hemorrhage. In those cases without a demonstrable lesion, the authors propose an acute development of systemic hypertension (secondary to cocaine) to be the probable pathophysiologic mechanism. They conclude that, because of the high incidence of abnormalities, angiography is warranted in cases of intracranial hemorrhage and cocaine abuse. Radiologic investigation is also the subject of a report in which four case studies of young individuals with histories of heavy cocaine abuse ("freebasing") precipitously develop acute symptoms of severe headache, disorientation, and stupor [13]. All four patients were discovered to have a subcortical hemorrhage on CT scan, and the findings on MRI and angiography were consistent with either vasculitis or an underlying cryptic malformation. Vasculitis has been a controversial subject where cocaine is concerned, although it has been well described as a complication of intravenous amphetamine use [14]. It was first described in 1970, and the original reports in the early 1970s involved almost exclusively cases of intravenous methamphetamine use although it was also seen in patients using heroin or ephedrine. The pathogenesis for this drug-induced vasculitis has been unclear but has been hypothesized to have an immunologic basis, possibly related to contaminants used to "cut" the heroin or amphetamines being injected. A case report by Kaye and Fainstat [15] described a 22-year-old male with a two-week history of intranasal cocaine use, who presented with right-sided headaches and transient visual blurring, followed by development of left hemisparesis and hemianesthesia. CT scan revealed a low-density right frontotemporal lesion consistent with infarction, and a carotid arteriogram was interpreted as compatible with vasculitis. Interestingly, in a subsequent letter to the editor appearing five months after the original report, Levine et al. [16] contest the diagnosis of vasculitis, instead suggesting that this was a case of subarachnoid hemorrhage, followed by cerebral vasospasm and infarction. Jacobs et al., [12] in their study referred to above, further discuss this subject in terms of understanding the mechanism for cocaine-induced cerebral ischemia. The two most likely mechanisms are felt to be *vasospasm* (either drug-induced or secondary to hypertension) or *vasculitis*. In their cases, the angiographic findings were generally noted to be narrowing or occlusion of major vascular structures at the base of the brain or of the middle cerebral artery, as opposed to the characteristic findings in *small vessels* previously reported as typical of vasculitis — narrowing, "beading" of vessels, and microaneurysms — and usually seen (as noted above) with amphetamines and phenylpropanolamine. In their series, Jacobs and co-workers found a predominance of basal ganglia and capsular infarcts similar to the usual pattern of lacunar infarcts associated with systemic hypertension. They also noted that many of the patients who developed cerebral hemorrhage and infarcts had other risk factors for increased incidence of stroke, such as history of hypertension, alcohol abuse, and smoking, suggesting that the presence of any of these could possibly place the cocaine addict at a greater risk for neurovascular sequelae.

Feinman [17] describes another case of a young, previously healthy male with an eight-year history of abusing cocaine who, after using crack for the first time, developed an acute encephalopathy and then a transient left hemiparesis, which resolved within 24 h. Feinman considers a possible diagnosis of necrotizing angiitis, which can be associated with drug abuse (in addition to its association with collagen vascular disease, hypersensitivity reactions, etc.). She proposes the possibility that this particular case could be due to that entity or to vasospasm as a *direct* effect of cocaine. Since 'crack' was the drug used in this case, and it usually is considered to be free of angiitis-producing contaminants, the conclusion reached is that it was more likely a case of direct cerebral vasoconstriction. This mechanism of vasospasm secondary to cocaine has also produced an array of other systemic complications, including myocardial infarction, renal infarction, and intestinal ischemia.

It is generally agreed that, in most instances of cocaine-related stroke and hemorrhage, the pathophysiologic mechanism is related to the drug's sympathomimetic effects. Support for this comes from the observation that amphetamines, LSD, PCP, methylphenidate, and phenylpropanolamine all share with cocaine the ability to alter vascular tone, and all have produced stroke [3]. The neuropharmacological mechanism is likely to be inhibition of norepinephrine, serotonin, and dopamine reuptake into the presynaptic terminal, producing an enhancement of sympathetic activity and resulting systemic hypertension. Caplan [18] discusses this as the usual mechanism underlying intracranial hemorrhage secondary to cocaine and a number of other intravenous drugs, but he also proposes another mechanism to explain intracranial hemorrhage after intravenous *injection* of pills made for oral use (such as injection of "T's and blues"). In the first situation, it is the *acute* rise in blood pressure in an otherwise normotensive individual that is the critical factor whereas, in the second case, there is an acute increase in cerebral blood flow after passage of a foreign body embolus that had been causing transient arterial obstruction ("reperfusion"). The foreign bodies in such cases could be substances such as talc, cornstarch, and other diluents added to drugs for intravenous injection. (Talc and other "fillers" are often found in tablets that are crushed, dissolved, and injected by drug addicts.) These two mechanisms, which are essentially very similar and represent in both cases an acute increase in blood flow in areas of normal or ischemic arterioles, probably explain most cases of intracranial hemorrhage secondary to drug abuse.

Although these are the most typical mechanisms for drug-induced stroke syndromes, Toler and Anderson [19] propose another possible mechanism, altered immune regulation, based on a case they describe of an intravenous cocaine user with a cerebral infarct who is discovered to have in his serum the presence of *lupus anticoagulant*, a specific antiphospholipid antibody that has been associated with hypercoagulable states and stroke. Although the patient had no known autoimmune disease, it appears that he had some kind of altered immune function. In fact, intravenous drug use has been associated with a number of immunological abnormalities, including elevated levels of gammaglobulins (IgG and IgM), false-positive serologies, hyperplasia of lymphoid tissues, increased incidence of anergy, and variations in serum complement level [19,20]. Clearly, a history of exposure to intravenous drugs can set the stage for the process of antigenic sensitization directed toward either the drug itself or the adulterant or vehicle. Besides cocaine, the phenomenon has been described with morphine, meperidine, and opium. Reexposure to the drug after a period of abstinence may be the precipitating event. Given the high frequency of IV drug use and immune alterations, this may not be a rare cause of stroke in this patient population.

In the postpartum period, cocaine has also been found to cause its devastating neurovascular complications. Mercado et al. [21] report the case of a

25-year-old female who had been abusing cocaine throughout her pregnancy and then developed a left frontoparietal hemorrhage in the immediate postpartum period. The episode was triggered by a period of hypertension and a grand mal seizure. Mechanism for the hemorrhage was unclear as angiography was negative, but the authors suggest it could have been secondary to either transient hypertension or cerebrovascular spasm, with local ischemia and necrosis leading to hemorrhage. The case is an interesting one since it brings cocaine exposure into the differential diagnosis of hypertension and seizures occurring in the postpartum period. More typically, this symptom complex is suggestive of pre-eclampsia/eclampsia which, like cocaine, can produce vasospasm and occasionally subarachnoid hemorrhage [21].

Just as cocaine can cause its deleterious effects on a pregnant woman, not surprisingly, it can also lead to serious neurovascular and other effects in the unborn fetus and, in fact, perinatal complications have been well documented. Pregnancy outcomes have generally been found to be worse in women using cocaine than in women using opiates, [3] with a higher incidence of spontaneous abortions and cases of abruptio placentae. Infants born to cocaine-using mothers have tended to be small for gestational age and have a higher incidence of reduced head circumference. Also, maternal cocaine use may place the fetus at greater risk for tachycardia and hypertension and therefore cerebrovascular complications. Chasnoff et al. [22] report on such a case in a neonate born to a cocaine-using mother. The infant at 24 h of age developed an acute focal cerebral infarct, which may have been a hemorrhage or possibly a thromboembolism. The authors therefore advise the inclusion of cocaine in the differential diagnosis of perinatal cerebral infarction. A variety of other lesions have also been seen in cocaine neonates, including diffuse atrophy, deep brain cysts, and periventricular leukomalacia, in addition to hemorrhages in many locations [3]. The presumed pathophysiology is a cocaine-induced increase in maternal blood pressure, with reduced uterine blood flow and subsequent fetal hypoxemia. In addition to these more serious structural lesions, children born to cocaine mothers may show cognitive deficits and behavioral effects that may persist for up to two years.

To summarize the serious neurovascular complications of cocaine, the most important factor for the busy practitioner is awareness of their existence. In this era of epidemic cocaine use, one must remember to consider it as a potential etiologic factor in any patient, particularly a young, previously healthy one presenting with an acute neurologic insult. Individuals with other risk factors or with an underlying structural lesion such as congenital berry aneurysm or AVM seem particularly at risk. Also, the fact that these events can occur precipitously, idiosyncratically, and without relation to dose or duration of previous exposure makes them especially frightening since even a first-time user can be affected.

## Headaches and Other Complications of Cocaine

In addition to seizures and the neurovascular complications of cocaine just reviewed, a variety of other neurologic problems have been reported. Lowenstein et al. [5] conducted a large retrospective study aimed at elucidating these complications. They reviewed 996 emergency room visits and 279 hospital admissions of patients with complications of cocaine abuse seen at San Francisco General Hospital between 1979 and 1986. The number of cocaine-associated complications rose steadily each year during the study period, consistent with nationwide trends in cocaine use. The major complications reported in this study were seizures, focal signs and symptoms, headaches, transient loss of consciousness, tremor, and toxic encephalopathy.

Headaches are commonly reported in community treatment facilities and in callers to cocaine-help hotlines [3]. Because of their potential association with hypertension and strokes, they should of course be taken seriously, although usually patients with headaches and *no focal symptoms* have a benign course.

Three cases of new-onset migrainelike headache with temporal association to cocaine use were recently reported by Satel and Gawin [23]. Two of the cases resembled common migraine and one basilar migraine. The authors discuss the pathophysiology of migraine as being linked to serotonin dysregulation and the interesting fact that cocaine also affects serotonergic function by inhibiting reuptake. This leads first to an increase in serotonergic activity but later a suppression or down regulation of the system. The patients in this study all developed their migraine symptoms after a delay following cocaine use but then rapidly improved following readministration of the drug, consistent with the typical response of migraine headaches to serotonin-enhancing agents like ergotamine. In light of cocaine's short half-life and the pattern of symptoms here, it seems that they were "rebound" or withdrawal headaches but sufficiently severe to motivate the patients to comply with a treatment program for abstinence. Satel and Gawin conclude by suggesting that these cases represent an illustration of cocaine-induced neurologic symptoms that may be related to its effect on central serotonergic function.

Other neurologic signs reported by Rowbotham [3] include enhancement of physiologic tremor, vertigo, nonspecific dizziness, blurred vision, ataxia, and tinnitus. Focal abnormalities such as transient motor, sensory, or visual disturbances may occur and are of uncertain origin, although most likely they represent either transient ischemic events (due to vasospasm, as previously discussed) or seizure discharges. With intravenous heroin abuse, and possibly cocaine as well, numerous myelopathies have been reported, usually affecting the thoracic levels of the spinal cord, and here, too, the presumed mechanism has been transient ischemia in a region of poor vascular perfusion [20]. Tics and choreiform movements such as those that occur with amphetamines have not yet been reported with cocaine, nor has hemiballismus, which has been seen with intravenous heroin. The cases of transient loss of consciousness that have been reported may represent syncopal episodes related to brief disturbances of cardiac rhythm leading to cerebral hypoperfusion [5].

Another potentially very serious complication of cocaine use has been described by Kosten and Kleber [24] as a variant of the well-known neuroleptic malignant syndrome (NMS). They discuss seven cases of "fatal overdose" occurring at blood levels that are usually considered "safe." Since hyperthermia was a prominent feature in all these cases, the authors propose a complex pathophysiologic mechanism based on central dopaminergic control of thermoregulation. Typically, NMS occurs during treatment with neuroleptics, which are dopamine receptor antagonists, but it may also occur during withdrawal from dopamine agonists, suggesting that a *relative* decrement in dopamine activity may be the crucial factor for its development. Although most cocaine abusers do not initially have a primary central dopamine deficiency (though some may, as will be discussed in a later section of this chapter), they may develop a state of relative dopamine depletion during periods when the cocaine is rapidly washed out of the body and levels are *falling*. In Kosten and Kleber's case reports, the patients had hyperthermia, delirium, and agitation, followed later by rigidity and akinesia, a symptom constellation highly reminiscent of NMS. Hyperthermia has also been reported by others as a serious and sometimes fatal complication of cocaine, [25] and its mechanism is probably related to several factors, including a direct central dopamine-mediated effect, as well as the increase in heat production due to stimulation of motor activity and diminished heat dissipation due to vasoconstriction. Of course, other differential diagnoses of hyperthermia must always be considered, such as systemic infection, malignant hyperthermia, and heat stroke. In terms of treatment implications for the NMS variant, logically, neuroleptics would seem to be specifically contraindicated, as they could worsen NMS. (Remember: they would also be detrimental for their effect on seizure threshold.) Ironically, this specific postcocaine syndrome may require the use of a cocainelike substitute such as bromocriptine to reverse the hypothesized relative deficiency of dopamine following cocaine withdrawal [24]. Benzodiazepines might also be a useful treatment adjunct for the accompanying agitation.

## Neurological Complications of Intravenous Drug Abuse

An obviously important and certainly more familiar category of complications of *intravenous* drug abuse would include the entire realm of infectious disorders, which will be discussed here only briefly. Numerous bacteria can, of course, invade the CNS as emboli or abscesses, usually secondary to cardiac involvement from bacterial endocarditis [20]. The most commonly offending agents in this group are alpha-hemolytic streptococci, staphylococci, and Pseudomonas. Fungal infections can also spread in the same fashion, and here the usual agents belong to Phycomycetes, Aspergillus, Cladosporium, or Candida. Kasantikul et al. [26] report an interesting and unusual case of primary chromoblastomycosis of the medulla oblongata occurring as a complication of heroin addiction in a 20-year-old addict from Thailand. The clinical course was characterized by a sudden onset of progressive medullary dysfunction, followed by death within 12 days. The postmortem exam revealed mycotic granulomas due to chromoblastomycosis, strictly limited to the medulla and adjacent leptomeninges. This was a particularly unusual case in that the fungus itself is rare; only one previous case has been described in association with drug abuse, and usually brain abscesses are cerebral in location while, in this instance, it was bulbar. The most likely source was felt to have been a contaminated needle, water, or skin, and the route of infection was presumably via hematogenous spread. Rubin, [20] in his review of neurological complications of intravenous drug abuse, also mentions other infectious entities that have been reported, including tuberculous meningitis, cervical osteomyelitis, spinal epidural and subdural abscesses, and tetanus. The risk of tetanus in IV drug users seems to relate to contaminated paraphernalia, and it is probably the "cutting agent" quinine that favors growth of the organism *Clostridium tetani*. Cerebral complications from hepatitis can also naturally be quite severe and include seizures, hepatic encephalopathy, and coma.

No review of infectious complications of intravenous drug abuse would be complete without mention of AIDS, in which neurological manifestations are now becoming increasingly common and more frequently diagnosed. The most acute form of CNS involvement by the HIV virus is acute meningoencephalitis, but the most *common* one is the entity now called AIDS-dementia complex or chronic AIDS encephalopathy, which may affect at least half of all AIDS patients [27]. The usual clinical manifestations are chronic deterioration of cognitive and behavioral functions, apathy, and a flat affect. Other less common neurological complications of AIDS, which are reviewed by Fischer and Enzensberger, [27] include an atypical form of aseptic meningitis, a vacuolar myelopathy, and involvement of peripheral and cranial nerves. In addition, there are, of course, all the secondary opportunistic infections that occur in these patients, the most common in this group being CNS toxoplasmosis, cytomegalovirus, herpes, and cryptococcus. Finally, these individuals may develop central nervous system malignancies, usually primary lymphoma or systemic lymphoma involving the CNS.

In addition to neurological involvement of the *central* nervous system, a number of peripheral nervous system disorders can also develop in intravenous drug users, both infectious and noninfectious. Here the list includes brachial and lumbosacral plexitis (described after heroin injection), as well as cases of painless mononeuropathy occurring a few hours *after* heroin injection but *not* at the injection site, and polyneuropathy, both acute and chronic forms, often presenting as a Guillain–Barré syndrome [20]. Polyneuropathy can also be a complication of nutritional deficiencies (as with alcoholics) and, in this same category, there have been reports of myelopathy, specifically, subacute combined degeneration secondary to B-12 deficiency. Acute rhabdomyolysis, with myoglobinuria and possible renal failure, has also been associated with the injection of adulterated heroin; its symptoms are muscle tenderness, edema, and weakness of all extremities [20].

A new and interesting addition to the drugs of the 1980s is the chemical MPTP (1-methyl-4-phenyl-1,2,3,6-tetrahydropyridine), which is usually not directly sought after by the addict, but rather is obtained as an impurity from injected material. This drug produces a syndrome nearly identical to idiopathic parkinsonism, with features of rigidity, bradykinesia, resting tremor, gait disturbance, and loss of postural reflexes. What is particularly interesting about this syndrome is its mechanism, which seems to be a drug-induced cell-specific cytotoxicity. The substance is oxidized to $MPP^+$, which is taken up by dopaminergic neurons, leading to impaired neurotransmission. Symptoms appear subacutely after several weeks or months but can persist even for years, although without progression, suggesting a self-limiting toxic reaction [20].

## Neurological Complications of Solvent Vapor Abuse

Thus far, we have been discussing primarily cocaine (which, of course, is typically snorted intranasally or injected intravenously) and other substances used intravenously. Organic solvents constitute another class of drugs that have become a growing public health concern in the United States and elsewhere, particularly among young adults and children. "Solvent sniffers" choose inexpensive and readily available toluene-based products like spray paint and glue for their euphoria-inducing effects. *N*-hexane or toluene has actually replaced benzene (which is toxic to liver and bone marrow) as the number one organic solvent in paints, lacquers, and thinners. Toluene has been well documented to cause multi-focal neurologic disorders, [28] with most of the earlier literature documenting its acute effects. Hormes et al. [29] have now studied the residual neurologic damage in 20 patients with histories of chronic solvent abuse (greater than two years' duration). After a period of abstinence of four weeks or longer, the patients were assessed for neurological dysfunction, cognitive impairment, and neurobehavioral abnormalities. Of Hormes' sample, 65% had neurological impairment, with the CNS appearing to be selectively vulnerable and no evidence for peripheral neuropathy. The abnormalities varied from mild isolated cognitive impairment to severe dementia associated with such signs as cerebellar ataxia, corticospinal tract dysfunction, oculomotor abnormalities, tremor, deafness, and hyposmia. The most disabling and frequent feature was cognitive dysfunction, which was generally the type referred to as subcortical dementia, as seen with other toxic metabolic encephalopathies. Manifestations included apathy, poor concentration, impaired memory, visuospatial dysfunction, and impairment of complex cognition. The most common signs on neurological examination were cerebellar and pyramidal tract, and were present mostly in those cases who were also cognitively impaired. Abnormalities were also found in brainstem auditory-evoked response, CT scans (nonspecific diffuse atrophy), and EEGs (diffuse slowing, no epileptiform activity). It appears that the effects of these drugs are diffuse in the central nervous system and, although the exact mechanism of toluene's neurotoxicity is uncertain, the drug is lipophilic and may therefore affect lipid components of cell membranes or the myelin sheath [29]. Although no significant relationship was found in this study between type or duration of exposure and neurological impairment, it does seem that the most severely affected patients tended to have histories of heavy and prolonged use. No withdrawal symptoms were observed in this sample, presumably due to the long half-life of hydrocarbons, meaning slow elimination from the CNS. There was a tendency toward continued gradual improvement in those patients who remained abstinent for an extended period of follow-up.

## SUBSTANCE ABUSE COMPLICATING NEUROLOGICAL DISORDERS

As indicated in the introduction to this chapter, the area of substance abuse complicating primary neurological disorders seems to be much less studied than the topic of neurological disorders complicating substance abuse, which has just been reviewed. Certainly many, if not most, neurological diseases are capable of causing in their victims an inordinate amount of distress, both physical and psychological. Pain and disability are frequently a major part of these patients' lives, and one would therefore not be surprised to learn that this group of individuals is more susceptible to abusing alcohol and drugs, at first with the aim of relieving some of this pain and suffering. Later this abuse becomes a separate and autonomous problem, causing its own inherent pain and disability.

## Headaches and Substance Abuse

Headaches and other chronic pain syndromes are among the most common disorders seen by neurologists, and they are the most likely to lead to substance abuse disorders.

A large clinicoepidemiologic study from Italy of drug abuse in chronic headache sufferers examined all patients referred to a university headache center over a five-year period (1979–1984) to determine how many were drug abusers. Defining drug abusers as patients using instant-relief drugs every day for at least one year, the study reported that 5% of the patients met the criteria [30]. Most of the drugs used by these patients were combination analgesics containing three or more substances: caffeine was the most common "ingredient," followed by ergot, and numerous other drugs, including acetaminophen derivatives, salicylates, and barbiturates. Although other investigators have found a high proportion of migraine patients abusing morphinelike drugs, such was not the case in this study, though almost half of the drugs did contain barbiturates. During the last year of the study, all patients observed were hospitalized and *detoxified*; most had withdrawal symptoms within 48 h lasting 3–7 days. Symptoms consisted of severe headaches, nausea, vomiting, anxiety, and insomnia, *regardless* of the drugs patients had been using. At the end of treatment, all patients were either headache-free or considerably improved. The study determined drug abuse to be among the most important factors causing transformation from "episodic" to "chronic" headache pattern. Although previous studies (discussed below) consistently found ergot to be the most likely drug to cause chronic headache and addiction, this investigation revealed no significant difference between ergotamine and other drugs in terms of addiction potential. Elsewhere in the European literature, there is evidence supporting this notion that frequent use of *all* types of analgesics with or without ergotamine can paradoxically maintain chronic headache—an iatrogenic effect that physicians may be reluctant to recognize [31]. As noted above, Granella et al. [30] found that all instant-relief drugs were capable of inducing a withdrawal syndrome. The reasons for this may be psychological as well as pharmacological. The authors propose that a "rebound phenomenon may occur as a result of a functional exhaustion in the antinociceptive system related to an oversaturation of the receptors." [30] One of the interesting findings from this study is the suggestion that analgesics may be capable of transforming episodic headache into chronic headache and that abuse of these analgesics can certainly *sustain* chronic headache and transform it into one with different clinical manifestations. In an earlier review by Heyck, [32] possible reasons why the misuse of analgesics can perpetuate headache are discussed. He suggests that, in many cases, the initial "tension headache" is actually a symptom of depression for which analgesics give relief. Another group of patients Heyck mentions are the head injury cases, especially those undergoing extensive diagnostic evaluations and seeking legal counsel for "compensation." Generally, the histories of these patients reveal inadequate treatment except for the injudicious prescription by physicians of pain medications that *perpetuate* the headache for which patients are seeking treatment.

Still, in spite of the evidence cited above implicating all classes of analgesics as potentially abusable, ergotamine remains one of the prime offenders since it is, after all, the drug of first choice in the treatment of migraine headache [33]. Lippman [34] was probably the first to describe a characteristic headache resulting from prolonged use of ergot derivatives, which he called the "ergotamine headache." Subsequently, over a period of many years and after analysis of many case studies, a syndrome of ergotamine dependency has been defined and well described as a subtle but widespread clinical condition [35,33]. The syndrome begins with a history of typical *intermittent migraine*, followed by insidious increase in use of ergotamine tartrate and a parallel increase in frequency of the migraine. The onset of headache is usually within 24 h of the last dose of medication, and the headache is unresponsive to all other treatments. As in all dependency states, this one meets the typical criteria of predictable and irresistible use of the drug, as well as development of tolerance and withdrawal [35]. Progressive depression, sleep disturbance, and loss of well-being occur as accompanying symptoms. Saper [33] reviews the possible mechanisms for development of the syndrome and considers the *central* effects of ergotamine to be critical, including the drug's effects on brainstem vasomotor centers (locus ceruleus), cortisol secretion, and neurotransmitter functions within the brainstem and hypothalamus. Saper explains the accompanying sleep and depressive symptoms as possibly related to either an alteration of serotonin and norepinephrine function or impact on the hypothalamic-pituitary-adrenal axis. Supporting the latter notion, earlier studies demonstrated a significantly increased incidence of positive DSTs in headache patients using excessive amounts of ergot [36]. Another possibility, suggested by Lance, [37] relates to ergotamine's effect on locus ceruleus, which is to diminish the sensitivity of neurotransmitter or receptor functions with chronic use and, thereby during withdrawal, to cause a kind of "rebound hyperactivity," analogous to the abstinence syndromes occurring with alcohol, opiates, and nicotine.

An important aspect of this ergotamine-dependency syndrome is the transformation of the initially intermittent migraine into a *daily* headache which, although still responsive to ergot, is unresponsive to all other migraine treatments and preventative agents, strengthening the argument that it is physiologically a dependency headache with a different pathophysiology than the original migraine [33]. Not until the patient can successfully break the cycle and stop the ergot is the natural frequency of the migraine re-established. Also, at that point, the individual again becomes responsive to preventative agents such as beta-blockers, tricyclic antidepressants, and calcium-channel-blockers. Treatment of these patients during the dependency phase is naturally difficult and requires a compliant individual. Hospitalization is often necessary to facilitate the treatment process and to tide the patient through the period of acute withdrawal, which may last from two to four days during which the patient may require symptomatic treatment with phenothiazines, sedatives, and even narcotics. Saper indicates that clonidine may be indicated to help ease the withdrawal period [33]. Eventually, once the patient is completely stabilized, it may, in some cases, be possible to reinstitute ergotamine very cautiously and under close supervision for *acute* migraine only, with precise instructions for maximum use once per week. In these susceptible individuals, the original factors promoting abuse could easily recur; these include patients' *fear* of headaches, hence use of ergotamine "to avoid them," use for all types of headache and not just migraine as is appropriate and, lastly, encouragement by unwary physicians to employ ergotamine at the first sign of any headache. Patients must, of course, be instructed to guard against all these potential dangers.

Another important drug present in over-the-counter analgesic preparations but also in many of the foods and beverages we consume on a regular basis is, of course, caffeine. Although this drug is not considered a major problem in the area of substance abuse, recent investigations have questioned its indiscriminant use [38]. Evidence for dependency exists as there is development of tolerance to the CNS-stimulating effects and as withdrawal symptoms are certainly well documented and familiar to most heavy coffee drinkers. Heavy consumers or those ingesting more than 500 mg/day of caffeine (equal to 5–6 cups of brewed coffee) are probably dependent and may be impaired psychologically and/or in performance efficiency [38]. As described earlier, addiction to caffeine can specifically occur in headache patients (not only in coffee drinkers) because of the presence of this drug in so many analgesic compounds. Rainey [39] describes the case of a 59-year-old woman with chronic craniofacial pain and headaches, who presented to a dentist for evaluation. Detailed history uncovered a daily consumption of over 800 mg/day caffeine, taken in pills, coffee, tea, and cola. When the patient was told to *stop* all caffeine, she actually developed acute withdrawal but, subsequently, there was near-complete remission of the headaches, obviating the need for an expensive work-up and evaluation. It was felt that "the frequency of this patient's headaches during each day was caused by her dependency on caffeine and most likely a continuing need to maintain a certain blood level of caffeine to avoid withdrawal symptoms, which were forewarned by the onset of the headaches." [39] It sounds very reminiscent of the ergotamine story.

In isolated instances, headache sufferers may turn to more "serious" drugs than ergotamine, caffeine, or others contained in the usual analgesic compounds. Earlier in this chapter, mention was made of migraine occurring as a complication of cocaine abuse. Brower, [40] in a recent report, presents a case in which the sequence of events seems to be reversed, namely, cocaine abuse occurring secondary to migraine. He discusses the concept of the self-medication hypothesis, which asserts that certain individuals may initiate cocaine or other drug use in order to medicate themselves for an underlying psychiatric disorder [41]. In this particular case, the patient was a 29-year-old male with history of classic migraine beginning six years earlier. He initially used ergot and caffeine but then, at age 27, began smoking "freebase" cocaine "leading to immediate and complete relief of headache for only 15 minutes after which euphoria subsided and headache recurred." Gradually, the pattern of cocaine abuse intensified, and he began using it even in the absence of headache. (In this case, the cocaine was never alleged to *cause* headache as in those cases reported by Satel and Gawin [23]). The patient was treated on a substance abuse unit, withdrawn from cocaine, and ultimately retaught to use ergotamine for his migraine headaches. This was the first reported case of cocaine dependence in a migraine patient, although dependence on opioids and barbiturates has been well documented in the literature in patients with migraine and other chronic headache syndromes [42]. Brower indicates, in his case history, that although the headaches were important in initiating cocaine use, other factors later superseded in perpetuating the abuse, such as craving for the drug and the need to relieve the dysphoria occurring during withdrawal. He proposes dopaminergic mechanisms to be operative here, with the user attempting to restore (via use of cocaine) dysfunctional dopaminergic systems. An underlying biological vulnerability to develop dopamine dysfunction may be a significant factor explaining why some patients may be at risk for addiction, a concept that will be further explained below in reference to some other illnesses. Of course, serotonergic mechanisms could also be implicated since cocaine, like ergot, enhances serotonin activity and acts as a vasoconstrictor, possibly explaining its initial "therapeutic" effect. In terms of ultimate long-term treatment, antidepressants may eventually prove useful in this group of patients where migraine and cocaine abuse coexist (irrespective of which came first) since tricyclics have, of course, been beneficial in preventing migraine [43] and, more recently, they have been found useful in some cocaine-dependent patients [44]. An important treatment implication is that simply focusing on the primary underlying disorder (in this case, migraine) is insufficient in terms of the cocaine dependence since the latter inevitably becomes an autonomous disorder. A comprehensive drug-treatment/rehabilitation program is essential for these as well as other drug-addicted patients in order to address adequately the other perpetuating factors [10].

## Chronic Pain and Substance Abuse

Chronic pain is a frequent reason for psychiatric and for neurologic consultation. Headaches have just been discussed in this context, but also low-back and neck pains, joint pains, and neuralgias are frequently the reason for referral and initiation of drug-taking behavior. Gallagher et al. [45] review the phenomenon of nonnarcotic analgesic abuse, which is common in this patient population, and reports on some of its epidemiologic characteristics: higher incidence in women, especially housewives of low socioeconomic status and 30–60 years of age; higher incidence of positive family history of similar nonnarcotic analgesic abuse; presence of multiple psychosocial stressors; and greater tendency to abuse alcohol and narcotics in addition to the nonnarcotic analgesics. Maruta, [46] in a review of substance abuse by patients with chronic pain, indicates that analgesics, but also sedative/hypnotics, are the types of drugs most commonly abused by patients with chronic pain and that the major three factors that seem to interact in this patient population are pain, depression, and drug/alcohol dependence. Maruta discusses a number of factors that enable patients with chronic pain to develop drug abuse and thereby become resistant to management in pain treatment centers. There seem, in fact, to be specific drugs that reduce the success rate for patients in a pain-management program (such as codeine and oxycodone compounds), although drug dependency, in general, appears to be a predictor of negative outcome. Patients tend to emphasize the medical causes of their pain while minimizing the psychosocial ones, thereby justifying the continued "need" for medication. Physicians can often contribute to the problem as well; their reactions to these treatment-resistant patients may vary from overconcern to irritation and total lack of sympathy to feelings of frustration and incompetence. Obviously, physicians expressing these feelings may have difficulty changing the prescription pattern and may be indirectly enabling the drug dependence to continue [46]. Cases of *subtle* abuse can be the most problematic, as indicated by Maruta in his description of a case report of a patient with chronic low-back pain who was using excessive amounts of aspirin, propoxyphene, diazepam, and flurazepam, all prescribed by physicians. In the hospital, the patient was noted to have a mild organic mental syndrome, with minor impairments in cognitive functioning, which improved after he was taken off all the medications. Since these patients usually don't meet official diagnostic criteria for drug abuse or dependence, the diagnosis is often overlooked, with serious consequences, as in this case of prescription drug–induced organic brain syndrome. Of course, one of the major negative consequences of this kind of abuse and dependency is the unfavorable effect it has on treatment in pain-management programs, this despite increasing awareness of the problem and more attention to medication issues in the treatment [46].

Although, in most cases of nonnarcotic analgesic abuse, there is no significant physical illness except for that caused by the medication itself, there are, of course, exceptions, namely, those patients who do have a serious underlying disorder with disability. Gallagher et al. [45] report the case of a 66-year-old woman with a 10-year history of multiple sclerosis (wheelchair-bound) and 7-year history of chronic left arm pain leading to daily acetaminophen abuse (5–6 g/day). In this case, the patient suffered from some short-term memory impairment resulting from the MS, which tended to exacerbate the analgesic abuse, although the most significant factors were probably psychological. Difficulties coping with frustration, anger, and boredom caused by her disability, as well as interpersonal factors in her family relationships, were all playing a role in facilitating the analgesic abuse. Also noteworthy is the observation that, in large doses, acetaminophen is psychoactive and has some CNS-stimulating effects which, together with the pain relief, can act as a primary positive reinforcer. Still, the nonnarcotic analgesics, as a rule, do not produce euphoria or a sense of well-being as do the usual psychotropic drugs that cause addiction; hence, the motivation for drug-taking behavior is different in these patient groups. These individuals often use the medication as a tool for coping with physical, and sometimes mental, stress as much as those patients do who abuse prescription drugs for pain or anxiety [45]. The treatment of these patients is difficult and often requires extensive pain-management training in a specialized pain treatment center with a focus on behavioral-cognitive treatment strategies for helping patients cope with stress; frequently, family therapy is necessary as an adjunct, since family stresses often play a role in maintaining the drug abuse behavior, as in the case just described.

## Multiple Sclerosis, Other Neurological
## Disorders, and Substance Abuse

Multiple sclerosis is known to be associated with disturbances of mood. Both maniclike syndromes and depressions occur with increased frequency in MS patients compared to controls and other neurological disorders [47]. It is not surprising that such patients would also be subject to greater risk for developing problems with substance abuse in order to cope with their mood disturbances as well as their physical disabilities. The case reported by Gallagher et al. and previously discussed [45] certainly illustrates this phenomenon. Olivera et al. [48] has also described a 36-year-old patient with MS and recurrent depression and anxiety, as well as history of abuse of cocaine, cannabis, heroin, and other drugs since age 20. The quality of this patient's drug problem appeared to be related once again to attempts to self-regulate his emotional problems chemically, in this case with dangerous psychotropic drugs. The importance of diagnosing and treating anxiety and depression in MS is emphasized as a way of possibly preventing the development or exacerbation of drug-dependency behavior. It may after all be the accompanying psychiatric disorder and not the primary neurologic one that determines the development of substance abuse.

One would expect that patients suffering from any number of other neurological disorders, such as epilepsy, neoplastic diseases, and extrapyramidal disorders, to name a few, would also be at risk for secondary substance abuse for similar reasons as those patients just described with headaches, pain syndromes, and multiple sclerosis. Such is probably the case, although little has been written on most of these specific categories of illness except for sporadic case reports. One such report by Tack et al. [49] describes a young woman originally treated with L-DOPA for a poorly defined extrapyramidal neurological disorder, who developed an "addiction" to L-DOPA, using up to 2500 mg daily, with development of a paranoid psychosis and a *true* dyskinetic movement disorder. Withdrawal of the drug was difficult, resulting in parkinsonian symptoms and craving for L-DOPA because of its long-term effects on receptors in the dopaminergic system. L-DOPA has not previously been considered to be an abused drug, although the majority of patients treated with it do experience mild psychic effects described as "alerting" or "activating" [49]. The original symptoms for which this patient was prescribed the L-DOPA were described as "inversion of the left foot and a gait disturbance," which the authors felt to be a conversion disorder, and her underlying personality was considered an important predisposing factor promoting the addiction. This was an unusual case, in which an initially questionable neurological disorder accompanied by a psychiatric disorder lead to substance abuse which, in turn, produced a more definite neurologic disorder.

## Attention Deficit Disorder and Cocaine Abuse

Attention deficit hyperactivity disorder (ADHD), as it is now called, has been referred to by many other names but, regardless of what one calls it, the disorder is certainly a familiar entity, usually treated by pediatric neurologists and psychiatrists. Symptoms often persist into adulthood, and the disorder is then called the residual type or adult-ADD. In terms of underlying pathophysiology, a dopamine-deficient state has been found to be associated with ADHD, and dopamine agonists are sometimes used to treat this condition [50]. Cocaine is, of course, a dopamine agonist; however, although there is evidence that *acutely* it increases dopamine turnover in the CNS, during withdrawal, there is actually a decrease in dopamine activity, and dopamine depletion results from chronic cocaine abuse [51].

Four case reports of cocaine addition and residual ADD were recently described by Cocores et al., [52] in which the ADD way hypothesized to play an etiologic role in the cocaine abuse, based on the theory that the patients may have been self-medicating a dopamine-deficient state. Family and longitudinal studies have previously shown an association between ADD and alcoholism, [41] but this is the first report of a similar association with cocaine abuse. All four patients were treated with the dopamine agonist bromocriptine rather than with a more traditional stimulant such as dextroamphetamine or methylphenidate, preferring to avoid such euphorigenic agents in this addiction-prone population. They all allegedly responded well, with no sensory overload or euphoria, but with definite improvement in their ADD symptoms, such as irritability, impulsivity, and impaired concentration. It is suggested that cocaine abusers with an underlying history of ADD carry a double burden during withdrawal from cocaine — namely, their developmental dopamine deficiency (the ADD) *plus* the additional reduction of dopamine function secondary to withdrawal itself. Nevertheless, even patients without a history of ADD experience symptoms of irritability and poor concentration during withdrawal, possibly indicating a kind of temporary cocaine-induced ADD stemming from dopamine depletion. "Correcting" this dopamine deficiency could be helpful therapeutically as it was in these patients with bromocriptine, which may be a safe and effective treatment for adults with residual ADD and cocaine abuse. Further study is, of course, necessary to determine how frequently ADD really does occur as an underlying factor in cocaine abuse. Such research could explore the possibility that some cocaine abusers may be self-medicating an ADD state, just as the previously described patients with migraine headaches were also attempting to self-medicate with cocaine. An underlying vulnerability to dopamine dysfunction may be the common factor in both of these patient groups, as well as in other neuropsychiatric patients with such diagnoses as depression and anxiety. These may be patients at special risk for addiction to cocaine or other drugs.

## Cognitive Impairment and Substance Abuse

One additional, but extremely important, category of dual-diagnosis patient that cannot be overlooked is the group of cognitively impaired individuals with substance abuse. Deficits in neuropsychological functions are common among drug abusers and may occur independently of other psychiatric disorders [53]. Naturally, these deficits are usually assumed to be secondary to the substance abuse itself (and, in fact, they often are); however, one must not ignore the possibility that an individual with a primary neurocognitive impairment (from any cause) may also be susceptible to the lure of drugs and alcohol.

Meek et al. [53] have very recently conducted a study on an inpatient substance abuse unit to assess the initial level of neuropsychological functioning of this patient population and to determine if cognitive deficits can improve during treatment. They found impairment of neurocognitive functioning on admission in approximately two-thirds of the patients, with the most frequently compromised areas involving attention and memory, calculations, abstraction, ability to follow complex commands, and visuospatial skills. There was a statistically significant improvement prior to discharge in some of these deficits.

The implications for treatment are far-reaching, since patients with cognitive impairment may be limited in their capacity to comply with the educational and adaptational aspects of a comprehensive drug treatment program. In essence, some patients may simply lack the cognitive skills necessary to comply with the programs typically offered and, therefore, more flexibility may be necessary in planning these treatment programs to suit the needs of patients with varied intellectual capacities. Particularly when the cognitive deficits are subtle, as they often are, they may go unrecognized by staff, as opposed to the patient with more severe and obvious organic impairment. As mentioned above, some of these patients with cognitive impairment may have had a premorbid organic disturbance, such as brain injury or even mental retardation and, in fact, these patients seem to be particularly vulnerable to substance abuse. The brain-injured patient, for instance, may have a frontal lobe syndrome with symptoms of emotional liability and behavioral dyscontrol, leading to attempts by the individual to "treat" some of these problems with psychoactive drugs, which then may escalate into a pattern of abuse or dependence.

Westermeyer et al. [54] studied a cohort of mentally retarded substance-abusing patients and compared them to a mentally retarded control group of patients who were not substance abusers. Data from this study confirmed not only that substance abuse does occur in the mentally retarded population but that there are similar pathological substance use patterns as well as similar behavioral, psychological, and social problems. The most common drugs used were found to be alcohol, tobacco, cannabis, amphetamines, and cocaine. It was noted that the presence of *familial* substance abuse strongly differentiated the mentally retarded drug-using patients from the controls, which is very comparable to findings in nonretarded drug-abusing populations. Caretakers and those providing other services to the mentally retarded need to be alerted to the possibility of this problem since treatment is obviously required and the diagnosis may often be delayed. Because of the underlying organic deficit, these patients may be susceptible to smaller than usual amounts of drugs and may therefore develop abuse and dependency problems more readily than normals [54]. Once again, treatment requirements would also be different in this group, where an individual with alcohol or cocaine addiction could obviously not comply with the typical drug-rehabilitation programs without significant modifications being made in the programs to compensate for cognitive limitations.

## ALCOHOLISM AND EPILEPSY

Although a complete discussion of the many neurological complications of alcohol abuse is not to be included in this chapter, an exception will be made for the important subject of epilepsy and its relationship to alcoholism.

First, it is vital to realize that an association between alcoholism and epilepsy has long been suspected although the precise nature of this relationship remains unclear. Because of methodological problems, it has been difficult to determine with any precision either the prevalence of epilepsy among alcoholics or the prevalence of alcoholism among epileptic patients. In fact, the prevalence of any type of seizure in alcoholics has varied across studies from 0.6–15%, and most authors would agree that the prevalence of true epilepsy among alcoholics is at least triple that in the general population [55]. As for the rate of alcoholism among seizure patients, that, too, has ranged considerably, from 12–36% in different investigations. These are all higher rates than those found in the general population, suggesting that individuals with epilepsy may seek relief in alcohol for their psychological and social problems. Yet an early study by Lennox [56] of the frequency of alcohol use in patients with and without epilepsy found that patients with epilepsy did *not* use more alcohol than controls but that those who drank tended to drink heavily and that, among epileptic men, alcohol use increased with age.

One of the principal questions being asked by researchers and clinicians today is how much of a risk factor is alcohol use for occurrence of seizures in patients with preexisting epilepsy. Several studies have addressed this important question. The most sophisticated one, completed by Hoppener et al., [57] found *no* significant change in frequency of seizures in epileptic patients receiving alcohol when compared to controls and no change in EEG epileptiform activity. The authors concluded that in patients with epilepsy, social drinking had little effect on seizure frequency (or anticonvulsant blood levels, which were also measured in this study). One must conclude that, in the earlier literature, where an exacerbation of seizures was usually found in conjunction with alcohol use, the patients studied were not "social drinkers" but rather alcoholics consuming much larger quantities of alcohol. Numerous mechanisms have been proposed to account for the higher frequency of seizures observed in epileptics who drink heavily: a direct "stimulant" effect of alcohol (see below), a withdrawal effect, enhancement of anticonvulsant drug metabolism through hepatic enzyme induction, alterations in absorption of anticonvulsant drugs, noncompliance with prescribed treatment during periods of drinking, changes in sleep patterns with relative sleep deprivation, etc. [58] Any or all of these mechanisms may play a role in exacerbating seizure frequency. Also, the metabolic effects of alcohol, such as hypoglycemia, changes in acid-base balance, electrolytes, hydration, or vitamin deficiencies, can certainly affect seizure control.

The subject of alcohol as a risk factor for seizures in persons *without* a history of epilepsy is also very interesting. It remains controversial whether acute alcohol intoxication itself can precipitate a seizure. Probably it can, although very rarely, even in individuals who seem to have seizurelike symptoms while drinking. It is generally agreed that seizures in alcoholics are usually related to *withdrawal* of alcohol after a sustained period of intoxication rather than a form of "epilepsy" precipitated by alcohol [59]. Still, it is a curious fact that most alcoholics do *not* experience seizures, even during withdrawal, and it is not clear why this is so. A number of previously held beliefs about withdrawal seizures have been modified based on more recent studies. For instance, it is now apparent that partial or focal seizures may occur more frequently than originally suspected (perhaps in 20–25% of cases), large quantities or long duration of alcohol abuse may not be a prerequisite for seizure occurrence, the timing of withdrawal seizures may vary much more than previously assumed, and EEG correlates may not always include photo-induced phenomena [58]. It is generally agreed that patients experiencing exclusively alcohol withdrawal seizures ("rum fits") do not require any long-term anticonvulsant therapy. Recently, however, it has even come into question whether anticonvulsants are necessary as prophy laxis for alcoholics undergoing withdrawal in detoxification treatment programs since the incidence of withdrawal seizures is very low, in some studies as low as 1%. It is especially true that patients with no prior history of withdrawal or other types of seizures may not require any prophylactic anticonvulsant treatment [55].

A recent report by Ng et al. [60] has taken the subject of alcohol-withdrawal seizures one step further by alleging that the relation of seizures to alcohol use may be *dose-dependent*; in other words, these seizures may somehow be directly induced by the ingestion of alcohol, independently of alcohol withdrawal. Whether alcohol itself is directly epileptogenic remains highly controversial since the molecular mechanisms of alcohol-related seizures, of which many have been proposed, remain unclear [61]. Alcohol administration does cause alterations in membrane receptors that may have a role in the pathogenesis of epilepsy. Also, the concentration of glutamate (an excitatory neurotransmitter) and the number of postsynaptic glutamate receptors are increased in animal studies after long-term alcohol administration. Most recent research has focused on alcohol's effects on GABA, revealing that alcohol enhances the inhibitory effects of GABA while, during alcohol withdrawal, sensitivity to GABA inhibition is reduced. Concentrations of GABA have been found to be depressed in human cerebrospinal fluid (CSF) during alcohol withdrawal and, of course, GABAergic drugs such as benzodiazepines are well known to be effective in alcohol withdrawal and epilepsy. A number of other possible mechanisms by which seizures may be induced by alcohol have been proposed, including modulation of G-proteins and calcium channels, effects on cyclic nucleotides, and induction of endogenous beta-carbolines [61]. In short, this area remains wide open for research.

An additional related question being asked today is whether chronic alcohol abuse is itself a risk factor for the development of epilepsy; in other words, is there such an entity as "alcoholic epilepsy"? This term has been defined differently by various authors but should probably be reserved for patients with recurrent *unprovoked* seizures who happen also to be alcoholic. Just as with other causes of epilepsy, the underlying pathogenetic mechanism has not been determined. It has been suggested that there may be a correlation with cerebral atrophy seen on CT scan. In one series, atrophy was noted in 75% of patients with epilepsy attributed to chronic alcohol abuse [62]. Such patients have no prior history of epilepsy but first develop withdrawal seizures and often experience periods of status epilepticus along with signs of cerebral atrophy. The author suggests that, in these individuals, the extent of morphological deterioration may eventually reach a point at which seizures occur independently of alcohol consumption. Another widely held theory is that the propensity to head trauma in these patients may account for the increased frequency of epilepsy. As mentioned earlier, preliminary epidemiologic studies suggest that chronic use of alcohol is associated with a threefold increased risk for unprovoked seizures or epilepsy.

Finally, it must be emphasized that whatever the mechanism(s) accounting for the coexistence of alcoholism and seizures, the fact remains that these two conditions do coexist and that persons suffering from both alcoholism and epilepsy need to be monitored very carefully for seizure occurrence, especially the likelihood of status epilepticus. Hence, the clinician must not lose sight of the critical importance of taking careful methodological history for both of these conditions since the implications for treatment are certainly extensive.

## SUMMARY AND CONCLUSIONS

An enormous number and diversity of neurological complications can develop secondarily to substance abuse disorders. These complications run the gamut from seizures to strokes, headaches, focal symptoms, and even significant cognitive impairment. Similarly, as we have seen, many neurological disorders can lead to the development of secondary substance disorders and, again, the variety is great both in terms of specific type of drug and severity of abuse. In some instances, the abuse may have a pharmacological basis, as in cases of self-medication to correct a dopamine deficiency or serotonin dysfunction. More typically, a patient in physical and/or psychological distress is trying to find a way to relieve that distress by turning to drugs.

An important lesson to be learned is that, in dual diagnosis, the primary and secondary disorders must each be treated. Obviously, when a neurological complication occurs in a substance abuse patient, most physicians would recognize the need to treat that condition, along with the underlying substance abuse problem. If a cocaine addict suffers a stroke, few clinicians would ignore the stroke and choose only to treat the addiction. However, when the sequence is reversed, and the neurological disorder is primary, with secondary substance abuse, there may be a tendency to focus on only the underlying disorder. This would be a mistake, as the patient who *begins* using drugs to self-medicate depression, ADHD, or migraine often develops an *independent* substance abuse disorder requiring its own independent comprehensive treatment. It isn't realistic to believe or hope that aggressively treating only the migraine will make the cocaine addiction disappear. Dual diagnosis means dual treatment.

## REFERENCES

1. Abelson HI, Miller JD. A decade of trends in cocaine use in the household population. *Cocaine Use in America: epidemiological and clinical perspectives.* NIDA Research Monograph Series 61, Rockville Md.: National Institute of Drug Abuse. 1985:35–49.
2. Post RM, Weiss SRB, Pert A. Cocaine-induced behavioral sensitization and kindling: Implications for the emergence of psychopathology and seizures. *Ann NY Acad Sci* 198?: 292–308.
3. Rowbotham MC. Neurologic aspects of cocaine abuse. *West J Med* 1988; 149:442–448.
4. Lathers CM, Tyau LSY, Spino MM, Agarwal I. Cocaine-induced seizures, arrhythmias and sudden death. *J Clin Pharmacol* 1988; 28:584 593.
5. Lowenstein DH, Massa SM, Rowbotham MC, Collins SD, McKinney HE, Simon RP. Acute neurologic and psychiatric complications associated with cocaine abuse. *Am J Med* 1987; 83:841–846.
6. Matsuzaki M. Alteration in pattern of EEG activities and convulsant effect of cocaine following chronic administration in the rhesus monkey. *Electroenceph Clin Neurophysiol* 1978; 45:1–15.
7. Merriam AE, Medalia A, Levine B. Partial complex status epilepticus associated with cocaine abuse. *Biol Psych* 1988; 23:515–518.
8. Weiss SRB, Costello M, Woodward R. Chronic carbamazepine inhibits the development of cocaine-kindled seizures (abstract). *Soc Neurosci* 1987; 13:950.
9. Brust JC, Richts RW. Stroke associated with cocaine abuse. *NY State Med J* 1977; 77:1473.
10. Cregler LJ, Mark H. Cardiovascular dangers of cocaine abuse. *Am J Cardiol* 1986; 57:1185–1186.
11. Wojak JC, Flamm ES. Intercranial hemorrhage and cocaine use. *Stroke* 1987; 18:712–715.
12. Jacobs I, Rozler M, Kelly J, Klein MA, Kling GA. Cocaine abuse: Neurovascular complications. *Radiol* 1989; 170:223–227.
13. Nalls G, Disher A, Daryabagi J, Zant Z, Eisenman J. Subcortical cerebral hemorrhages associated with cocaine abuse: CT and MR findings. *J Computer Assisted Tomography* 1989; 13(1):1–5.
14. Cahill DW, Knipp H, Mosser J. Intracranial hemorrhage with amphetamine abuse. *Neurology* 1981; 31:1058–1059.
15. Kaye BR, Fainstat M. Cerebral vasculitis associated with cocaine abuse. *JAMA* 1987; 258(15):2104–2105.
16. Levine SR, Welch KMA, Brust JCM. Cerebral vasculitis associated with cocaine abuse or subarachnoid hemorrhage? *JAMA* 1988; 259(11):1648.
17. Feinman BN. Neurologic sequelae of cocaine. *Hospital Practice* 1/89; 97–104.
18. Caplan L. Intracerebral hemorrhage revisited. *Neurology* 1988; 38:624–627.
19. Toler KA, Anderson B. Stroke in an intravenous drug user secondary to the lupus anticoagulant. *Stroke* 1988; 19(2):274–275.

20. Rubin AM. Neurologic complications of intravenous drug abuse. *Hospital Practice* 4/87; 279–288.
21. Mercado A, Johnson G, Calver D, Sokol RJ. Cocaine, pregnancy, and postpartum intracerebral hemorrhage. *Obstet Gynecol* 1989; 73(3):467–468.
22. Chasnoff IJ, Bussey ME, Savich R, Stack CM. Perinatal cerebral infarcts and maternal cocaine use. *J Pediat* 1986; 108:456–459.
23. Satel SL, Gawin FH. Migraine-like headache and cocaine use. *JAMA* 1989; 261(20):2995–2996.
24. Kosten TR, Kleber HD. Rapid death during cocaine abuse. A variant of the neuroleptic malignant syndrome? *Am J Drug Alcohol Abuse* 1988; 14(3):335–346.
25. Campbell BG. Cocaine abuse with hyperthermia, seizures, and fatal complications. *Med J Austral* 1988; 149:387–389.
26. Kasantikul V, Shuangshoti S, Sampatanukul P. Primary chromoblastomycosis of the medulla oblongata: Complication of heroin addiction. *Surg Neurol* 1988; 29:319–321.
27. Fischer PA, Enzensberger W. Neurological complications in AIDS. *J Neurol* 1987; 234:269–279.
28. Lazar RB, Ho SU, Melen O, Daghestani AN. Multifocal central nervous system damage caused by toluene abuse. *Neurol* 1983; 33:1337–1340.
29. Hormes JT, Filley CM, Rosenberg NL. Neurologic sequelae of chronic solvent vapor abuse. *Neurol* 1986; 36:698–701.
30. Granella F, Farina S, Malferrari G, Manzoni GC. Drug abuse in chronic headache: A clinicoepidemiologic study. *Cephalalgia* 1987; 7:15–18.
31. Isler H. A hidden dimension in headache work: Applied history of medicine. *Headache* 7/1986; 27–29.
32. Heyck H. Headaches and drug dependence. *Panminerva Medica* 1982; 24:151–153.
33. Saper JR. Ergotamine dependency — A review. *Headache* 1987; 27:435–438.
34. Lippman CW. Characteristic headache resulting from prolonged use of ergot derivatives. *J Nerv Ment Dis* 1955; 121:270–273.
35. Saper JR, Jones M. Ergotamine tartrate dependency: Features and possible mechanisms. *Clin Neuropharmacol* 1986; 9(3):244–256.
36. Saper JR, Jones JM. Hypothalamic-pituitary-adrenal disturbances in ergotamine rebound headache: Clinical and mechanistic implications (abstract). *Headache* 1985; 25:163–164.
37. Lance JW. *Mechanisms and Management of Headache*. 4th ed., Boston: Buttersworths; 1982.
38. Gilliland K, Bullock W. Caffeine: A potential drug of abuse. *The Addictive Behaviors*. New York: Haworth Press, 1984:53–73.
39. Rainey JT. Headache related to chronic caffeine addiction. *Texas Dent J* 7/1985; 29–30.
40. Brower KJ. Self-medication of migraine headaches with freebase cocaine. *J Subst Abuse Treatment* 1988; 5:23–26.
41. Khantzian EJ. The self-medication hypothesis of addictive disorders: Focus on heroin and cocaine dependence. *Am J Psychiatry* 1985; 142:1259–1264.

42. Langemark M, Olesen J. Drug abuse in migraine patients. *Pain* 1984; 19:81–86.
43. Lance JW. The pharmacothcrapy of migrainc. *Med J Austral* 1986; 144:85 88.
44. Gawin FH, Kleber HD, Byck R, Rounsaville BJ, Kosten TR, Jatlow PI, Morgan C. Desipramine facilitation of initial cocaine abstinence. *Arch Gen Psychiat* 1989; 46(2):117 121.
45. Gallagher RM, Stewart FI, Weissbein T, Weissbein A. Non-narcotic analgesic abuse: A common biopsychosocial problem. *Gen Hosp Psychiatry* 1988; 9:102–107.
46. Maruta T. Substance abuse by patients with chronic pain. *Curr Psychiat Ther* 1982; 155–160.
47. Martin MJ, Black JL. Neuropsychiatric aspects of degenerative diseases. In: *Textbook of Neuropsychiatry*. Hales R, Yudofsky S, eds. American Psychiatric Press, 1987:262.
48. Olivera A, Fero D, Evans M. Major depression, anxiety, and substance abuse in a multiple sclerosis patient: Diagnosis, treatment, and outcome. *J Clin Psychiatry* 1988; 49:2.
49. Tack E, De Cuypere G, Jannes C, Remouchamps A. Levodopa addiction, a case study. *Acta Psychiatr Scand* 1988; 78:356–360.
50. Wender PH. Minimal brain dysfunction, an overview. In: *Psychopharmacology: A Generation of Progress*. Lipton MA, DiMascio A, and Killam KF, eds. New York: Raven Press, 1978:1429–1435.
51. Dackis CA, Gold MS. New concepts in cocaine addiction: The dopamine depletion hypothesis. *Neurosci Biobehav Rev* 1985; 9:1–9.
52. Cocores JA, Davies RK, Mueller PS, Gold MS. Cocaine abuse and adult attention deficit disorder. *J Clin Psychiatry* 1987; 48(9):376–377.
53. Meek PS, Clark HW, Solana VL. Neurocognitive impairment: the unrecognized component of dual diagnosis in substance abuse treatment. *J Psychoactive Drugs* 1989; 21(2):153–160.
54. Westermeyer J, Phaobtong T, Neider J. Substance use and abuse among mentally retarded persons: A comparison of patients and a survey population. *Am J Drug Abuse* 1988; 14(1):109–123.
55. Chan AWK. Alcoholism and epilepsy. *Epilepsia* 1985; 26(4):323–333.
56. Lennox WG. Alcohol and epilepsy. *Q J Stud Alcohol* 1941; 2:1–11.
57. Hoppener RJ, Kuyer A, van der Lugt PJM. Epilepsy and alcohol: The influence of social alcohol intake on seizures and treatment in epilepsy. *Epilepsia* 1983; 24:459–471.
58. Hauser WA, Ng SKG, Brust JCM. Alcohol, seizures, and epilepsy. *Epilepsia* 1988; 29(Suppl. 2):S66 S78.
59. Victor M, Brausch C. The role of abstinence in the genesis of alcoholic epilepsy. *Epilepsia* 1967; 8:1–20.
60. Ng SKG, Hauser WA, Brust JCM, Susser M. Alcohol consumption and withdrawal in new-onset seizures. *NE J Med* 1988; 319(11):666–673.
61. Simon RP. Alcohol and seizures. *NE J Med* 1988; 319(11):715–716.
62. Avdaloff W. Alcoholism, seizures, and cerebral atrophy. *Adv Biol Psychiatry* 1979; 3:20–32.

# 6

## Substance Abuse and Mood Disorders

**Charles Ciolino**

*Fair Oaks Hospital, Overlook Hospital, and The Summit Medical Group, Summit, New Jersey*

The coexistence of substance abuse and mood dysfunction can present diagnostic and treatment challenges for the clinician. Uncertainty about the etiological relationships between the substance abuse and the affective symptomatology can lead to difficulty in adequately diagnosing the patient: Is the presenting depression the result of the substance abuse, or is the substance abuse the patient's attempt to self-medicate the depression? Are they coexisting independent conditions? Treatment choices may also be uncertain: Should the substance abuse and mood disorder be treated concurrently, or should one be treated prior to the other? Should psychotropic medications be used?

As an example of the interrelationships between substance abuse and mood disorder, Schuckit [1] has described five factors that may contribute to the confusion between alcoholism and affective disorder:

1. Depressive/dysphoric symptoms can be caused by alcohol in most people.
2. Temporary serious depression can follow prolonged drinking.
3. During primary affective episodes, particularly during mania, drinking can escalate.
4. Depressive symptoms and alcohol problems can coexist in other psychiatric disorders.

5.  Alcoholism and affective disorder can coexist independently in a small proportion of patients.

This chapter will explore the relationship between substance use and mood disorders and will present clinical presentations of affective symptomatology with various substances. Issues of genetics, epidemiology, biological markers, and treatment will be discussed in greater depth in other chapters of this book.

## RELATIONSHIPS BETWEEN SUBSTANCE USE AND MOOD DISORDERS

Two approaches to differentiating substance abuse from mood disorders are the primary-secondary distinction and the transient-persistent distinction.

In the primary-secondary dichotomy, [2] chronology of symptoms determines which disorder is primary. For example, if substance abuse predated the onset of affective symptoms, then primary substance abuse with secondary mood symptoms would be diagnosed.

The use of a resource person (relative or close friend) who has observed the patient over a period of time can help overcome the difficulty in gathering data adequate to make this distinction [3,4].

Generally, substance abuse is primary, with secondary affective symptomatology. For example, one-third of alcoholic patients may experience symptoms of secondary depression at some point during the course of their illness [5]. However, the prevalence rate of primary depression in male alcoholics has been reported as 2–3% [6]. For chronic drinkers of either sex who exhibit symptoms of both depression and alcoholism, the diagnosis is alcoholism and not primary affective illness in approximately 90% of these patients [7]. However, in alcoholic patients with primary depression, more impairment was found than in those with concurrent or secondary depression [8].

In addition, even for those patients with a primary substance use disorder, secondary affective symptoms may contribute to relapse to substance use after a period of abstinence has been achieved [9].

The transient-persistent dichotomy described by Kranzler and Liebowitz [10] may also be useful in understanding psychiatric symptoms that appear in association with substance use. The transient state includes affective symptoms that are acute and last, at most, for only a few weeks. While symptom intensity may be high, it is not sustained. Symptoms may be secondary to substance withdrawal. Thus, treating the withdrawal or allowing sufficient passage of time with continued abstinence generally leads to resolution of these transient affective symptoms.

For example, in a study of 191 alcoholics by Brown and Schuckit, [11] although 42% of primary alcoholics entering treatment appeared significantly depressed, these depressive symptoms resolved quickly, and only 6% were depressed at four weeks into treatment.

On the other hand, persistent affective symptoms in a substance abuser last for periods of weeks to months and are much less likely to resolve spontaneously without treatment. There is a greater likelihood that these states may become chronic, with greater resultant morbidity and mortality.

In order to make more accurate diagnoses of primary affective disorders in substance abusers, observations over a two- to four-week substance-free period have been recommended in the psychiatric evaluation of alcoholics [12,13] and opiate abusers [14]. A longer drug-free period (up to two months) has been suggested for cocaine abusers [15,16] prior to diagnosis of primary affective illness.

## SELF-MEDICATION HYPOTHESIS

A long-standing notion in psychiatry has been that substance abuse is often the product of psychopathology, resulting in the patient's attempt to "self-medicate" dysphoric symptoms [17,18]. However, some controlled studies have tended to limit this view by demonstrating that substance abuse and withdrawal reactions often exacerbate dysphoric symptoms. Studies on the effects of stimulants, [19–21] benzodiazepines, [22] opiates, [23] and alcohol [24] have sometimes failed to substantiate the self-medication hypothesis. However, Casteneda and colleagues [21] did demonstrate that users of central nervous system (CNS) depressants, such as alcohol and opiates, reported relief of their psychiatric symptoms with substance use. They also found that CNS-stimulant (cocaine) use resulted in aggravation of psychiatric symptoms. Dependence on cocaine persisted despite a perceived drug-induced aggravation of dysphoric symptoms, which would tend to dispute the self-medication hypothesis in this situation.

Studies of alcohol use in patients with primary depressive disorders indicate that 70–80% of patients with severe depression do not escalate their alcohol intake [1,25]. The majority of patients with major depressive disorders either decrease their alcohol use or maintain a similar pattern of drinking, perhaps because of their recognition that drinking intensifies dysphoric symptoms [4].

## ALCOHOL AND DEPRESSIVE SYMPTOMS

Alcoholics are likely to present for treatment with moderately severe levels of depression and, for the majority of these primary alcoholics, secondary depressive symptoms tend to remit by the second week of treatment and continue to decrease more gradually with three or four weeks of abstinence [26]. Dysphoric mood (depressed mood, guilt, feelings of worthlessness, anhedonia, and irritability) may dominate the clinical presentation of recently detoxified alcoholics; these depressive symptoms are the ones that generally change most rapidly. Vegetative symptoms (insomnia, motor retardation, somatic symptoms, sexual dysfunction, weight loss, diurnal variation) appear to be the affective symptoms most resistant to change over the first month of alcohol abstinence [26].

Depressed alcoholics report more previous treatment for substance abuse, withdrawal symptoms, marital problems, and unemployment, as well as a higher incidence of early morning drinking, than those alcoholics without depression [27]. A detached interpersonal style and alienated self-image also characterize this group of depressed alcoholics [28].

It has been reported that when depression is combined with alcoholism, the outcome is poorer for men than for women [29]. Alcoholics reporting depression during periods of sobriety return to drinking more frequently than those with normal mood [30].

The occurrence of depression in alcoholics who maintain sobriety has also been investigated. A survey of Alcoholics Anonymous members who maintained sobriety for at least five years revealed that depression occurred in 15%, with a mean onset of symptoms at 35 months of sobriety [31].

Biological markers have been used to help distinguish a primary alcoholic with secondary depression from a primary depressive disorder patient with secondary alcoholism [32]. Sleep patterns have been used to help differentiate these two entities. A shortened latency for the first rapid eye movement (REM) episode has been documented in patients with severe primary depression [33]. Primary alcoholics and primary alcoholics with secondary depression, however, tend to have longer than average latencies (90 min), while primary depressives and primary depressives with secondary alcoholism have short REM latencies (45 min) [32]. The status of the cholinergic system has also been found to help differentiate primary alcoholics from primary depressives. Primary alcoholics are generally less sensitive to cholinergic agonists (such as physostigmine) than normal controls, while primary depressives will be more sensitive [32].

Alcohol abstinence is associated with a decrease in urinary-free cortisol (UFC) excretion, even in a distinct subgroup of alcoholic patients with persistent depression [34]. However, measures of UFC do not appear to be useful adjuncts in the early identification of depression in primary alcoholic patients [34].

The thyrotropin-releasing hormone (TRH) test and dexamethasone suppression test (DST) have been reported to have some degree of diagnostic predictive value with respect to major depression [35,36]. However, the TRH test and DST may not be sufficiently specific to confirm the diagnosis of major depression in alcoholic patients because chronic alcoholic abuse may also cause endocrine abnormalities, either directly or indirectly, secondary to coexistent hepatic dysfunction [37].

## ALCOHOL AND MANIC SYMPTOMS

In a study of substance abuse in 60 bipolar patients, 25% were found to abuse one or more drugs, with alcohol, cannabis, and cocaine accounting for 82% of the drug abuse [38]. While it appears that the prevalence of alcoholism among bipolar patients is not higher than that found in the population, [39] problem drinking may complicate the clinical picture of at least 20% of acutely manic patients [40,41]. Bipolar patients are at greater risk for increased alcohol intake during the manic phase of their illness [42] and during the hypomanic phase of cyclothymia [43].

Comparison of bipolar alcoholic patients and unipolar alcoholic patients suggests that bipolar patients, particularly those who were older, functioned at a better level during a 2-yr follow-up period, had a previous history of longer periods of abstinence, and maintained more frequent contact with Alcoholics Anonymous [44]. In addition, bipolar patients, when compared to unipolars, are more likely to be episodic drinkers and less likely to report impairment in their marital relationships, social activities, and work patterns because of drinking [44].

## STIMULANTS AND AFFECTIVE SYMPTOMS

Acute administration of central nervous system stimulants, such as amphetamines and cocaine, produces euphoria, increased vigor, arousal, and improved mood in normal volunteers, while repeated administration and use of higher doses can have an adverse effect on mood [45]. Stimulant abusers, in the course of self-administration of the drug, may initially experience mood-elevating effects but subsequently experience symptoms of depression [46,47].

Chronic cocaine use often results in a three-stage abstinence syndrome, with prominent transient mood symptoms [15]. The initial stage, often occurring hours after cessation of drug use, includes agitated depression, followed by fatigue and a desire for sleep. The second stage, occurring 1–6 days later, presents with worsening dysphoria, anhedonia, anxiety, and drug craving. The third stage, generally up to 10 weeks and sometimes significantly longer, is characterized by periodic drug craving and euthymic mood [15].

A similar clinical pattern has been noted in amphetamine withdrawal. Peak depressive symptoms are noted about 48–72 hr after cessation of amphetamine intake [48]. However, cases have been reported of chronic high-dose stimulant abusers, particularly intravenous amphetamines users, who have persistent drug craving, and persistent depressive symptomatology, particularly anergia and anhedonia, that do not remit even after abstinence of more than 10 years [49,50]. Animal studies have documented occasional dopaminergic neuronal degeneration with chronic stimulant administration, [51] perhaps providing a mechanism for chronic dysphoria in some abstinent stimulant abusers.

## OPIATES AND AFFECTIVE SYMPTOMS

Opiates acutely decrease anxiety and somatic preoccupation and acutely elevate mood, while chronic use may produce increases in depression, anxiety, social isolation, and motor retardation [23]. Dackis and Gold [52] diagnosed 25% of their detoxified heroin addicts as having major depression, while finding 62% of their detoxified methadone patients to have major depression. Prolonged opiate withdrawal (such as from methadone) may result in changes in CNS homeostasis, which sometimes results in an organic affective syndrome, with depression as its major feature.

Comparison of depressive symptoms in heroin addicts and alcoholics indicates that these two groups may be differentiated by their types of depressive symptomatology. Steer and colleagues [53] found that alcoholics described themselves as feeling more like failures and having more somatic preoccupation than heroin addicts, whereas heroin addicts reported more weight loss and loss of libido.

## OTHER DRUGS AND AFFECTIVE SYMPTOMS

### Sedative-Hypnotics

Sedative-hypnotic drugs, particularly benzodiazepines, are widely abused alone or together with other drugs. Treating depressed individuals with these medications may result in iatrogenic sedative dependence [54]. Sedative withdrawal may resemble depression when associated with dysphoric and vegetative symptoms and may result in depression severe enough to warrant antidepressant therapy [54,55].

Acute administration of sedative-hypnotics generally produces effects similar to those seen with alcohol administration, including decreased anxiety and euphoria [56]. However, depression, as well as increased anxiety and hostility, may be observed as paradoxical effects of sedative-hypnotics [57].

## Phencyclidine

Chronic administration of phencyclidine (PCP) can lead to a clinical presentation of increased symptoms of dysphoria, irritability, and anxiety [58]. Chronic PCP abusers may also exhibit emotional lability, social incompetence, overt impulsiveness, poor social judgment, poor attention span and concentration, poor interpersonal relationships, and social maladjustment. Abstinence from PCP and initiation of appropriate treatment may gradually reverse these characteristics [59]. PCP-induced depression has been found to be associated with poor outpatient clinic attendance and increased suicide risk. Hospitalization of these PCP-induced depressed patients has been beneficial [60].

## Cannabis

Cannabis intoxication may produce affective symptoms, such as psychomotor retardation, decreased concentration, decreased libido, paranoia, and guilty rumination, that may confound the evaluation of depression [54]. Chronic, high-dose cannabis users may exhibit an amotivational syndrome characterized by diminished goal-directed activity, apathy, inability to master new problems, and deterioration of personal habits [61]. The concept of an amotivational syndrome in chronic cannabis users is controversial, however, and other reports have failed to validate this syndrome [62,63].

## Solvents

Jacobs and Hamid-Ghodse, [64] in their study of 47 adolescent male solvent abusers (inhaling gas lighter fuel, glue, or paint thinner), found that significantly more solvent abusers were depressed than a comparison group that did not abuse solvents. Seventy percent reported that they inhaled solvents because they were depressed, thus implicating the use of solvents as self-medication. Underlying depressive traits may predispose vulnerable adolescents to solvent abuse. Assessment and, if necessary, treatment of possible depression should be considered when solvent abuse is identified.

## CONCLUSION

Substance abuse and mood dysfunction can coexist in various ways. Mood dysfunction may be secondary to primary substance abuse; substance abuse may be secondary to a primary mood disorder; or both conditions may coexist independently. The most common presentation appears to be primary substance abuse with secondary affective symptomatology. A clinical implication of this finding is that the affective symptoms may often be transient phenomena that may resolve with continued abstinence from the offending substance. However, persistent affective symptoms presenting in a substance abuser after a period of abstinence may require treatment with appropriate medication and psychotherapy. Specific treatment issues will be discussed in subsequent chapters.

Knowledge of possible clinical presentations of affective symptomatology with various substance abuse disorders, including withdrawal reactions and mixed substance abuse, can be useful to the clinician in the evaluation and management of dual-diagnosis patients.

## REFERENCES

1. Schuckit MA. Genetic and clinical implications of alcoholism and affective disorder. *Am J Psychiat* 1986; 143:140–147.
2. Goodwin DW, Guze SB. *Psychiatric Diagnosis*. New York: Oxford University Press, 1980.
3. Schuckit, MA. The clinical implications of primary diagnostic groups among alcoholics. *Arch Gen Psych* 1985; 42:1043–1049.
4. Schuckit, MA, Monteiro MG. Alcoholism, anxiety and depression. *Br J Addiction* 1988; 83:1373–1380.
5. Schuckit MA. Alcoholic patients with secondary depression. *Am J Psychiat* 1983; 140:711–714.
6. Winokur G, Rimmer J, Reich T. Alcoholism IV. Is there more than one type of alcoholism? *Br J Psychiat* 1971; 118:525–531.
7. O'Sullivan K, Williams P, Daly M. A comparison of alcoholics with and without coexisting affective disorder. *Br J Psychiat* 1983; 143:133–138.
8. Powell BJ, Read MR, Penick EC, et al. Primary and secondary depression in alcoholic men: An important distinction. *J Clin Psychiat* 1987; 48:98–101.
9. Marlatt GA. Relapse prevention: Theoretical rationale and overview of the model. In: Marlatt, GA, Gordon JR eds. *Relapse Prevention*. New York: Guilford Press, 1985.
10. Kranzler HR, Liebowitz NR. Anxiety and depression in substance abuse: Clinical implications. *Med Clinics North Amer* 1988; 72(4):867–885.
11. Brown SA, Schuckit MA. Changes in depression among abstinent alcoholics. *J Stud Alcohol* 1988; 49:412–417.
12. Nakamural MM, Overall JE, Hollister LE, Radcliffe E. Factors affecting outcome of depressive symptoms in alcoholics. *Alcoholism: Clin Exper Res* 1983; 7:188–13.
13. Dackis CA, Gold MS, Pottash ALC, Sweeney DR. Evaluating depression in alcoholics. *Psychiat Res* 1986; 17:105–109.
14. Dackis CA, Pottash ALC, Gold MS, Annitto W. The dexamethasone suppression test for major depression among opiate addicts. *Am J Psychiat* 1984; 141:810–811.
15. Gawin FH, Kleber HD. Abstinence symptomatology and psychiatric diagnosis in cocaine abusers: Clinical observations. *Arch Gen Psychiat* 1986; 43:107–113.

16. Weiss RD, Griffin ML, Mirin SM. Diagnosing major depression in cocaine abusers: The use of depression rating scales. *Psychiat Res* 1989; 28:335–343.

17. Institute of Medicine. Psychopathology related to alcohol abuse. In: *Causes and Consequences of Alcohol Problems*. Washington, D.C.: National Academy Press, 1987.

18. Khantzian E. The self-medication hypothesis of addictive disorders: Focus on heroin and cocaine dependence. *Am J Psychiat* 1985; 142:1259–1264.

19. Fischman MW, Schuster CR. Cocaine self-administration in humans. *Fed Pros* 1982; 41:241–246.

20. Griffith JD, Cavanaugh J, Held J, et al. Dextroamphetamine: Evaluation of psychotomimetic properties in man. *Arch Gen Psychiat* 1972; 26:97–100.

21. Castaneda R, Galanter M, Franco H. Self-medication among addicts with primary psychiatric disorders. *Compr Psychiat* 1989; 30:80 83.

22. Griffiths RR, Bigelow GE, Liebson I. Differential effects of diazepam and pentobarbital on mood and behavior. *Arch Gen Psychiat* 1983; 40:865–873.

23. Meyer RE, Mirin SM. *The Heroin Stimulus. Implications for a Theory of Addiction.* New York: Plenum Press, 1979.

24. Tamerin JS, Mendelson JH. The psychodynamics of chronic inebriation: Observations of alcoholics during the process of drinking in an experimental group getting. *Am J Psychiat* 1969; 125:866–899.

25. Mayfield DG. Alcohol and affect: Experimental studies. In Goodwin DW, Erickson CK eds. *Alcoholism and Affective Disorders*. New York: S.P. Medical and Scientific Books, 1979.

26. Brown SA, Schuckit MA. Changes in depression among abstinent alcoholics. *J Stud Alcohol* 1988; 49:412–417.

27. Pary R, Lippmann S, Tobias CR. Depression and alcoholism: Clinical considerations in management. *Southern Med J* 1988; 81(12):1529–1635.

28. McMahon RC, Davidson RS. An Examination of depressed vs. nondepressed alcoholics in inpatient treatment. *J Clin Psychol* 1986; 42:177–184.

29. Rounsaville BJ, Zelig SD, Babor TF et al. Psychopathology as a predictor of treatment outcome in alcoholics. *Arch Gen Psychiat* 1987; 44:505–513.

30. Westermeyer J, Neider J. Depressive symptoms among native American alcoholics at the time of a 10-year follow-up. *Alcoholism: Clin Exp Res* 1984; 8:429–439.

31. Behar D, Winokur G, Berg CJ. Depression in the abstinent alcoholic. *Am J Psychiat* 1984; 141:1105–1107.

32. Overstreet DH, Janowsky DS, Rezvani AH. Alcoholism and depressive disorders: Is cholinergic sensitivity a biological marker? *Alcohol Alcoholism* 1989; 24:253–255.

33. Shiromani P, Gillin JC, Henricksen SJ. Acetylcholine and the regulation of REM sleep. *Ann Rev Pharmacol Toxicol* 1987; 27:137–156.

34. Irwin MR, Risch SC, Brown SA et al. Urinary free cortisol excretion in depressed alcoholic patients. *Biol Psychiat* 1988; 24:213–216.

35. Carroll GJ, Feinberg M, Greden JF et al. A specific laboratory test for the diagnosis of melancholia: Standardization validation, and clinical utility. *Arch Gen Psychiat* 1981; 38:15–22.

36.  Gold MS, Pottash ALC, Extein I et al. Diagnosis of depression in the 1980s. *JAMA* 1981; 245(15):1562–1564.
37.  Dackis CA, Pottash ALC, Bailey J et al. The specificity of the Thyrotropin Releasing Hormone (TRH) Test and Dexamethasone Suppression Test (DST) for major depressive illness in alcoholics. In: *Problems of Drug Dependence.* Research Monograph Series #43, 1983.
38.  Miller FT, Busch F, Tanenbaum JH. Drug abuse in schizophrenic and bipolar disorder. *Am J Drug Alcohol Abuse* 1989; 15:291–295.
39.  Schwarz L, Fjeld SP. The alcoholic patient in the psychiatric hospital emergency room. *QJ Stud Alcohol* 1969; 30:104–111.
40.  Stenstedt A. A study in manic-depressive psychoses. *Acta Psychiatr Neurol Scand* (Suppl) 1952; 79:3011.
41.  Dunner DL, Hensel BM, Fieve RR. Bipolar illness: Factors in drinking behavior. *Am J Psychiat* 1978; 136:583–585.
42.  Reich LH, Davies RK, Himmelhoch JM. Excessive alcohol use in manic-depressive illness. *Am J Psychiat* 1974; 131:83–85.
43.  West AP. Lithium treatment of depressed alcoholics: A hypothesis. *Am J Psychiat* 1983; 140:814.
44.  O'Sullivan K, Rynne CJ, Miller J et al. A follow-up study on alcoholics with and without co-existing affective disorder. *Br J Psychiat* 1988; 152:813–819.
45.  Johanson CE, Uhlenhuth EH. Drug preferences in humans. *Fed Proc* 1982; 11:2.
46.  Fischman MW, Schuster CR. Cocaine self-administration in humans. *Fed Proc* 1982; 41:241–246.
47.  Griffith JD, Cavanaugh J, Held J. Dextroamphetamine: Evaluation of psychotromimetic properties in man. *Arch Gen Psychiat* 1972; 26:97–100.
48.  Jaffe J. Drug addiction and drug use. In: Gilman AG, Goodman LS, Rall TW eds. *The Pharmacological Basis of Therapeutics.* (7th ed.). New York: Macmillan, 1985: 532–581.
49.  Schuster CR, Fischman MW. Characteristics of human volunteering for a cocaine research project. In: Adams EH and Kozel NJ eds. *Cocaine Use in America: Epidemiologic and Clinical Perspectives.* NIDA Research Monograph 61. Rockville, Md.: Dept of Health and Human Services, 1985: 158–170.
50.  Utena H. Behavioral aberrations in methamphetamine intoxicated animals and chemical correlates in the brain. *Prog Brain Res* 1966; 21:1902.
51.  Seiden L. Neurochemical toxic effects of psychomotor stimulants. Presented at the 23rd Annual Meeting of the American College of Neuropsychopharmacology, San Juan, PR, Dec 12, 1984.
52.  Dackis CA, Gold MS. Depression in opiate addicts. In: Mirin SM ed. *Substance Abuse and Psychopathology.* Washington, D.C.: American Psychiatric Press, 1984:20–40.
53.  Steer RA, Beck AT, Shaw BF. Depressive symptoms differentiating between heroin addicts and alcoholics. *Drug Alcohol Dependence* 1985; 15:145–150.
54.  Dackis CA, Gold MS, Estroff TW. Inpatient treatment of addiction. In: Karasu TB ed. *Treatments of Psychiatric Disorders.* (Vol. 2). Washington, D.C.: American Psychiatric Association, 1989: 1359–1379.

55. Olajide D, Lader M. Depression following withdrawal from long-term benzo-diazepine use. A report of four cases. *Psychol Med* 1984; 14:937.

56. Khantzian EJ, McKenna GJ. Acute toxic and withdrawal reactions associated with drug use and abuse. *Ann Intern Med* 1979; 90:361–372.

57. Hall RC, Zisook S. Paradoxical reactions to benzodiazepines. *Br J Clin Pharmacol* 1981; 11:995–1045.

58. Mello NK. Control of drug self-administration: The role of aversive consequences. In: Petersen RC, Stillman RC eds. *PCP: Phencyclidine Abuse: An Appraisal*. Washington, D.C.: National Institute on Drug Abuse Research Monograph 21, 1978.

59. Daghestani AN, Schnoll SH. Phencyclidine abuse and dependence. In: Karasu TB ed. *Treatment of Psychiatric Disorders*. (Vol. 2). Washington, D.C.: American Psychiatric Association, 1989:1209–1218.

60. Caracci G, Migoni P, Mukherjee S. Phencyclidine abuse and depression. *Psychosomat* 1983; 24:932–933.

61. Stefanis C, Boulougouris I, Liakos A. Clinical and psychophysiological effects of cannabis in long-term users. In: Braude MC, Szara S. *Pharmacology of Marijuana*. New York: Raven Press, 1976.

62. Carter WE. *Cannabis in Costa Rica: A Study of Chronic Marijuana Use*. Philadelphia Institute for the Study of Human Issues, 1980.

63. Brady JV, Fotin RW, Fischman MW et al. Behavioral interactions and the effects of marijuana. *Alcohol, Drugs and Driving* 1986; 2:93–103.

64. Jacobs AM, Hamid-Ghodse A. Depression in solvent abusers. *Soc Sci Med* 1987; 24:863–866.

# 7

## Substance Abuse and Anorexia Nervosa and Bulimia Nervosa

**Michael M. Newman**

*Fair Oaks Hospital, Summit, New Jersey*

During the last decade, considerable attention has focused on comorbidity in patients with anorexia nervosa and/or bulimia nervosa. For the most part, the emphasis has been on the relationship between affective illness and eating disorders. With as many as 75% of patients with an eating disorder having a lifetime diagnosis of major depression, [1,2] the term "dual diagnosis" applied to this patient population has largely been understood as the presence of both an eating disorder and depression. Recognizing an association between these two disorders has clearly helped researchers to design protocols examining the etiology and treatment of anorexia and bulimia nervosa.

While the comorbidity of substance abuse and eating disorders has also been well documented, this subject has clearly not received the same kind of attention as has the relationship between affective illness and eating disorders.

## ALCOHOLISM AND ANOREXIA NERVOSA

The association between eating disorders and alcoholism was noted by Crisp, [3] who reported that 4 of 11 anorectics who regularly binged and purged had problems with alcohol. More than 10 years later, Eckert and co-workers, [4] reported on 105 anorectic patients from a multicenter study and found that 7 (6.7%) of those patients had "problems with alcohol."

Although that figure does not suggest a preponderance of alcohol abuse in anorectic patients, the clinical data on those 7 patients are noteworthy. When compared with those anorectics without an alcohol history, patients with anorexia nervosa and alcoholism were more likely to have a history of kleptomania, frequent bingeing behavior, and purging behaviors, as well as a greater number of previous hospitalizations. Thus, there was a suggestion that alcoholism was present in anorectic patients who had other factors associated with a poor prognosis.

Subsequent studies examining the significance of binge eating in anorectic patients also found that bulimic anorectics compared with restricting anorectics were more likely to have a history of alcohol problems. Garfinkel and co-workers [5] studied 73 restricting anorectics and 68 bulimic anorectics and found that 20.4% of the bulimic anorectics versus 4.8% of the restricting anorectics had a history of weekly alcohol use. Similarly, the bulimic anorectics were more likely to have a history of stealing, self-mutilation, and suicide attempts. Strober [6] confined his study to adolescents admitted to the hospital for anorexia nervosa and found that 23% of the bulimic anorectics versus none of the restricting anorectics reported alcohol use.

In summary, alcoholism may be a common finding in bulimic anorectic patients. In addition, bulimic anorectics tend to have disturbances of impulse control, including stealing, self-mutilative acts, and suicide attempts and, when compared with restricting anorectics, have more history of affective illness, [5,7] and a worse prognosis for recovery [8].

## ALCOHOLISM AND BULIMIA NERVOSA

The first reports noting the association between bulimia and alcohol abuse were those that compared restricting anorectics with bulimic anorectics. Clearly, increased prevalence of alcohol abuse was one of the distinguishing features of the bulimic group [4-6]. In the mid-1980s several investigators began to report on large series of patients who were of normal weight, binged and purged, and had a diagnosis of bulimia.

In an early report in which 34 cases of bulimia were reviewed, [9] 41% of the patients reported drinking alcohol several times per week, and 5 of the 34 (14.4%) reported daily alcohol use. Hatsukami et al. [10] reported that, in a series of 108 bulimic patients, 12% had a past history of alcohol abuse, but only 1.9% reported current alcohol abuse. A total of 16.8% reported having a history of daily alcohol use for a period of at least one month at some point in their lives. Mitchell and co-workers [11-13] reported on 275 bulimic patients who presented for evaluation at a specialty eating-disorder program, 23% of whom acknowledged a history of alcohol abuse. In one controlled study, the National Institute of Mental Health Diagnostic Interview Schedule was administered to patients with a lifetime history of bulimia, patients with major depression, and normal control subjects [1]. A lifetime diagnosis of alcohol abuse or dependence was present in 36% of the bulimic patients versus 21% of the women with major depression and 11% of the controls. Bulik [14] compared 35 bulimic women with 35 normal controls. Alcohol abuse was present in 48.6% of the bulimics compared with 8.6% of the controls, and alcohol dependence was present in 22.9% of the bulimics versus none of the controls.

Other studies, however, have not found as high an association between bulimia and alcohol abuse. Johnson and co-workers [15] reported on 316 patients who had written to request information from an eating-disorder program. Included in the information sent was a questionnaire that subjects were asked to complete. As less than 10% of that population reported daily drug or alcohol use, the authors concluded that drug and alcohol use was not prevalent. A similar conclusion was reached by the authors of a British study, [16] in which none of the 35 patients referred for treatment of bulimia gave a history "suggestive of dependence" on alcohol or drugs. Neither of those studies mentioned the frequency of alcohol use or whether there were alcohol-related problems; it is quite possible that, with a more complete history, a greater number of patients would have met criteria for a diagnosis of alcohol abuse. Also, there may be differences between patients who write to request information and those who actually present for treatment. Walsh and colleagues [2] reported that 14% of 50 patients who sought treatment for bulimia had a history of alcohol abuse.

The association between alcohol use and binge eating has also been noted in nonpatient populations. Killen and co-workers [17] studied 646 tenth-graders. Based on self-report questionnaires, 10.3% of the students were classified as bulimic, and 10.4% were classified as purgers (induced vomiting and/or laxative use without binge eating). When compared with the rest of the students, the bulimics and purgers reported significantly higher cigarette and marijuana use and more frequent bouts of drunkenness. While bulimics and normals were similar in the number that reported drinking several times per month (10% vs. 7.7%), 23.2% of the purgers reported that they drank alcohol at least several times per month.

In summary, the studies of normal weight patients with bulimia are similar to those of bulimic anorectics. In both these patient groups, there appears to be a significant degree of alcohol abuse.

## DRUG ABUSE AND EATING DISORDERS

The current data on drug abuse in patients with anorexia nervosa are sparse. Whether this reflects a relatively low prevalence is simply not known. Most of the reports including large series of patients were written before the recent rise in cocaine abuse, and it would not be surprising to learn that a significant number of patients use cocaine to control their appetite and avoid weight gain.

In 1980, Garfinkel and co-workers [5] reported that 11.6% of 73 restricting anorectics compared with 28.6% of 68 bulimic anorectics reported a history of ever having used a "street drug." In another more recent report, that same group [18] reported that use of street drugs was present in 19% of restricting anorectics and 40% of bulimic anorectics. Strober, [6] in his series of 44 patients admitted to a hospital for anorexia nervosa, found no patients with a history of drug use. Two other reports included small series of patients. In one, 3 of 9 bulimic anorectics had a history of drug abuse [2] and, in another, 5 of 16 restricting anorectics and 13 of 25 bulimic anorectics had a lifetime history of drug abuse [19–21].

The evidence demonstrating an association between bulimia and drug abuse is considerable. In a series of 101 bulimics, 30.7% reported a lifetime history of daily stimulant use for a period of at least one month. In an expanded series of 275 bulimics, [12] diet pills were used several times per week by 34.1% of the bulimics, and 17.7% reported a history of treatment for chemical dependency. In another study, 36% of 121 patients with bulimia versus 21% of 24 female patients with major depression had a lifetime diagnosis of drug abuse or dependence [1].

Powers and co-workers [22] compared diagnoses of substance abuse in 30 bulimics obtained by clinical interview with those from structured diagnostic interviews. In the former, two bulimics reported cocaine abuse, one reported cannabis abuse, and one reported cannabis dependence. When administered the Structured Clinical Interview for DSM-III-Patient Version a total of 14 patients had a diagnosis of psychoactive substance abuse.

Somewhat lower figures were reported for drug abuse by Walsh and colleagues, [2] who found that 3 of 34 (9%) bulimics had a history of drug abuse. In that same study, 3 of 7 (43%) bulimics had a history of anorexia nervosa, and 3 of 9 (33%) of bulimic anorectics.

Unfortunately, little can be found in the literature concerning the timing of the onsets of the substance abuse and eating disorder or concerning significance of having the two disorders. One study deals with 85 patients hospitalized on a substance abuse specialty unit undergoing concurrent treatment for alcohol and/or drug abuse and eating disorders. In that group, 60% reported that the onset of their eating disorder preceded their substance abuse, 23% had substance abuse prior to their eating disorder, 8% reported simultaneous onset, and 9% were uncertain [25]. The extent to which drugs may have been used by the patients who developed their substance abuse after their eating disorder to limit food intake is a matter for speculation. Hatsukami and co-workers [23] compared bulimic patients with bulimia only, bulimia and substance abuse, and bulimia and affective illness. The bulimics with substance abuse had a higher rate of diuretic abuse and previous psychiatric inpatient treatment compared with the other two groups. Both comorbid groups had a higher incidence of suicide attempts, more social problems, and a greater rate of overall treatment than the group with bulimia only.

## FAMILY STUDIES

Studies assessing substance abuse in families of patients with anorexia nervosa and/or bulimia nervosa have included retrospective chart reviews, information provided by patients, and interviews with first-degree relatives. The data can best be interpreted by examining mothers and fathers of subgroups of eating disorder patients. In an early study of families of anorectics conducted by Halmi and Loney, [24] 12.8% of fathers and 2.1% of mothers were found to have alcohol problems. There was no differentiation made between restricting and bulimic anorectics. Strober et al. [26] interviewed the parents of 35 restricting anorectics and 35 bulimic anorectics. While the prevalence of alcoholism ranged from 3% to 9% in the parents of the restricting anorectics as well as the mothers of the bulimic anorectics, 29% of the fathers of the bulimic anorectics had a significant history of alcoholism. Similar findings were obtained in retrospective chart review of 43 patients hospitalized for anorexia nervosa and bulimia [27]. In that second study, 2.9% of the mothers and 30.2% of the fathers were found to be alcoholic.

Families of patients with bulimia without anorexia nervosa also appear to have significant substance abuse problems. In a series of 34 bulimics, 17 reported alcoholism in at least one first-degree relative, and 7 reported having fathers who were alcoholic [9]. Similarly, Herzog et al. [28] reported 10 of 30 bulimics who had a history of alcoholism in at least one family member, and Beary et al. [29] reported 35% of 20 bulimics who had at least one first-degree relative treated for alcoholism. Mitchell et al. [11] studied 275 bulimic patients and found that 37.1% had a family history of drug abuse in at least one first-degree relative. Patients with a positive family drug history were significantly more likely to have had a history of prior treatment for alcohol and/or drugs (27% vs. 12.3%) and more likely to have had problems with drugs or alcohol (43.1% vs. 29.2%).

One study, however, has yielded somewhat contradictory results. Hudson et al. [21] assessed a total of 420 first-degree relatives of 89 eating-disorder patients. A total of 12.8% of the relatives were found to have a history of substance abuse. The highest rate of substance abuse was found in families of patients with both anorexia nervosa and bulimia, in which a rate of 18.2% was present. The somewhat lower prevalence of substance abuse compared to other studies may, in part, be due to the method by which information was collected: in approximately one-third of the sample by interviewing family members and in two-thirds of the sample by interviewing only the patients.

## EATING DISORDERS IN SUBSTANCE ABUSE PATIENTS

Recently, several reports have begun to appear in the literature suggesting that eating disorders may be present in a significant number of substance abuse patients. Beary et al. [29] studied 20 consecutive women admitted for alcohol abuse and found that 35% had a previous major eating disorder. In another study in which 27 alcoholic women were interviewed about their drinking and eating habits, [30] 11 (40%) reported a present or past history of major binge eating. The bulimic alcoholics, compared with the alcoholics without an eating disorder, were significantly younger, weighed more, and reported a younger age of onset of drinking problems. Interestingly, the bulimic alcoholics were less likely to have a family history of alcoholism. The authors also reported that there was a tendency for the alcoholism to develop after the onset of eating-disorder symptoms.

Jonas et al. [31] administered a structured clinical interview to 259 consecutive callers to the National Cocaine Hotline and found that 32% of the callers met criteria for a diagnosis of anorexia nervosa and/or bulimia. Of the sample with bulimia, 44% were men, suggesting an unusually high association between substance abuse and eating disorders in men. Lastly, Marcus and Halmi [32] interviewed 30 consecutive female admissions to a substance abuse unit and found that 47% met criteria for anorexia nervosa and/or bulimia nervosa.

## POLYSUBSTANCE ABUSE AND EATING DISORDERS

Surprisingly little has been written about polysubstance abuse in patients with eating disorders. For the most part, researchers have simply noted "alcohol" and/or "substance abuse," with little elaboration, especially failing to include the extent to which multiple diagnoses were present in the same patient. An exception is the report by Hatsukami et al. [23] describing substance abuse in bulimic patients. The authors noted that, of the 34 patients with substance abuse and an eating disorder, 55.9% had alcohol abuse, 35.3% had alcohol and drug abuse, and 8.8% abused drugs but not alcohol.

Newman and co-workers [33] studied the extent of polysubstance abuse in admissions to a specialized eating-disorders treatment unit. Information regarding drug and alcohol use was obtained by clinical interview with patients admitted over a six-month period. A total of 34 patients were studied: 8 had a diagnosis of anorexia nervosa (3 of whom were also diagnosed with bulimia nervosa), 24 had a diagnosis of bulimia nervosa (4 of whom had a previous history of anorexia nervosa), and 2, who restricted their food intake and purged, were diagnosed as having an eating disorder not otherwise specified.

In that same study, at time of admission, 13 patients had a dual diagnosis of an eating disorder and substance abuse. An additional 3 patients had a past history of substance abuse, which was in remission. Of those 16 patients, 8 were diagnosed with bulimia nervosa, 4 with bulimia nervosa and a past history of anorexia nervosa, 1 with anorexia nervosa, 2 with anorexia nervosa and bulimia nervosa, and 1 with eating disorder not otherwise specified.

With regard to patterns of substance abuse in the study by Newman and colleagues, 4 reported single drug use, and 12 reported multiple drug use. The latter group had an average of three substances of abuse. Current cocaine abuse was reported by 8 patients and a past history of cocaine abuse by 4 patients. Of note, although the sample size is obviously small, is the fact that 3 of 4 patients with a diagnosis of bulimia nervosa and past history of anorexia nervosa also had a history of cocaine abuse. Current alcohol abuse was reported by 9 patients, with an additional 2 patients reported a past history of alcohol abuse. With regard to the sequence of the onset of the eating and substance abuse disorders, 9 patients were clearly able to distinguish the onset of the eating disorder prior to the substance abuse disorder, 5 patients reported abusing at least one substance prior to the onset of their eating disorder, and 2 patients reported concomitant onsets of the two disorders.

In summary, the study by Newman and co-workers replicates the studies demonstrating significant substance abuse in patients with eating disorders. Furthermore, it is not uncommon for patients with eating disorders to have a history of multiple drug use.

## SUMMARY

A review of the literature demonstrates that as many as one-third of patients who present for treatment of an eating disorder may have a significant history of substance abuse. Little research to date has focused on the nature of the relationship between these two disorders other than to document their comorbidity. There is the suggestion in one study that, based on their having a greater number of psychiatric hospitalizations, [23] eating-disorder patients who also have a history of substance abuse have a worse prognosis than those with no such history of drug and alcohol use. Why, other than because drugs such as cocaine and amphetamines suppress appetite, women with eating disorders appear to be as high a risk as they are to develop substance abuse remains to be answered. It is not uncommon for bulimic women to report that bingeing and purging relieve feelings of anxiety and tension, [12] and they may be turning to drugs for similar reasons. In terms of clinical treatment, it is clear that a detailed drug history with drug screening is essential when a patient is evaluated for anorexia nervosa or bulimia nervosa. In addition, treatment for substance abuse must be an integral part of the treatment of a patient diagnosed with an eating disorder and a drug or alcohol problem.

## REFERENCES

1.  Hudson JI, Pope HG, Jonas JM, Yugelman-Todd D. Family history study of anorexia nervosa and bulimia. *Br J Psychiatry* 1983; 142:133–138.
2.  Walsh BT, Roose SP, Glassman AH, Gladis M, Sadik C. Bulimia and depression. *Psychosom Med* 1985; 47:123–130.
3.  Crisp AH. The possible significance of some behavioral correlates of weight and carbohydrate craving. *J Psychosom Res* 1967; 11:117–131.
4.  Eckert ED, Goldberg SC, Halmi KA, Casper RC, Davis JM. Alcoholism in anorexia nervosa. In: Pickens RW, Heston LH, eds. *Psychiatric Factors in Drug Abuse*. New York: Grune and Stratton, 1979.
5.  Garfinkel PE, Moldofsky H, Garner DM. The heterogeneity of anorexia nervosa: bulimia as a distinct subgroup. *Arch Gen Psychiatry* 1980; 37:1036–1040.
6.  Strober M. The significance of bulimia in juvenile anorexia nervosa: An exploration of possible etiologic factors. *Int J Eating Disorders* 1981; 1:28–43.
7.  Casper RC, Eckert ED, Halmi KA, Goldberg SC, Davis JM. Bulimia: Its incidence and clinical importance in patients with anorexia nervosa. *Arch Gen Psychiatry* 1980; 37:1030–1035.
8.  Russell G. Bulimia nervosa: An ominous variant of anorexia nervosa. *Psych Med* 1979; 9:429–448.
9.  Pyle RL, Mitchell JL, Eckert ED. Bulimia: A report of 34 cases. *J Clin Psychiatry* 1981; 42:60–65.
10. Hatsukami D, Eckert E, Mitchell JE, Pyle R. Affective disorders and substance abuse in women with bulimia. *Psych Med* 1984; 14:701–704.
11. Mitchell JE, Hatsukami D, Pyle R, Eckert E. Bulimia with and without a family history of drug abuse. *Addict Behav* 1988; 13:245–251.

12. Mitchell JE, Hatsukami D, Eckert ED, Pyle RL. Characteristics of 275 patients with bulimia. *Am J Psychiatry* 1985; 142:482–485.
13. Mitchell P. Heroin-induced vomiting (Letter). *Am J Psychiatry* 1987; 144:249–250.
14. Bulik CM. Drug and alcohol abuse by bulimic women and their families. *Am J Psychiatry* 1987; 144:1604–1606.
15. Johnson CL, Stuckey MK, Lewis LD, Schwartz DM. Bulimia: A descriptive survey of 316 cases. *Int J Eating Disorders* 1982; 2:3–16.
16. Fairburn CG, Cooper PG. The clinical features of bulimia nervosa. *Br J Psychiatry* 1984; 144:238–246.
17. Killen JD, Tatlor CB, Telch MJ, Robinson TN, Maron DJ, Saylor KE. Depressive symptoms and substance use among adolescent binge eaters and purgers: A defined population. *Am J Publ Health* 1987; 77:1539–1541.
18. Garfinkel PE, Garner DM, O'Shaughnessey M. The validity of the distinction between bulimia with and without anorexia nervosa. *Am J Psychiatry* 1985; 142:581–587.
19. Hudson JI, Pope HG, Yurgelun-Todd D, Jonas JM, Frankenburg FR. A controlled study of lifetime prevalence of affective and other psychiatric disorders in bulimic outpatients. *Am J Psychiatry* 1987; 144:1283–1287.
20. Hudson JI, Pope HG, Jonas JM, Yurgelun-Todd D. Phenomenologic relationship of eating disorders to major affective disorder. *Psychiat Res* 1983a; 9:345–354.
21. Hudson JI, Pope HG, Jonas JM, Yurgelun-Todd D. Family history study of anorexia nervosa and bulimia. *Br J Psychiatry* 1983b; 142:133–138.
22. Powers PS, Coovert DL, Brightwell DR, Stevens BA. Other psychiatric disorders among bulimic patients. *Compr Psychiatry* 1988; 29:503–508.
23. Hatsukami D, Mitchell JE, Eckert ED, Pyle R. Characteristics of patients with bulimia only, bulimia with affective disorder, and bulimia with substance abuse problems. *Addict Behav* 1986; 11:399–406.
24. Halmi KA, Loney J. Familial alcoholism in anorexia nervosa. *Br J Psychiatry* 1973; 123:53–54.
25. Filstead WJ, Parella PP, Ebbitt, J. High risk situations for engaging in substance abuse and binge eating behaviors. *J of Studies of Al* 1988; 49:136–141.
26. Strober M, Salkin B, Burroughs J, Morrell W. The validity of the bulimia-restrictor distinction in anorexia nervosa: Parental personality characteristics and family psychiatric morbidity. *J Nerv Ment Dis* 1982; 170:345–351.
27. Collins GB, Kotz M, Janesz JW, Messina M, Ferguson T. Alcoholism in the families of bulimic anorectic. *Cleveland Clin Quart* 1985; 52:65–67.
28. Herzog DG. Bulimia: The secretive syndrome. *Psychosomat* 1982; 23:481–487.
29. Beary MD, Lacey JH, Merry J. Alcoholism and eating disorders in women of fertile age. *Br J Addict* 1986; 81:685–689.
30. Lacey JH, Moureli E. Bulimic alcoholics; some features of a clinical subgroup. *Br J Addict* 1986; 81:389–393.
31. Jonas JM, Gold MS, Sweeney D, Pottash ALC. Eating disorders and cocaine abuse: A study of 259 cocaine abusers. *J Clin Psychiatry* 1987; 48:47–50.

32. Marcus RN, Halmi KA. Eating disorders in substance abuse patients. American Psychiatric Association New Research. Abstract NR 248, 1988.
33. Newman MM, Le Maire M, Gold M. Axis II and substance abuse in eating disorders. Presented at the 143rd Annual Meeting of the American Psychiatric Association New Research. Abstract NR 538, 1990.
34. Rivinus TM, Biederman J, Herzog DB, Kemper K, Harper GP, Harmatz JS, Houseworth S. Anorexia nervosa and affective disorders: a controlled family history study. *Am J Psychiatry* 1984; 141:1414–1418.

# 8

# Marijuana and Psychopathology

**A. James Giannini**

*The Ohio State University, Columbus, Ohio*

The psychopathology of marijuana comes as much from the marijuana itself as from drugs that are used to adulterate or boost its effects [1]. More than 400 potentially psychoactive ingredients have been isolated from the three most common marijuana plants, *Cannabis indica*, *Cannabis sativa*, and *Cannabis americana* [2]. Approximately 65 of these ingredients are cannabinoid compounds [2,3]. The most important compound cannabinoid is delta-9-tetrahydrocannabinol, which is most commonly called THC [3]. THC is unusual in that, unlike most psychoactive substances, it lacks an amino nitrogen. It is THC that produces most of the effects commonly seen with marijuana abuse. These include drowsiness, a dreamlike state, visual misperceptions, decreased attention span, depersonalization, derealization, decreased reaction time, and decreased coordination [4].

Substances that are commonly taken with marijuana include phencyclidine, heroin, and cocaine [5]. All these substances tend either to enhance or add to the desirable psychoactive effects of marijuana. In increasingly common circumstances, marijuana is soaked in solvents to increase its potency. These solvents include formaldehyde, insecticides, and kerosene [6]. The affect of all these combinations and adulterants is to add paranoid psychoses to the list of untoward effects of marijuana abuse.

Finally, chronic marijuana abuse is associated with feelings of anxiety and depression. When these symptoms occur, many abusers tend to cushion their "down" feelings with alcohol, cocaine, or amphetamine. Thus, the effects of these drugs are added to the affects of marijuana [7].

## HISTORY

The first written mention of marijuana was documented approximately 3,000 years ago in the *Herbal* of Chen Nung, a Chinese emperor and amateur biologist [8]. Ancient Egyptians in the Middle Kingdom recorded the use of marijuana by the armies of the Scythian invaders. The Israelite King Solomon mentioned marijuana in his *Song of Songs* [9].

In classical civilization, Homer recorded in the *Iliad* the gift of marijuana given by Telemachus to Helen. The Greek physician Galen noted its being used to treat otitis media, while Hippocrates is thought to have referred to it in a surviving fragment. Its use was later recorded in the *Thousand and One Nights* of Haroun Al-Rashid [10]. In the thirteenth century, the Persian warlord Naguib Ad-Din was able to recruit large numbers of soldiers for his mercenary army by intoxicating them with hashish and then spiriting them away from their villages. From his use of hashish-intoxicated troops, we derived the word "assassin." [11,12]

Marijuana has existed in the United States since pre-colonial days. Its first recorded use in the United States was in 1611 in Jamestown, Virginia, where it was grown as a commercial fiber. In the eighteenth century, tincture of marijuana was sold in Philadelphia by John Biddle. Its use was endorsed by, among others, Dr. Benjamin Rush, [13] a founder of American psychiatry. Illustrations of the marijuana plant were seen extensively in John Tenniel's plates for Lewis Carroll's first editions of *Alice in Wonderland* and *Through the Looking Glass* [14,15].

The idea of marijuana as a recreational drug was introduced to the United States by U.S. troops who had participated in the American invasions of Latin America in the early twentieth century. In 1937, the Marijuana Tax Act was passed, and marijuana abuse was outlawed. As a result of social pressure exerted by such books as Charles Reich's *The Greening of American* and by political pressure from various lobbying groups, the Comprehensive Drug Abuse and Prevention Control Act of 1970 reduced the penalties for possession of small amounts of marijuana [16].

## DERIVATION

Marijuana is a generic name for a number of drugs derived from the cannabis plant. Marijuana is a mixture of dried leaves and flowers of the cannabis plant. Hashish is the resin secreted by the leaves of the cannabis plant. Hash oil is a distillate of the entire plant.

## MODE OF USAGE

Marijuana is most commonly smoked in the form of a cigarette or with a water pipe. Hashish can be either smoked or eaten. It is sometimes prepared with baked goods, such as the brownies used in Peter Sellers' film, *I Love You, Alice B. Toklas*. Hashish can also be dissolved in alcohol to form tincture of marijuana. Hash oil can be sprinkled on marijuana, tobacco, or oregano and then smoked.

## CHEMISTRY

As mentioned above, the major psychoactive compound found in marijuana is delta-9-tetrahydrocannabinol. Some psychoactively important compounds include cannabinol and cannabolic acid. Cannabinol is an active derivative of delta-9-THC, which spontaneously forms in vitro. These three compounds tend to act as sedatives. Most of the other cannabinoids have been little studied [17].

## DIRECT PSYCHOPATHOLOGY OF MARIJUANA

The effects of marijuana vary according to the emotional status of the abuser. Acute effects differ from chronic effects. Also, there seems to be a withdrawal state in marijuana abuse with distinct symptoms different from those seen in states of active abuse.

### Acute Abuse

Acute abuse is associated with a state resembling delirium. Spatial and depth perceptions are distorted although true hallucinations are rare. There are also perceptual illusions of time dilation. Depersonalization and derealization are often accompanied by tactile hallucinations. These latter distortions, in some cases, progress to panic or paranoid ideation and, occasionally, psychosis. Marijuana abusers, at least subjectively, report hyperacusis, hyperacuity, and increased creative free-form thinking. This tends to produce magical and illogical thinking. Thought process is marked by tangentiality, defects in the spheres of immediate and intermediate memory, and decreased estimation [18–20].

### Chronic Abuse

Changes associated with chronic marijuana abuse occur in the areas of thought, mood, and personality. The changes in thought tend to be grouped as either "organic" or "psychotic." The presentation of "organic" marijuana users can range from the presentation of the characters in a Cheech and Chong movie to that of a nursing home resident. Marijuana abusers tend to be apathetic and poorly motivated. Their attention span is quite short, and they are easily distracted. They have difficulty in following conversations, simple written material, and television programs. As a result, they tend to be isolated from persons and events in their immediate environment because they can grasp concepts only partially. They tend to misperceive the meanings of conversation. This serves only to introvert further an individual who already suffers from chemically induced social isolation. There is an inability to maintain a continuous stream of thought, so that responses to stimuli tend to be inappropriate and erratic. Personal habits generally deteriorate, and there is marked decrease in personal hygiene, which can be associated with urinary and fecal retention. Besides producing these effects, chronic use of THC reduces the insight necessary to correct this pathological behavior [18,20–22].

Psychotic symptoms sometimes occur in association with organic symptoms or sometimes occur in place of them. The most common psychotic signs are derealization, depersonalization, and magical thinking. Often, psychotic abusers feel that they have peculiar insights into the human condition. They develop theories on nearly every subject which, however, appear nonsensical to those around them. Gradually, they become very suspicious and guarded. This suspiciousness can become increasingly hostile until psychotic paranoid persecutory delusions emerge. Because the abusers cannot understand those around them and are not understood by them, their paranoid delusions are reinforced. Long-term persecutory delusions sometimes generate delusions of grandeur. They tend to make the abuser more insufferable and further isolated. The hyperacusis and hyperactivity associated with acute ingestions is reinforced by chronic stimulation of THC, so that true auditory and visual hallucinations emerge. These hallucinations are the type that usually reinforce paranoid themes. Haptic hallucinations also intensify and tend to be the focus of irritation. The auditory hallucinations, in some instances, are accompanied by delusions of alien thought insertion and mind reading or other telepathic capabilities [19,23].

## Mood Disorders

In addition to changes of thought capability, the mood of the abusers can be altered by chronic abuse. Both depression and anxiety are seen. Unfortunately, the response of most abusers is to medicate themselves further with more marijuana. THC-fueled anxiety presents with the classic fight response. Physical concomitants include tachycardia; pupillary dilation; blushing; profuse sweating over the back, axillary, and pubic areas; and a peculiar perceived scrotal tightening. Objectively, there is increased dumping of free-fatty acid into the peripheral circulation and activation of histamine-1 receptors to produce more gastric hydrochloric acid [24].

The result of all these changes is perceived as anxiety. In response, the abuser tends to be tense and overreactive to mild changes in environment. There is an excessive response to changes or mild stressors. If anxiety persists, the patient may complain of headaches which are relieved by caffeine but not by acetaminophen or aspirin. Akathisia is relieved not only by high levels of physical activity but also by ingestion of alcohol, barbiturates, methaqualone or tranquilizers. Occasionally, specific phobic responses such as agoraphobia, acrophobia, and claustrophobia develop. They can be accompanied by terror when the phobic abuser is placed in a stress situation [18].

A depression usually develops with chronic abuse. This particular depression is virtually indistinguishable from that of a major depressive disorder. It has a suicide rate that is two to four times greater than that of primary depression [25]. The usual expected complaints of perceived helplessness, perceived hopelessness, worthlessness, and general sadness are usually seen. The neurovegetative signs of difficulty falling asleep, nocturnal sleep disturbance, early morning awakening, diurnal mood variation, apathy, anorexia, diminished sexual desire and response, low-back pain, and decreased bowel movements are all seen. Appetite is disturbed, and there is sometimes globus hystericus and, rarely, pica. Males tend to have problems with potency and ejaculation, while females complain of diminished frequency and intensity of orgasm as well as dyspareunia [26].

Concentration is usually quite diminished and accompanied by lack of ambition. There is generalized psychomotor retardation, with fatigue and apathy. This is accompanied by perceived diminution of bodily strength and endurance. The normal generalized aches and pains of daily life tend to be exaggerated. There is much guilt over previous transgressions. This guilt can reach delusional proportions. These delusions, however, are different from those of the marijuana psychosis in that the focus is on guilt or somatic deterioration. As in the case of marijuana psychosis, there is a tendency to self-medicate with marijuana. This self-medication, in turn, generates a vicious spiral, and the depression is aggravated [18,23,26].

## Withdrawal Symptoms

A withdrawal syndrome definitely occurs with this continuance of marijuana use. Associated symptoms include anxiety and depression, which can either occur independently or aggravate a previously existing mood disorder. Sleep tends to be disturbed, with many frightening dreams and nightmares.

These dreams are caused by increased duration of REM-phase sleep. Appetite is much diminished, and there is a weight loss that can encompass 15–20% of the body weight over a 30–60 day period. The patient is hyperirritable, with gross resting tremors, extreme diaphoresis, nausea, and akathisia. There is a potential for measured violence during withdrawal. The individual tends to be hypervigilant and overreactive to loud noises or abrupt environmental changes. Even such mild stimulants as caffeine can have an exaggerated effect. The startle reflex is exaggerated, and there is prolonged reactive pupillary dialation.

## CHRONIC ABUSE—PHYSIOLOGY

It is currently believed that the effects of marijuana involves regulation of the catecholamine and indolamine systems. Anatomically, the hypothalamus, limbic system, mamillary tract, interior thalamus, amygdala, nucleus accumbens, and pars compacta are all involved in generating the effects of marijuana. These anatomical areas are responsible for information processing, pleasure, emotional response, appetite, and libido [27,28].

The major involved system is that of the primary pleasure centers. An essential feature of the primary pleasure systems is the ventral tegmental area, which is directly stimulated by marijuana. This area receives projections from the lateral hypothalamus. Messages are then transferred from the ventral tegmentum and pars compacta to the nucleus accumbens. In this manner, emotional homeostasis is maintained. Marijuana disrupts this homeostasis by introducing the need for THC. This creates false hunger, which is greater than that for sex or food but not greater than that for water [29].

A second system disrupted by marijuana is the Papez circuit, which amplifies memory within an emotional matrix. In this system, memories are transferred from the hippocampus through the hypophlamic mamillary bodies to the anterior thalamus. From the anterior thalamus, fibers ascend to the cingulate gyrus. From here, they project to the retrosplenial cortex to descend to the hippocampus. In this way, a closed reverberating circuit is achieved. In this bidirectional pathway, new memories are processed for storage and invested with an emotional overlay. Marijuana thus acts to amplify the pleasurable memories associated with periods of intoxication so that a self-perpetuating positive reinforcement is achieved [30,31].

It appears that marijuana's effects on the reward system tend to be dopaminergic. The actions in the Papez circuit involve changes in cholinergic neurons. Since REM-stage sleep is affected, it is probable that serotonergic activity is also altered.

## DETOXIFICATION

Detoxification in the acute setting rarely involves pharmacological intervention. If there is a large amount of agitation, hydroxyzine 25 to 50 mg PO or IM may be effective. Metabolism may be increased by giving the patient a hot shower or bath. Further enhancement can be provided by caffeine either through IM caffeine benzoate or through ingestion of caffeine beverages. Haloperidol 5 mg IM is useful for treatment of psychotic states or isolated hallucinations or delusions. While there has been no reliably recorded case of overdose in adults, a possible overdose with ingested marijuana in children should be treated aggressively. Support respiration and maintain blood pressure with Levophed, 2 ampules per 250 cc of 0.45 normal saline. Titrate this solution against the blood pressure [18,32].

## TREATMENT AND REHABILITATION

A rehabilitation program should offer isolation from high-risk social situations and events with a program that also reintegrates into the social setting. During the inpatient phase of the treatment program, the focus should be on milieu and group therapy. This way the comments and intervention of the abuser's peers can be utilized to deal with misperceptions and rationalizations. Staff intervention should focus on reality testing and integration into the social aspect of the ward structure. Reality testing would be the province of the psychiatrists. During the latter phases of the hospitalization, insight-oriented or goal-directed therapy can also be useful. A key intervention can be produced by the occupational therapist, who can work with the patient toward developing a drug-free life-style. Strenuous physical therapy under the direction of the physical therapist will assist the patient in working toward recovering bodily integrity. As the time for discharge approaches, the family or significant others should be included in the therapy protocol. They can form the bridge that allows patients to find their place in the non-sheltering outside community [1,33].

To encourage patients to reject the drug subculture, examine their behavior, avoid reinforcement toward drug abuse, and develop drug-free friendships, the Narcotics Anonymous program should be consulted. The familiar 12-step program can be useful for all these purposes. Those close to the patient should also be encouraged to attend Nar-Anon to buttress the results of Narcotics Anonymous. If possible, the patient should also attend an after-hours rehabilitation program under the supervision of a psychiatrist. Such programs as Chemical Abuse Centers, Inc., in the Midwest or After Five in New England can allow the patient to maintain an independent life-style while focusing on a drug-free existence. In these programs, the employer and family, as well as Narcotics Anonymous, are used as the three supportive legs to keep the patient from relapsing. Multiple family sessions, counseling with previously impaired counselors, and peer-group therapy are all organized around the work schedule. This provides an entire menu of resources that can be utilized in resisting the pressures of visual, social, and emotional stimuli [29,34].

## MARIJUANA COMBINATES AND ADULTERANTS

Marijuana's effects can be enhanced by using opiates, phencyclidine, or cocaine. Opiates are frequently smoked with marijuana or hashish. They are used to enhance the feelings of euphoria and giddiness. When used on a less than occasional basis, they provide no particular treatment problem. Physiologically, they serve to reinforce the pleasure circuits of the brain. If heroin or other opiate derivatives are used on a chronic basis, addiction may occur. This addiction needs to be treated with a separate detoxification protocol. Give clonidine 17 mg/k of body weight in four divided doses on the first day of detoxification, with a gradual decrease until the patient is totally detoxified over a 7–10 day period. During the inpatient phase of marijuana treatment, it should be noted that the blockage of positive reinforcement by positive memory experiences will be particularly difficult in the opiate/marijuana-abusing patient [1,35].

Phencyclidine, unlike the opiates, inhibits rather than reinforces the memory circuit. As an anticholinergic drug, phencyclidine disrupts the transmission of new data from the reticular activating substance to the hippocampus [36]. Phencyclidine, however, does increase the anxiety, thought disorder, paranoia, and irritability associated with marijuana. When phencyclidine is used on more than an occasional basis, desipramine 200–250 mg/day should be prescribed to treat the withdrawal dysphoria [37]. Since most abusers are amnestic for all or part of their phencyclidine intoxication periods, there tends not to be memory reinforcement by stimuli [38]. Acute psychosis does not respond well to phenothiazines. Since phencyclidine is a DA-2 agonist, the DA-2 antagonist haloperidol is recommended. Dosages of 5 mg IM or PO usually suffice [39].

When cocaine is used with marijuana, there is an enhancement of exhilaration and euphoria. Cocaine is a very powerful stimulator of the primary pleasure circuits and thus reinforces the relationship between drug-related stimuli and recalled associations. If the patient has used large amounts of cocaine, detoxify acutely with bromocriptine 0.625–2.5 mg three to four times a day. Detoxify on a declining schedule over a three- to four-week period to avoid long-term reinforcement. Add desipramine 200–250 mg qd, and maintain this latter medication for three to eight months. When marijuana, phencyclidine, and cocaine are all abused, the treatment is identical to that of cocaine [37,10].

## DIAGNOSTIC GROUPS ABUSING MARIJUANA

For several centuries, marijuana has been prescribed and used as a treatment for menstrual cramps and premenstrual syndrome. Indeed, Queen Victoria of England was a sufferer from cramping who used marijuana on advice of the royal physicians, including Sir William Gull. Since the lay literature has popularized and legitimated the use of marijuana for this purpose, one can expect to see at least a small but definite population of patients with either premenstrual cramping or premenstrual syndrome who have included marijuana as one of their home remedies. In this abusing population, physicians should be alert for complaints of cramping or cyclic exacerbations of irritability. There will also be periods of easy fatigability, episodic bulimia, and physical symptoms such as periodic breast tenderness, headaches, arthralgia, myalgia, and bloating and weight gain [41].

In the upper Appalachian region, marijuana is combined with asthmador as a home remedy. Asthmador (*Lobelia cardinalis*) is grown throughout Appalachia and also sold in health food stores and rural roadside stands throughout the United States. It is a cholinergic drug at low levels of intake and an anticholinergic drug at higher levels. Combined with marijuana, it can induce vivid visual hallucinations, photodermititis, which has been misdiagnosed as agoraphobia, and periods of intense inattention, which have been erroneously diagnosed as petit mal. Occasionally, hypotension results. Rarely, grand mal seizures occur shortly after smoking the asthmador-marijuana combination. This can be treated with diazepam 5 to 10 mg by slow IV push [18].

Upper-middle-class manics have been reported to abuse marijuana when the manic high becomes unpleasant. Anxiety disorders have also been treated with marijuana. The poor results of this self-treatment protocol apparently have not discouraged anxiety-prone patients from repeating their experimentation [1].

Populations experiencing isolation or ennui, such as college students, adolescents, and the military are all at risk for marijuana abuse. These populations have in common feelings of dysphoria, detachment, reduced social involvement, and highly interactive workdays followed by minimally interactive social time. Marijuana brings the lonely individual in contact with an alternative subculture that provides social connectedness. The drug itself filters out the perceived negative situations and provides its own rationale for positive feedback.

Because of social attitudes, it is difficult to bring the marijuana abuser to treatment. Denial of a link between drug and symptoms is common. The perception of marijuana as a safe "soft" drug still persists. In many cases, marijuana magnifies underlying psychopathology rather than introducing new symptoms. As a result, even the medical personnel who may have referred the patient may fail to see any direct link [42]. In particular, it is difficult to convince the patient, the family, or referring physician that psychosis is a result of marijuana. The passive acceptance of marijuana by society as a whole and the active proselytization of marijuana by the patients' social group may further undermine the role and mission of the therapist [43]. Key symptoms such as depression and psychosis can be sorted out and attacked in sequence. Judicious use of antipsychotics, plus an aggressive use of reality-oriented therapy in an outpatient setting, should be pursued in the paranoid or otherwise psychotic individual. Withdrawal symptoms require support. It is at this time that the abuser is most likely to discontinue withdrawal therapy. The team approach emphasizing intense occupational therapy and strenuous physical therapy allows the patient to derive feelings of achievement and satisfaction while minimizing emotional and physical withdrawal symptoms. The depression and ennui associated with the withdrawal phase can continue long past the acute withdrawal. Support groups are mandatory. The isolation that propels the marijuana abuser must not be allowed to recur. Structured outpatient treatment settings that encourage the patients' independence at work and in the family should provide a part of the continued treatment. Narcotics Anonymous should also be used as a lifelong treatment modality that brings the patient emotional and social support to maintain a drug-free life-style.

## REFERENCES

1.  Giannini AJ, Slaby AE. *Drugs of Abuse*. Oradell, NJ: Medical Economics, 1989.
2.  Turner CE, Elsohly MA, Boeren EG. Constituents of cannabis sativa. *J Nat Prod* 1980; 43:164–234.
3.  Hollister LE, Gillespie HK, Olson A, Lindgren J. Do plasma concentrations of delta-9-THC reflect the degree of concentration? *J Clin Pharmacol* 1981; 21:1715–1725.
4.  Braff DL. Impaired speed of visual processing in marijuana intoxication. *Am J Psychiatry* 1981; 138:613.
5.  Giannini AJ. PCP: Detecting the abuser. *Med Aspects Human Sexuality* 1987; 21(1):100–112.
6.  Spector I. *AMP—A new form of marijuana. J Clin Psychiatry* 1988; 46:498–499.

7. Adams PM, Brown B, Hagerstrom G, Portnoy L. Marijuana, alcohol and combined effects on the course of recovery. *Psychopharmacol* 1978; 56:81–86.
8. Winek CL. Historical aspects of marijuana. *Clin Toxicol* 1977; 10:243.
9. *The Living Bible.* London: Coverdale House, 1971.
10. Burton RF. *The Thousand Nights and a Night.* London: MacMillan, 1889.
11. Sykes P. *A History of Persia. Vol. I.* London: Oxford University Press, 1921.
12. Lawrence TE. *Seven Pillars of Wisdom.* Garden City, NY: 1926.
13. Rush B. *Autobiography.* GW Corner, Ed. Princeton, NJ: Princeton University Press, 1948.
14. Carroll L. *Alice's Adventures in Wonderland.* London: MacMillan, 1865.
15. Carrol L. *Through the Looking Glass and What Alice Found There.* London: MacMillan, 1871.
16. Morison SE. *The Oxford History of the American People.* New York: Oxford University Press, 1965.
17. Machuulam R. Marijuana chemistry. *Science* 1970; 168:1159–1172.
18. Giannini AJ, Slaby AE. *Handbook of Overdose and Detoxification Emergencies.* New Hyde Park, NJ: Medical Examination/Excerpta Medica, 1985.
19. Giannini AJ. *Biological Foundations of Clinical Psychiatry.* New York: Elsevier/Medical Examination, 1986.
20. Turner CE. Cannabis: The plant, its drugs and their effects. *Aviat Space Med* 1983; 54:368.
21. Tennant FS, Groesbeck CJ. Psychiatric effects of hashish. *Arch Gen Psychiatry* 1972; 27:1433–1436.
22. Estroff TW, Gold MS. Psychiatric aspects of marijuana abuse. *Psychiatr Annals* 1986; 16:221–224.
23. Negrote JC, Lawson TR, Sbriglio R, Giannini AJ. Physiological adverse effects of cannabis. *CMAJ* 1973; 108:195–199.
24. Poddar MC, Dewey WL. Effects of cannabinoids on catecholamine uptake and release. *J Pharmacol Exp Ther* 1981; 214:63–69.
25. Jones RT, Benomitz N, Bachman I. Clinical studies of cannabis tolerance and dependence. *Ann NY Acad Sci* 1976; 282:210–234.
26. Millman RB, Sbriglio R. Patterns of use and psychopathology in marijuana abuse. *Psychiatr Clin N Amer* 1986; 9:533–545.
27. Miller NS, Dackis CA, Gold MS. The relationship of addiction, tolerance and dependence to alcohol and drugs: A neurochemical approach. *J Substance Abuse Treatment* 1987; 4:39–44.
28. Tunving K. Psychiatric aspects of cannabis use. *Acta Psychiatrica Scand* 1985; 72:209–217.
29. Nauta WJH. Hippocampal projections and related neural pathways in the rat. *Brain* 1958; 81:319.
30. Papez JW. A proposed mechanism of emotion. *Arch Neurol Psychiatry* 1937; 38:725–730.
31. Yakovlev PI. Motility, behavior and the brain. Organization and neural coordinates of behavior. *J Nerv Ment Dis* 1948; 107:313–317.

32. School SH, Daghestan AN. Treatment of marijuana abuse. *Psychiatr Ann* 1986; 10:249–254.
33. Nakken C. *The Addictive Personality*. Center City, MN: Hazelden, 1988.
34. Schaffer B. *Is It Love or Is It Addiction?* Center City, MN: Hazelden, 1987.
35. Gold MS, Pottash ALC, Sweeney DR, Kleber HD. Opiate withdrawal using clonidine. *JAMA* 1980; 243:343–347.
36. Castellani S, Giannini AJ, Adams PM. Phystostigmine and haloperidol treatment of acute phencyclidine intoxication. *Am J Psychiatry* 1982; 139:508–509.
37. Giannini AJ, Malone DM, Giannini MC, Loiselle RH. Treatment of chronic cocaine and phencyclidine abuse with desipramine. *J Clin Pharmcol* 1986; 26: 211–216.
38. Castellani S, Giannini AJ, Adams PM. Effects of naloxone, metenkephlin and morphine or phencyclidine induced behavior in the rat. *Psychopharmacol (Berlin)* 1982; 78:76–80.
39. Giannini AJ, Eighan MS, Giannini MC, Loiselle RH. Comparison of haloperidol and chlorpromazine in the treatment of phencyclidine psychosis: Role of the DA-2 Receptor. *J Clin Pharmacol* 1984; 24:202–204.
40. Giannini AJ, Billet TA. Bromocriptine-desipramine protocol in cocaine detoxification. *J Clin Pharmacol* 1987; 27:549–562.
41. Yamaguchi K, Kandel DB. Patterns of drug use from adolescence to young adulthood. *Am J Pub Health* 1984; 74:673–681.
42. Miller NS, Giannini AJ. The medical model of addiction. *J Psychoact Drugs* 1990; 22:83–85.
43. Miller NS, Giannini AJ, Gold MS, Philomena JA. Drug abuse and drug testing: Medical, legal and ethical issues. *J Substance Abuse Treatment* 1990; 8: 231–239.

# 9

## Studies of Prevalence of Dual Diagnosis in Psychiatric Practice

**Marc Galanter and Ricardo Castaneda**

*New York University School of Medicine, New York, New York*

This chapter reviews the literature on the epidemiology of patients presenting for general psychiatric treatment who are also substance abusers and of those substance abusers in treatment who also have associated psychiatric disorders. A considerable portion of patients seen in emergency rooms, as much as half in some settings, are substance abusers, and over a third of general psychiatry admissions have been found to present problems materially influenced or precipitated by substance abuse. Substance abuse is also frequently found among psychiatric inpatients. Psychiatric disorders, on the other hand, are highly prevalent in all subpopulations of substance abusers.

Diagnostically, it can be difficult to differentiate general psychiatric and addictive syndromes: primary and secondary affective disorder from consequences of long-term substance abuse, cognitive sequelae of abuse from psychotic symptoms pictures, antisocial personality disorder from behavior disorders due to abuse patterns, and self-medication patterns from primary general psychiatric syndromes.

Treatment studies are often focused on concomitant psychotherapeutic management for patients being treated for addiction. Often, emphasis is placed on pharmacotherapy for enhancing outcome in the dually diagnosed. Qualitatively new options tailored to this population still remain to be studied, however, as do the changes necessary in the treatment system to assure proper long-term management.

Relatively little information is available on the proper diagnosis and treatment of substance abuse in patients who present with other psychiatric problems. Despite this, there is a growing recognition among clinicians that patients treated for nonaddictive psychiatric illness often have their rehabilitation compromised by alcohol or drug abuse [1]. Although treatment facilities are generally segregated into separate units for general psychiatric disorders and substance abuse, it is becoming increasingly clear that many general psychiatric patients require coordinated treatment for combined disorders.

Patients with combined addiction and psychiatric disorders present to a variety of different clinical settings, including general psychiatric facilities and treatment units for alcoholism and other drug abuse.

Patients in the first group come to the attention of treating parties as they enter the mental health "portal" of the health systems and are distinguished from the patients who come through the addiction treatment "portal" for alcohol and drug problems and are then found also to have psychiatric disorders.

## PREVALENCE OF ADDICTIVE DISORDERS AMONG PATIENTS PRESENTING FOR TREATMENT OF PSYCHIATRIC DISORDERS ACCORDING TO PLACE OF PRESENTATION

There are no data available for the prevalence in the general population of combined general psychiatric and substance abuse disorders. The most exacting and recent assessment of the prevalence of psychiatric disorders in the population overall is the Epidemiologic Catchment Area study, carried out in three metropolitan areas in 1980–1982, where the following six-month prevalence rates were found, on average [4]. Altogether, alcohol and drug abuse were found in 6.4% of this population (5.0% for alcohol and 2.0% for drugs, respectively). Comparable figures for schizophrenia and for affective disorders were 1% and 5.2%, respectively. Not surprisingly, substance abusers, characterized by denial of their illness, were poor consumers of treatment services. Only one in seven (13.6%) was likely to have made mental health visits during the previous six months, whereas almost half (46.7%) of those with schizophrenia and a third (31.4%) with affective disorder had been seen by mental health professionals during the same period.

As we shall see, patients with schizophrenia and affective disorders constitute a sizable portion of all persons treated in the mental health system who have difficulties with substance abuse. In order to ascertain the magnitude of the dual-diagnosis problems, the presentation of such patients, as reported in the literature, will be considered in several different settings. The mental health portal includes: the emergency room, the general hospital psychiatric unit, the veterans' hospital, the public psychiatric facility, and the private psychiatric hospital; the addiction treatment portal includes: clinical facilities for the treatment of alcoholism, methadone maintenance programs, and other drug abuse treatment settings. Because patients present differently in each of these settings, each is instructive with regard to the manifestations of the syndrome of dual diagnosis.

## The Emergency Room

Of the wide range of patients present in the emergency rooms of general hospitals, only a minority are admitted to inpatient services for acute care. In order to ascertain the fate of alcoholics in this group, Schwartz and Field [5] followed the routing of alcoholic patients who presented at an emergency room in a large public general hospital by examining clinicians' evaluations of a series of alcoholic patients ($N = 305$). Half (49%) of these alcoholics were sent home from the ER, with or without clinic referral. Of the 39% who were admitted, one-third were sent into regular psychiatric units, having presented with acute problems meriting care in an acute psychiatric unit. In the setting studied by Schwartz and Field, these latter patients were more often black, probably, these authors speculated, because blacks were more likely to treat their psychoses with alcohol rather than to seek traditional psychiatric care. In a similar study of consecutive emergency cases ($N = 174$), Treier and Levy, [6] using patient self-reports, found that fully 35% of their sample had alcohol-related, and 15% drug-related, admissions.

In a more detailed evaluation, Atkinson [7] had house officers complete a research questionnaire on 503 patients seen in a psychiatry emergency service, so that each patient was evaluated to ascertain the importance of alcohol and drug abuse in his admission. Some measure of substance abuse was found relevant to precipitating the presentation in over half the cases, with alcohol alone in 20%, drugs alone in 21%, and both together in 12% of the admissions. When cases were reviewed by diagnosis, it was found that alcohol or drug use played a role among 53% of transient situational disorder, 29% of schizophrenics, and 20% of affective disorders. The studies noted here drew on either clinician assessment or patient report. None was based on data from urinalyses for drugs of abuse, although this technique has recently been found to be a valuable diagnostic tool, as will subsequently be seen. Nonetheless, even without such verification, it is amply clear from these findings that the emergency service is an important site for case finding with regard to combined psychiatric and addictive disorder. If there were hospital-based services specifically designated for such problems, it is likely that a good number of emergency patients would be referred there.

## The Psychiatric Acute Inpatient Service

The most severely disordered of psychiatric patients generally begin their care with admission to general hospital psychiatric units. How often is this course necessitated by circumstances related to alcohol and drug use? Crowley et al. [8] carefully evaluated 50 consecutive patients admitted to an adult psychiatric ward making use of clinical assessments, psychometric measures, and serum and urine analyses for drugs of abuse. By these means, they found that 18% of these admissions would probably not have entered the hospital if not for a drug or alcohol problem, and an equal number had a substance abuse problem that contributed substantially to their admission. Both these groups were more likely to be diagnosed as character disorders than the balance of the patients, whose admissions were unrelated to drugs.

Urinalyses were positive most frequently for sedatives (24%), followed by alcohol (10%), narcotics (6%), and antipsychotics (3%). (It should be noted that the study by Crowley et al., done in the early 1970s, predated the recent rise in cocaine abuse.) Significantly, urinalyses revealed that the patients themselves often did not report the nature of their current drug use to interviewing physicians, which underlines the importance of multiple sources of information.

Profiles on the Minnesota Multiphasic Personality Inventory suggested less psychosis and more sociopathy among the drug/alcohol-precipitated group of admissions. These patients apparently manifested less severe ancillary pathology than the other admissions and were apparently hospitalized for drug-related symptoms primarily. Indeed, the authors point out that the alcohol/drug group had originally tried to remedy their own difficulties, such as dysphoria and marital problems, through intoxication, but these intoxicants were now more the cause of such problems than a result.

The findings of this study are complemented by those of two others. Ritzler et al. [9] found that patients in a psychiatric inpatient service with more acutely debilitating diagnoses, such as schizophrenia and other psychoses, were less likely to be heavy drinkers than patients with diagnoses of personality disorder or neurosis. In addition, the issue of social problems associated with substance use among patients on psychiatric services was examined by Davis, [10] who used standardized interview schedules after admission to study a population of psychiatric inpatients ($N = 170$) and outpatients ($N = 130$). He found that 63% of the males and 49% of the females had a history of heavy use of alcohol or drugs, although these findings were not generally apparent in admission histories or hospital notes. Over half of those patients who used substances heavily (65% of the males and 45% of the females) experienced deleterious social consequences from their use.

It is difficult to differentiate whether social problems are a cause of drug abuse or a sequela. For example, Westermeyer and Walzer, [11] in their study of patients ($N$ = 100) between the ages of 15 and 25 who were admitted to the psychiatric unit at the University of Minnesota Hospitals, defined 39% of them as heavy drug users. In comparison to other admissions, these patients were more often unemployed, divorced, or separated. They had experienced more problematic social events, such as felonies or truancy, and had more impaired social resources, such as family discord. Westermeyer and Walzer point out, however, that the problematic social behavior, in some cases, predated drug use and, in others, followed it.

Altogether, these findings strongly suggest that substance abuse plays a prominent role in precipitating the admissions of a large portion, perhaps a third, of patients in acute psychiatric services. Furthermore, relevant patterns of drugs use are not necessarily ascertained in clinical interviews at the time of admission and are generally not picked up in the hospital unless intoxication or withdrawal characterizes patients' presentations.

## Veterans Hospitals

Veterans Administration hospitals house a population at considerable risk for substance abuse. Many veterans abused alcohol or drugs while in the military service, and subsequently found that the opportunity existed for continuing substance abuse while they were hospitalized at VA facilities. McLellan et al., [12] for example, found that half (49%) of a sample of VA patients ($N$ = 156) hospitalized for psychiatric problems acknowledged that alcohol or drug use had been a "problem" for them at some point. These patients were more likely to have used *drugs* than alcohol if they had been hospitalized *during* the Vietnam era and more likely to have had a problem with alcohol if hospitalized before that time. Importantly, almost a third (30%) of the overall sample indicated that they had used alcohol or drugs at least three times weekly during their stay in the hospital, thereby reflecting the considerable access of patients to substances of abuse in this typical veterans' facility.

Alterman and associates conducted a number of studies on substance use and abuse in veterans' hospitals [13–15]. We shall consider their findings in relation to alcohol first. With the aid of nursing staff on wards not allocated to substance abusers, they were able to identify 9.5% of schizophrenics among hospitalized patients (101 of 1063) who carried a secondary diagnosis of alcoholism [13]. Of this group, 55% were reported to be drinking during their hospitalization, and most all of them (46% of the total) were known to become intoxicated. In addition, half were seen to have drinking-related problems interfering in their (47%) and management (53%) in the hospital. In the Alterman study, problem drinkers tended to be younger than the remainder of the schizophrenic population and were more likely to be black and to be paranoid.

In another study, Alterman et al. [14] evaluated general psychiatric patients in a VA psychiatric hospital ($N = 979$) and excluded those on designated substance abuse units. Altogether, one-quarter carried a primary (11%) alcohol-related diagnosis (ARD) or a secondary or tertiary (13%) one. Altogether, 9% of the patients were reported to be drinking in the hospital although, interestingly, most of the drinkers came from the sizable group of patients who carried neither primary, secondary, nor tertiary ARD. Alterman and co-workers point out that the patients' drinking in the hospital seriously compounded their psychiatric problems and was likely to yield a much poorer treatment diagnosis.

Alterman et al., [15] also examined drug problems in the VA in another study, using reports by nursing staff. Altogether, 40% of patients ($N = 533$) on acute and subacute psychiatric units had a history of alcohol abuse, and an additional 18% had a history of either drug or combined drug and alcohol problems. Furthermore, a majority of those patients with drug problems (58%) were illicitly using drugs in the hospital. Compared to nonusers, drug users tended to be younger, were more likely to be black, and showed the same incidence of schizophrenia (83%). Half of the drug users were taking drugs three or more times a week, with almost all (96%) using marijuana and half (48%) the users drinking alcohol. As with the alcohol users, negative attitudes toward treatment were commonly found among these drug abusers, along with cliquishness, secretiveness, and the need for greater supervision.

These considerable rates of alcohol and drug use in the VA hospital bode poorly for patients whose substance abuse problems go untreated while they are in the hospital. Their attitudes are poor, and the likelihood for abuse upon discharge is considerable. As with patients in acute general hospitals, the need for proper attention to alcohol and drug problems among general psychiatric patients is underlined in these studies.

## Public Psychiatric Hospitals

Public psychiatric hospitals typically admit patients whose mental illnesses are acutely disruptive, severely debilitating, or life-threatening. Because of this, their populations are revealing with regard to the relationship between substance abuse and severe mental illness. One early study drew on statistical reports on internees in facilities operated by the Department of Mental Hygiene of New York State [16]. Admissions between 1951 and 1960 in 18 hospitals revealed a notable finding in relation to patients who had psychoses due to alcohol. Whereas the number of admissions overall had declined over the course of this period, the number of patients admitted for psychosis due to alcohol had increased (from 6.8 to 8.1 per 100,000). An examination of this population of alcoholic psychotics revealed that the large majority (82.5%) were from metropolitan areas and that the incidence of alcoholic psychosis among blacks was almost four times that among whites. Significantly, however, these were not the only patients whose admission may have been precipitated by alcohol use, as it was found that approximately 17% of all admissions overall were known to be "intemperate users of alcohol."

These findings are augmented by McCourt et al., [17] who studied patients at Boston State Hospital. Only 30% of this sample ($N = 115$) were given a diagnosis of alcoholism, but more than half (57%) had at least one trouble area due to drinking, and a quarter (24%) of the patients themselves reported that they were alcoholics. The authors concluded that although state mental hospitals have many diagnosed alcoholics, they may indeed have many more admitted under other diagnoses.

Similar results were found in a study conducted on patients admitted to psychiatric facilities in North Carolina [18]. Two samples were evaluated, one in a state hospital ($N = 100$) and the other in a veterans' hospital ($N = 320$); in both, the incidence of alcoholism was found to be 24%. The breakdown among alcoholics by primary diagnosis was manic depressive 33%, schizophrenic 22%, and psychoneurotic and depressive 20%. The authors comment with some pessimism on the plight of treating physicians, pointing out that they often respond "with disgust" to individuals who use alcohol excessively. On the other hand, if they were to respond with compassion, recognizing alcoholism as an illness, they might, according to the authors, experience undue optimism, referring the patients to Alcoholics Anonymous in hope of a positive outcome, only to find that the patients responded poorly.

Admissions precipitated by drugs of abuse were also studied in a population of diagnosed drug abusers ($N = 12$) who were admitted to Bellevue Psychiatric Hospital, a large acute public psychiatric facility in New York City. In this study, Hekimian and Gershon [19] grouped patients by their primary drug of abuse. All were admitted in either a psychotic, toxic, or withdrawal state and represented overall approximately 5% of admissions to the hospital. Those whose admissions were precipitated by heroin (20%) were most often diagnosed as sociopathic, and their admissions were generally related to toxic or withdrawal states. On the other hand, admissions precipitated by marijuana (7%) amphetamines (20%), or psychedelic (42%) were generally diagnosed as schizophrenic; these latter patients typically had a preexisting history of psychotic symptoms that were exacerbated by the drug of abuse, reflecting the considerable vulnerability of more seriously disturbed patients exposed to substances of abuse with psychotomimetic potential. Additional patients (12%) were admitted for use of barbiturates, cocaine, glutethimide, and other drugs.

The difference in severity of pathology among groups using different drugs was also evident in that only a small number (19%) of heroin addicts required further hospitalization after their Bellevue admission, whereas marijuana abusers required it in half the cases. The authors emphasize that over half the patients in the marijuana, amphetamine, and psychedelic group were considered schizophrenic or were treated for this condition before they resorted to their drug use. This underlines the puzzling but compelling interrelationship between drug abuse and psychopathology in certain schizophrenic patients, along with the need to clarify what impact the combination has on the course of these patients' illness.

## Private Psychiatric Hospitals

Drug use and attendant psychopathology are clearly affected by culture and subculture. This is seen in the case of private psychiatric hospitals, which typically cater to a more affluent and better-educated population than public facilities do. It is particularly evident in the patterns of drug use that emerged in the counterculture era, which peaked in the early 1970s. For example, an evaluation by Sherans et al. carried out on patients 25 or younger at the Institute of Living in Hartford, Connecticut, revealed a population ($N = 167$) that was almost exclusively white, from middle- and upper-middle-class socioeconomic backgrounds [20]. Most of these patients (73%) had used marijuana, and fully half (52%) had used LSD or other hallucinogens. An appreciable number has also used amphetamines (62%), barbiturates (44%), and narcotics (34%). Altogether, 74% of the patients studied had used one of these drugs. Significantly, of those who had used a given drug, about half had used it at least 30 times (45–68% for the various drugs, respectively) had used each one at least 30 times. The use of any drug before the age of 15 was probably a predictor of more serious subsequent involvement, in particular, eventual use of barbiturates and narcotics. Sherans and co-workers observed that, for these adolescents, drug use was in part a way of coping with life's difficulties and intrapsychic stress but one that, in actuality, only created further conflict.

Sherans et al. did not examine the relationship between drug use and the circumstances precipitating admission. It is clear, however, that, during the counterculture era, considerable psychopathology was precipitated by psychotomimetics per se. A considerable decline in use of this category of drugs has, however, taken place since then. For example, federal surveys on high school drug use [21] show that the incidence of hallucinogen use among students within the last 12 months had declined by almost half (from 11.2% in 1975 to 6.5% in 1984). Reports are available, however, on the incidence of psychopathology by hallucinogens during the period when they were more popular [22–24].

The use of drugs among patients admitted to private facilities during the counterculture era is further evident in a study of patients ($N$ = 224) admitted to Hillside Hospital, a private psychiatric institution in New York City. Cohen and Klein [25] reported a sixfold increase in the incidence of illicit drug use between 1960 and 1967 (from 5 to 31%). They were able to study a sample of 70 abusers from 1967 patients; they divided them into 39 "extreme" drug users, characterized by almost habitual use of two or more drugs, and 31 mild to moderate abusers. Drug abusers, on the whole, tended to have a higher IQ than other patients at the hospital ($\overline{X}$ = 113 vs. 103), reflecting the culture of the time. Marijuana, amphetamine, and LSD were the most commonly abused drugs. Notably, the large majority (85%) of the extreme drug users were diagnosed as having character disorders, with only a small number (5%) of schizophrenics among them. Corresponding figures for the mild to moderate drug users showed a considerably greater incidence of schizophrenia, with 58% diagnosed as having character disorders and 26% as schizophrenic; those for the controls showed an even greater proportion of schizophrenics (46% and 40%). Again, these findings reflect the incidence of character disorders among patients admitted with histories of drug use. Based on these findings, Cohen and Klein suggest that, for these young, middle-class psychiatric patients, involvement in illicit drugs was part of a subculture that encouraged drug use as well as promiscuous sexual activity.

In 1970–1971, patients at the same hospital, aged 15 to 25, were studied to ascertain their use of illicit drugs *during* the hospital stay [26]. Whereas the previous study was conducted retrospectively by chart review, this one drew on weekly urinalyses carried out over an average course of 27 weeks, beginning at admission. Analyses were done only for barbiturates, amphetamines, and narcotics, however, because of the limitations of the technology available at the time. At admission, 52% of patients had urine positive for one of these drugs and, over the course of their stay in the hospital, 60% were positive for barbiturates (53%), amphetamines (24%) or narcotics (13%) at one time or another. Since no patient was found to use narcotics more than five times or amphetamines more than seven, the authors speculate that the more heavily addicted patients may well have left the hospital early. They further pointed out that, in order to ascertain the episodic use of drugs in the hospital, it is necessary to do multiple testing on at least 10 occasions. They suggest that, because of possible interactions between psychotropic medication and drugs of abuse, urine testing should be considered as a general policy among hospitalized patients.

## Some Observations

Given the apparent magnitude of the dual-diagnosis problem, it is notable that there are so few recent studies on the epidemiology of this syndrome. There are no published data on prevalence of dually diagnosed patients in the general population, and only a few of the studies on patients in the general psychiatric population cited there were published since 1980. Nonetheless, there is considerable need for further empirical observations. In the first place, we know little about the relationship between the nature of dual diagnosis in the general population relative to how it presents at treatment facilities. Furthermore, more sophisticated diagnostic instruments that have been developed in recent years, such as Diagnostic Interview Survey, have yet to be applied to dually diagnosed populations for more accurate psychiatric assessment. Because of this, little is known about the relative utilization of mental health services for this syndrome, or the need for services.

Because of changes in the kinds of drugs abused by the general public, it is important that the epidemiology of specific drugs abused be examined. Such trends in drug use are illustrated by the considerable decline in psychomimetic use in recent years, and the increase in cocaine use — particularly in the "crack" form. This latter agent, because it allows for rapid onset of action at high doses of freebase cocaine, generates a major onslaught on the mental health of persons who are already psychiatrically disabled.

Dually diagnosed patients are generally found to have a lower incidence of schizophrenia and major depressive disorder than other general psychiatric patients. Conversely, other patients are more likely to be diagnosed as having character disorder. Why is this? It may be that the more severely disabled patients lack social skills that are necessary to sustain a drug abuse habit. Alternatively, patients with a less debilitating diagnoses may be vulnerable to drug-induced crises of adaptation, which precipitate the need for psychiatric treatment. Furthermore, it may be that drug-seeking is one manifestation of character disorder and the complex adaptive problems it precipitates.

Studies on chronic-stay facilities such as private psychiatric hospitals and veterans' hospitals illustrate that psychiatric patients are prone to using drugs during their hospitalization so long as the opportunity presents. It is likely that such patients use drugs to an appreciable extent when engaged in ambulatory care, too. Little attention has been paid to assessing psychiatric sequelae of this problem and the impact of rehabilitation, and almost none has been paid to the specialized treatment necessary to address such patterns of abuse. Given the findings reported here, however, it is reasonable to assume that an appreciable portion of morbidity and treatment failure among chronic psychiatric patients is due to their ongoing patterns of drug and alcohol abuse.

## PREVALENCE FOR PSYCHIATRIC DISORDERS AMONG PATIENTS PRESENTING FOR TREATMENT OF ALCOHOLISM AND OTHER SUBSTANCE ABUSE ACCORDING TO PLACE OF PRESENTATION

### Alcoholism: Community Surveys and Treatment Facilities

The reported prevalence of psychiatric disorders in alcoholic populations is very high. In the available literature, the rates of psychopathology among alcoholics in treatment (usually in detoxification units), for example, range from 50% [27] and 60% [28] to 77%, [29] and even 98% [30] and are comparable to a lifetime rate of associated psychopathology of 87% reported by Rounsaville [31] in opiate addicts. Such high prevalence of psychopathology in alcoholics, however, is not only observed in detoxification units. In fact, one community survey yielded similar results. In the only investigation that has focused on frequency of alcoholism and other psychiatric diagnoses in a community, Weissman and Myers [32] reported on a community survey conducted in 1975–1976. Using systematic research and diagnostic criteria, the sample included respondents interviewed during a longitudinal survey of a community mental health center catchment area in New Haven, Connecticut. During the third wave of this longitudinal study initiated in 1967, only 510 persons were evaluated. Thirty-four subjects were identified as ever having been alcoholic, representing a lifetime rate of alcoholism of 6.7%. Of these, 24, or 71%, had been diagnosed, at some point in their lives, as having at least one psychiatric disorder, including a major depressive episode (44%), minor depression (15%), depressive personality (6%), and bipolar illness (5%). Six, or 18%, of the alcoholics had been given psychiatric diagnoses other than depression. Interestingly, these diagnoses were not mutually exclusive: 32% of the subjects had received only one of these four diagnoses at some point in their lives, 12% had been given two, and 9% had received three. In another paper focusing on depression, [27] Weissman and Myers remark that the depressive syndrome in alcoholics in heterogeneous and includes unipolar, bipolar, primary, and secondary depressions as well as depressive personality. Their results show that although not all alcoholics are depressed, many do meet RDC-DSM-III criteria for major depression, and Weissman and Myers stress that systematic diagnostic assessment of alcoholics is required. We will later review the issue of diagnostic criteria for depression in alcoholics.

## Alcoholism Treatment Facilities

A large study by Mendelson et al., [33] based on chart review of 10,558 hospitalized patients, investigated the prevalence of medical and psychiatric disorders among subjects admitted for primary alcoholism to 13 hospitals located in eight different states. Only general categories of mental disorders are given, yet at least 40% of all discharge diagnoses were psychiatric diagnosis, mostly neuroses (25%), personality disorders (17%), and other nonpsychotic mental states. Psychotic disorders were diagnosed in 6.5% of the sample.

A more rigorous report on the prevalence of lifetime psychiatric diagnoses in alcoholics is one by Hesselbrock et al. [29] on 321 alcoholic men and women admitted to three hospitals for alcohol detoxification in 1985. Using strict DSM-111 criteria and the NIMH Diagnostic Interview Schedule, they assessed the lifetime psychiatric diagnoses among 231 men and 90 women. The frequency of psychiatric diagnoses varied according to gender. Among men, antisocial personality disorder was found in 49% of the sample and easily constituted the most prevalent diagnosis, followed by drug abuse, which was diagnosed in 45%, major depression in 32%, and phobias in 20%. Among women, major depression was the most prevalent lifetime psychiatric diagnosis. In fact, more than half (52%) had suffered from this disorder. Other diagnoses in women included phobias in 44%, other substance abuse in 38%, and antisocial personality disorder in 20%. Other less frequent diagnoses in both groups included panic disorder 10%, mania 4%, and schizophrenia 2%.

The study by Hesselbrock and co-workers revealed the following gender-related results regarding onset. The men in this study had been abusing alcohol twice as long as the women had. While, in the women, most psychopathology preceded the onset of alcoholism, in men, just the opposite occurred, with the exception of antisocial personality disorder and panic disorder. Also of note is the fact that gender and presence of specific psychopathologies modified both the course and the symptom picture of alcoholism. In general, women showed a later onset of regular intoxication and dependence than men. Phobia in both men and women antedated the onset of alcohol abuse.

### VA Alcohol Detoxification Units

Similar lifetime rates of psychopathology have been reported in VA detoxification units. In 1982, Powell et al. [34] found that, in a group of 570 alcoholic veterans, almost two-thirds fulfilled criteria for one or more additional psychiatric diagnosis. The lifetime rates for these diagnoses were: depression 42%, mania 20% antisocial personality disorder 20%, substance abuse 17%, and anxiety disorders such as panic disorder, phobia, and obsessive compulsive disorder, each 10%. Schizophrenia was diagnosed in 4% of the sample. Fourteen percent had only one psychiatric diagnosis, 14% had 2, 14% had 3 or 4, and 6% had met criteria for 5 or more at some point in their lives.

*Diagnosing Depression in Alcoholics*

The issue of depression in alcoholism deserves individual scrutiny. Available reports on the prevalence of depression among alcoholics vary from 3% [35] to 98% [30]. This striking discrepancy arises from the different diagnostic criteria for depression adopted in each investigation. This is clearly illustrated in a study by Keeler et al. [36] on 35 hospitalized and recently detoxified alcoholics, in which the instruments used to diagnose depression included clinical assessment and the following scales: the Hamilton Depression Rating Scale, the Zung Self-Rating Depression Scale, and the MMPI. The prevalence of diagnosis of depression ranged from 8, 65 to 71% as shown in Table 1. It is apparent from the study that the choice of diagnostic criterion or scale used determines the prevalence of diagnosis of depression in any given alcoholic population. Moreover, the Hamilton, Zung, and MMPI scales are not diagnostic in themselves, a relevant issue in view of the potential for unnecessary antidepressant treatment.

The study results replicate findings from other investigations. For example, Winokour et al. [35] found a similar prevalence of depression (3%) in detoxified alcoholics when diagnoses were made through clinical assessment alone. Rosen [37] and Weingold et al. [38] reported similar rates of depression using the depression scale of MMPI (43%), and the MMPI and Zung (66%), respectively. The study also emphasizes that prevalence discrepancies stem from depressive symptoms from alcoholism, different diagnostic criteria, and the effects of sample bias from demographic factors such as ethnicity, social standing, region, and method of subject location.

**Table 1**  The Prevalence of Depression Among Recently Detoxified Alcoholics According to Keeler et al. [19]

| | | Score | |
|---|---|---|---|
| Diagnostic instrument | Diagnosed as depressed, % | Mean | SD |
| Clinical diagnosis | 8.6 | | |
| Hamilton DRS | (20 + )  28 | 13.2 | 7.4 |
| Zung Self-Rating Depression Scale | (44 + )  66 | 49.8 | 12.2 |
| MMPI or Zung | 69 | | |

*Prevalence of Anxiety Disorders, Including Phobic Disorders, in Alcoholics*

We have already mentioned that, in multihospital survey, [33] most alcoholics studied were classified under the heading "neurosis," a poorly defined term that suggests anxiety disorders. In another study already reviewed, [29] lifetime prevalence of anxiety disorders varied with sex, with 20% men, and 44% of women diagnosed as anxious. In studies conducted at VA detoxification units, lifetime prevalence of phobic disorders was 10%. In these studies, [29,34] phobia, in both men and women, predated the onset of alcoholism.

One study [39] systematically determined the prevalence of DSM-III (SCID) anxiety disorders among inpatient alcoholics in three university-affiliated hospitals (*N* = 84). Subjects were rated for DSM-III anxiety disorders using the Structured Clinical Interview for DSM-III (SCID). The prevalence of anxiety disorders (22.6%) was reported to be higher than that expected for the general population (2–4%) as rated by past history on the SCID. Among 19 anxious patients, 15 had only one of the following disorders: simple phobia, 3 subjects; generalized anxiety, 5; post-traumatic stress disorder 2; panic disorder and agoraphobia without panic attacks only one subject. Interestingly enough, 12 of the 19 anxious patients also reported that their alcoholism followed the onset of their respective anxiety disorders.

In an early report on the prevalence of agoraphobia and social phobia among 102 alcoholics admitted for detoxification, Mullaney and Trippett [40] found that 33 subjects of the sample had disabling agoraphobia and/or social phobia, and 37 had "borderline phobic symptoms." Again, the majority of phobic conditions preceded the onset of alcoholism. The diagnosis of phobia was made by clinical assessment and the use of self-rating scales such as the Survey of Social Inadequacy, the Fear Survey Schedule, and the SCL-90. Another study [41] on a sample (*N* = 60) of hospitalized alcoholics used unpublished questionnaires to diagnose anxiety disorders. Over half the sample were rated as having agoraphobia and/or social phobia. Twenty-one subjects were found to have only mild phobias, and 11 were felt to have severe phobias.

## TREATMENT CENTERS FOR BOTH ALCOHOLISM AND OTHER DRUG ABUSE

There is only one study available on a population of alcoholics and other substance abusers. [42] The objective of Ross and co-workers' study was to determine the prevalence of lifetime and current psychiatric disorders in patients seeking treatment for alcoholism and/or other substance abuse problems. Subjects in the study included 260 men and 241 women. Information was obtained using the NIMH Diagnostic Interview Schedule (DIS), and psychiatric diagnoses were computer-generated according to DSM-III criteria. The majority (58%) of the subjects were alcoholic; only 18% were drug abusers only; and 18% were both alcoholic and substance abusers. Fully four-fifths (78%) had a DIS lifetime psychiatric disorder in addition to substance abuse, and two-thirds (65%) had a current DIS mental disorder. Eighty-four percent met sampled criteria for at least one psychiatric disorder exclusive of substance abuse in their lifetime, and 68% had a current disorder with symptoms manifest in the past month. Additionally, 43% had two or more current psychiatric diagnoses in addition to any substance abuse disorder. The most common lifetime psychiatric disorders (fully meeting diagnostic criteria) were antisocial personality disorder 47%, phobias 26%, psychosexual dysfunctions 24%, major depression 20%, and dysthymia (depressive personality) 9%. The diagnosis of generalized anxiety disorder was found to have unsatisfactory reliability but, even when anxiety was excluded from the data, four-fifths of the weighted sample were given a lifetime DIS psychiatric diagnosis in addition to alcoholism or other drug abuse. The number of lifetime DIS diagnoses per patient was 4.8; the number of current DIS diagnoses was 3.4. Those patients in the study with both alcoholism and at least another substance abuse disorder had a much higher prevalence of lifetime psychiatric disorders than other patients. Moreover, patients with alcoholism and other addiction were almost certain also to meet criteria for an additional psychiatric diagnosis. No differences were found in the prevalence of psychiatric disorders between patients with alcohol problems only and those with a drug problem only. It is also of note that patients who abused both alcohol and another substance were the most psychiatrically impaired. Those subjects who abused either barbiturates/sedatives/hypnotics, amphetamines, or alcohol were the most likely to have DIS mental disorder.

Regarding the relative ages of onset of addictive and psychiatric disorders, the authors report that the beginnings of antisocial personality disorder always preceded the onset of alcohol or other drug abuse. The onset of drug abuse was more likely to follow that of anxiety disorders (excluding generalized anxiety), schizophrenia, and major depression. However, a large minority (23–40%) developed these psychiatric disorders subsequently to substance abuse. The presence of a disorder in any class increased the odds of having another disorder in almost any other class, either currently or earlier in their lifetime. Interestingly, while the presence of alcohol dependence was inversely related to the odds of having another drug-related diagnosis, the presence of drug abuse increased the odds of having almost any other drug-related diagnosis.

Finally, the severity of alcohol abuse and other substance abuse was the best predictor of the occurrence of an associated psychiatric disorder. This,

Ross et al. suggest, may imply that many of psychiatric symptoms could be secondary to addiction. It is also possible that psychopathology and alcohol and other substance abuse tend to be correlated for various other reasons, such as self-medication on their mutual relationship to stress.


## PSYCHIATRIC DIAGNOSIS OF OPIATE ADDICTS

Reports on the psychopathology of opiate addicts repeatedly suggest that the most frequent diagnosis in this population is that of personality disorder (50-90%). Psychotic disorders are reported to range from 0 to 20%, depending on the setting, and neurotic disorders range from 0 to 14% [43]. As in all other attempts at comparing prevalence studies of associated psychopathologies, we find discrepant diagnostic criteria as the main source of variance in prevalence rates. Although studies applying strict, standardized criteria generally document a prevalence of associated psychiatric diagnoses in about one-third of different populations of opiate addicts (Weissman), the most recent studies [31,43] report a much higher prevalence, 87 and 93%, respectively. Rounsaville et al., [31] for example, in a study of 583 opiate addicts engaged in a multimodality treatment program, found the following lifetime rates of psychiatric disorders: depression 54%, alcoholism 34.5%, antisocial personality disorder 26.5%, intermittent depression 19%, labile personality 16.5%, phobic disorder 9.6%, generalized anxiety disorder 5.4%, schizotypal personality disorder 8.4%, minor depression 8.4%, and hypomanic disorder 6.6%. There were considerable variations in the observed prevalence rates of some disorders across sociodemographic variables; women, for example, had higher rates of depression, cyclothymia, bipolar illness, panic disorders, and phobias. Men were more likely to be given a diagnosis of antisocial personality disorders. Younger addicts had higher rates of intermittent depression. Depression also, was most common in whites, followed by Hispanics and then blacks. Whites also had the highest rate of generalized anxiety disorder. Hispanics showed the highest frequency of intermittent depression and schizoaffective depression and the lowest rates of hypomania and bipolar illness. Whites also had the lowest rates of phobic disorders.

One of the most striking findings of this study was that 70.3% of the sample had a current psychiatric diagnosis, and 86.9% met diagnostic criteria for at least one psychiatric disorder other than drug abuse at some time in their lives. More than half (52%) had two or more diagnoses in addition to drug abuse. The great majority of psychiatric disorders in this sample were accounted for by chronic or episodic depressive disorders, antisocial personality disorder, and alcoholism.

Khantzian and Treece, [43] using DSM-III criteria, also investigated the prevalence of current psychiatric disorders among 133 narcotic addicts. Subjects in the study came from a variety of sources, including two methadone maintenance clinics, a residential treatment facility, and the community (these subjects were not involved in treatment). While 60% of the subjects met criteria for affective disorder, only 17% had other Axis 1 diagnosis, and 23% received no Axis 1 diagnosis at all. The observed rate of 50% of the subjects diagnosed as having depression in this investigation is comparable to that reported by Rounsaville et al. [31] in their study already reviewed. Regarding the prevalence of character pathology, one-third of the sample had antisocial personality disorder; another third had other personality disorders; and the remaining third did not meet criteria for any Axis II diagnosis. Of the sample, 77% met criteria for one or more diagnoses on Axis 1, and 65% met criteria for an Axis II diagnosis. Ninety-three percent met criteria for either an Axis I or Axis II diagnosis, and 49% had diagnoses on both axes. Only one diagnostic category was related to demographic variables. Patients with anxiety disorder were slightly younger than other patients (27 to 30 years, respectively). Subjects with affective disorders had a higher mean polydrug index than patients with other diagnoses. Patients with personality disorders, antisocial personality, in particular, had a higher polydrug index than the rest of the sample. Multiple substance abuse was very frequent; in fact, 47% had a concurrent DSM-III diagnosis of another addiction, and 86% had a history of a secondary alcohol or other drug abuse.

## REFERENCES

1. Sundram CJ. *The Multiple Dilemmas of the Multiplied Disabled*. Albany, NY: New York State Commission of Quality of Care for the Mentally Disabled, 1986.
2. Gottheil, E (Section Ed.). Combined alcohol and drug abuse problems. In: Galanter M ed. *Recent Developments in Alcoholism* IV. New York: Plenum Press, 1986:3–106.
3. Meyer RE. *Psychopathology and Addictive Disorders*. New York: Guilford Press, 1986.
4. Myers JK, Weissman MM, Tischler GL, Holzer CE. Six-month prevalence of psychiatric disorders in three communities 1980 to 1982. *Arch Gen Psychiatric* 1984; 41:959–967.
5. Schwarz L, Field SP. The alcoholic patient in the psychiatric hospital emergency room. *Quart J Stud Alc* 1969; 30:104–111.
6. Trier TR, Levy RJ. Emergent, Urgent and Elective Admissions. *Arch Gen Psychiat* 1969; 421:423–430.

7. Atkinson R. Importance of alcohol and drug abuse in psychiatric emergencies. *Calif Med* 1973; 118:1–4.
8. Crowley TJ, Chesluk D, Dilts S, Hare R. Drug and alcohol abuse among psychiatric admissions. *Arch Gen Psychiat* 1974; 30:13–20.
9. Ritzler BA, Strauss JS, Vanord A, Kokes RF. Prognostic implications of various drinking patterns in psychiatric patients. *Am J Psychiatry* 1977; 134(5): 546–549.
10. Davis DI. Differences in the use of substances of abuse by psychiatric patient compared with medical and surgical patients. *J of Nerv and Men Dis* 1984; 172(11):654–657.
11. Westermeyer J, Walzer V. Sociopathy and drug use in a young psychiatric population. *Dis Nerv Syst* 1975; 36:673–677.
12. McLellan AT, Druley KA, Carson JE. Evaluation of substance abuse problems in a psychiatric hospital. *J of Clin Psychiatry* 1978; 39:425–430.
13. Alterman AI, Erdlen FR, McLellan AI, Mann SC. Problem drinking in hospitalized schizophrenic patients. *Addictive Behaviors* 1980; 5:273–276.
14. Alterman AI, Erdlen FR, Murphy E. Alcohol abuse in the psychiatric hospital population. *Addictive Behaviors* 1981; 6:69–73.
15. Alterman AI, Erdlen DL, Laporte DJ. Effects of illicit drug use in an inpatient psychiatric population. *Addictive Disorders* 1982; 7:231–242.
16. Moon LE, Patton RE. The alcoholic psychotic in the New York State mental hospital. *Quart J Stud Alc* 1963; 24:664–681.
17. McCourt WF, Williams AF, Schneider L. Incidence of alcoholism in a state mental hospital population. *Quart J Stud Alcohol* 1971; 32:1085–1088.
18. Parker JB, Meiller RM, Andrews GW. Major psychiatric disorders masquerading as alcoholism. *South Med J* 1960; 53:560–564.
19. Hekiman LJ, Gorshon S. Characteristics of drug abusers admitted to a psychiatric hospital. *JAMA* 1968; 205:125–130.
20. Sherans CR, Fitzgibbons DJ. Drug use in a population of youthful psychiatric patients. *Am J Psychiatry* 1972; 128:1381–1387.
21. Johnston LD. Use of licit and illicit drugs by American's high school students, 1975–1984. DHHS Publication (No. ADM) 85-1394, 1985.
22. Hensala J, Epstein L, Blacker L. LSD and psychiatric inpatients. *Arch Gen Psychiat* 1967; 16(5):554–559.
23. Blumenfld M, Glickman L. Ten months experience with LSD users admitted to county psychiatric receiving hospital. *New York State J Med* 1967; 67:1849–1853.
24. Vardy MM, Kay SR. LSD psychosis or LSD-induced schizophrenia? *Arch Gen Psychiat* 1983; 40:877–883.
25. Cohen M, Klein DF. Drug use in a young psychiatric population. *Am J Orthopsychiatry* 1970; 40:448–455.
26. Blumberg AG, Cohen M, Heastan AM, Klein DF. Covert drug abuse among voluntary hospitalized psychiatric patients. *JAMA* 1971; 217:1659–1671.
27. Weissman MM, Myers JK. Clinical depression in alcoholism. *Am J Psych* 1980; 137:3, 372–373.

28. Fowler RC, Liskow BI, Tanna VL. Psychiatric illness and alcoholism. *Alcoholism* 1977; 1:125–128.
29. Hesselbrock MN, Meyer RE, Keener JJ. Psychopathology in hospitalized alcoholics. *Arch Gen Psych* 1985; 42:1050–1055.
30. Shaw JA, Donley P, Morgan DW. Treatment of depression in alcoholics. *Am J Psychiatry* 1975; 132:641–644.
31. Rounsaville BJ, Weissman MM, Kleber H, Wilber C. Heterogeneity of psychiatric diagnosis in treated opiate addicts. *Arch Gen Psychiatry* 1982; 39:161–166.
32. Weissman MM, Myers JK, Harding PS. Prevalence and psychiatric heterogeneity of alcoholism in a United States urban community. *J Stu Alcohol* 1980; 41,7, 672–681.
33. Mendelson JH, Babor TF, Mello NK. Alcoholism and prevalence of medical and psychiatric disorders. *J Stud Alcohol* 1986; 47,5:361035.
34. Powell BJ, Penick EC, Ekkehard O, Bingham SF, Rice AS. Prevalence of additional psychiatric syndromes among male alcoholics. *J Clin Psychiatry* 1982, 43:10:404–407.
35. Winokour G, Rimmer J, Reich T: Alcoholism IV: Is there one type of alcoholism? *Br Psychiatry* 1971; 118:525–531.
36. Keeler MH, Taylor CJ, Miller WC. Are all recently detoxified alcoholics depressed? *Am J Psychiatry* 1979; 136:4B:S86 588.
37. Rosen AC. A comparative study of alcoholic and psychiatric patients with the MMPI. *Q J Stud Alc* 1960; 21:253–266.
38. Weingold HP, Lachin JM, Bell AH. Depression as a symptom of alcoholism: Search for a phenomenon. *J Abnor Psychol* 1968; 73:195–197.
39. Weiss KJ, Rosemberg DJ. Prevalence of anxiety disorder among alcoholics. *J Clin Psychiatry* 1985; 46:3–5.
40. Mullaney JA, Trippett CJ. Alcohol dependence and phobias, clinical description and relevance. *Brit J Psychiat* 1979; 135:565–573.
41. Smail P, Stockwell T, Canter S, Hodgson R. Alcohol dependence and phobic anxiety states. 1.A prevalence study. *Brit J Psychiatry* 1984; 144,53–47.
42. Ross HE, Glaser FB, Germanson T. The prevalence of psychiatric disorders in patients with alcohol and other drug problems. *Arch Gen Psychiatry* 1988; 45:1023–1031.
43. Khantzian EJ, Treece C. DSM-III psychiatric diagnosis of narcotic addicts. *Arch Gen Psychiatry* 1985; 42:1067–1071.

# 10

## Diagnosing Dual Diagnosis Patients

### Charles R. Norris, Jr. and Irl L. Extein

*Fair Oaks Hospital at Boca/Delray, Delray Beach, Florida*

## INTRODUCTION

The concept of the dual-diagnosis patient is an old one taking on new meaning in the era of a biopsychosocial approach. On the surface, making a dual diagnosis is fairly straightforward as we see many patients with psychiatric symptomatology who also abuse drugs and alcohol. However, questions of diagnostic primacy and treatment focus are controversial. In the past, traditional psychiatrists minimized the chemical dependency while emphasizing treatment of the psychiatric and emotional components, whereas the traditional addiction treatment community minimized the psychiatric symptomatology while emphasizing the treatment of the chemical dependency [1]. Both suggested that treatment of one would take care of the other. Today's biopsychosocial psychiatrist strives to treat the "whole" patient by synthesizing wisdom from the past with today's growing knowledge [2].

In this chapter, we will attempt to delineate the criteria for making each diagnosis using DSM-III-R [3]. We will also look at how the criteria may overlap, not only confusing the diagnostic picture but also the significance in terms of treatment. There are many articles being written today about primary versus secondary depression and how that relates to addictions, reminding one of the old question: Which came first, the chicken or the egg? [4,5] Once both chemical dependency and a psychiatric disorder such as depression are present, one tends to feed on the other. Clearly, the more one becomes depressed, the more one drinks or drugs to try to copy with the emotional pain, and the more one drinks or drugs, the more problems occur that increase the stress and deepen the depression.

## INITIAL EXAMINATION

### Clinical History

We begin with a new patient by obtaining a detailed clinical history, not only from the individual patient but also, whenever possible, from family or friends who often are better historians. The family's denial, coupled with the addict's tendency to manipulate, cover up, and lie, may distort the history.

When we start out with a new patient, we use an open-ended question approach, such as: "What kind of things have been going on in your life that led you to come for treatment today?" Higher-functioning, cooperative patients will often give much of the necessary history, requiring the clinician simply to listen carefully. We find that patients frequently identify themselves as either coming for addiction treatment or by presenting a psychiatric symptom such as depression or anxiety. Once the patient has presented his own understanding of what is going wrong in his life, then we begin to focus with more specific questions to gather details that may originally have been missed. For example, if a patient sees himself as an addict, he may initially deny being depressed but, on closer questioning, give many of the vegetative signs of depression, including periods of suicidal ideation. Because of the propensity to self-medicate, he may rarely allow himself to be in touch with underlying feelings of depression for more than a few hours. When the patient is aware of depressive symptomatology, he may have attributed, sometimes correctly, the various symptoms to the addiction. There is clear-cut overlap that makes differential diagnosis challenging at best. For example, classical vegetative signs of depression, such as change in sleep pattern and appetite; decreased energy, concentration, and sex drive; anhedonia; and feelings of hopelessness, helplessness, and suicidal ideation all can be covered over or minimized by an addict using cocaine. Cocaine will alter sleep patterns; cause loss of weight and appetite; decrease energy during the "crash" period; decrease concentration while "high"; and decrease sex drive in chronic use. Most chronic cocaine users report loss of interest in activities, family, and job and eventually begin feeling hopeless, helpless and, at times, suicidal.

A good clinical history includes a family history with specific questions about members in the family that may have had alcohol or chemical dependency problems, as well as questions about psychiatric problems. Detailed questions about physical problems in the patient's medical history and in the family history are important. Frequently, a history of cirrhosis can lead the patient to realize that "grandpa" was an alcoholic. Ask if the relative had a problem from drugs or drinking too much. The patient may not yet understand or accept that these problems imply addiction or alcoholism. Questions about social and developmental history should include questions about childhood traumas, physical abuse, parental divorce, school experiences, military and work experiences, and relationships. Detailed history about previous use of other substances, amounts, and responses are also worthwhile clinical information. Many patients will deny an alcohol problem but admit drinking a "six-pack" each night.

Schuckit, [6] has emphasized the importance of what he dubbed "timeline history." Essentially, he emphasized the importance of trying to establish which problem came first and to what degree. Asking about drug-free periods may reveal affective symptomatology and help establish a primary diagnosis of depression. Unfortunately, many patients started using and abusing substances very early without any lengthy periods of sobriety.

## Laboratory Studies

Medical work-up begins with a good physical examination, followed by a set of routine screening laboratory studies. We typically start with an SMA-23, CBC, electrolytes, thyroid profile, RPR for syphilis, urinalysis, B-12, folate, magnesium (for alcoholics), chest x-ray and EKG. If the patient has been a needle drug user, an active homosexual, or a heterosexual with multiple partners, we check a hepatitis profile and, after gaining written authorization, HIV for antibodies. We do an EEG in view of the multiple neurological insults related to addiction. If there is a history of head trauma with unconsciousness or a history of seizures, we order an MRI scan and consider neurological consultation.

Two laboratory tests, in particular, have been proposed as biological markers for major depression: the dexamethasone suppression test (DST) and the thyrotropan-releasing hormone (TRH) stimulation test. These tests can be useful, with certain caveats, in dual diagnosis of the substance abuser. The DST can be a useful marker for major depression in alcoholics if utilized in the post-detoxification period. One study of 15 nondepressed alcoholics without liver disease showed 20% DST nonsuppression during detox, with no cases of nonsuppression after three weeks of sobriety.

The TSH response to TRH tends to be blunted in many alcoholics, even after long periods of sobriety. Hence, the TRH test is not a useful marker for major depression in alcoholics, though it still may be used to identify hypothyroidism if an augmented TSH response is noted [7,8]. The DST has been shown to correlate with major depression in detoxified heroin and methadone addicts.

## Psychological Testing

Psychological testing may also offer useful insights into underlying psychopathology in chemical dependency patients. Once again, waiting a reasonable period of time after detoxification often maximizes the benefits from such testing. We routinely[14] use the Beck Depression Inventory and a full battery of neuropsychological and psychological tests in appropriate patients.

## CLINICAL OBSERVATION

While history, physical examination, and laboratory studies are being completed, along with psychological testing, we are clinically observing the patient. Chemical dependency patients in a structured treatment setting will often begin to show clearing of their psychiatric symptomatology within several weeks of detoxing from their substance of choice. This depends to some degree on the substance. In our experience, methadone patients are the most likely to have major depression after detox, followed by cocaine addicts, with alcoholics the least likely. Waiting allows differentiations between states of intoxication and physiological withdrawal versus other organic or psychotic presentations. Ideally, four weeks would elapse before making psychiatric diagnosis; however, for various reasons, three to ten days is more practical. If neuroleptics are necessary for acute agitation, their long-term use needs to be constantly reassessed.

Making a chemical dependency diagnosis of the psychiatric or medical patient may be suggested by a serum or urine drug screen. Asking specifically and directly about consumption, substance use and medicine are also important. Other lab results, such as elevated liver enzymes and especially GGTP, may give clues. Good physical exams may pick up needle marks, perforated nasal septum, or the physiological changes noted above. A high suspicion for drug-related symptoms is important, such as considering that chest pains in young, otherwise healthy males may suggest cocaine abuse. Further history from family and friends may verify suspicions. These clinical techniques are similar to those described by researchers such as Rounsaville and Kranzler, [9] who discuss various ways to assess dual diagnosis. They review a variety of techniques that include self-reports such as the Beck Depression Inventory, the use of structured versus unstructured interviews, and describe screening and diagnostic interviews. Mirin et al. [10] describe a

280-item questionnaire "designed to get demographic data, quantitate the extent and duration of drug and alcohol use and assess current social adjustment periods." They also utilize a 90-item Symptom Distress checklist, the Beck Depression Inventory, the Hamilton Rating Scale, and family history gathered by a unit social worker using a structured clinical interview for all available first-degree relatives.

We are now going to review the DSM-III-R criteria for substance abuse and dependence, followed by review of DSM-III-R criteria for commonly seen psychiatric pathology in chemical dependency. DSM-III-R is the Diagnostic and Statistical Manual of Mental Disorders, Third Edition, Revised [3]. It is published by the American Psychiatric Association as the current accepted standard for making psychiatric diagnosis in America. DSM-III-R makes a distinction between psychoactive substance abuse disorders and psychoactive substance–induced organic mental disorders such as intoxication and withdrawal states. There are two main categories under psychoactive substance abuse, dependence and abuse. The following section lists the diagnostic criteria for psychoactive substance dependence.

## PSYCHOACTIVE SUBSTANCE DEPENDENCE [3]

### Diagnostic Criteria

At least three of the following criteria indicate substance dependence:

Substance often taken in larger amounts or over a longer period than the person intended.

Persistent desire or one or more unsuccessful effort to cut down or control substance use.

A great deal of time spent in activities necessary to get the substance (e.g., theft), taking the substance (e.g., chain smoking), or recovering from its effects.

Frequent intoxication or withdrawal symptoms when expected to fill major role obligations at work, school or home (e.g., does not go to work because hung over, goes to school "high", intoxicated while taking care of his or her children), or when substance use is physically hazardous (e.g., driving when intoxicated).

Important social, occupational, or recreational activities given up or reduced because of substance use.

Continued substance use despite knowledge of having a persistent recurrent social, psychological, or physical problem that is caused or exacerbated by use of substance (e.g., keeps using heroin despite family arguments about it), cocaine-induced depression, or having an ulcer made worse by drinking.

Marked tolerance: Need for markedly increased amounts of the substance (i.e., at least a 50% increase) in order to achieve intoxication or desired effect, or markedly diminished effect with continued use of this same amount.

Characteristic withdrawal symptoms* (see specific withdrawal syndromes under Psychoactive Substance–Induced Organic Mental disorders).

## Analysis

As we study the diagnostic criteria for substance dependence, we see that there is a combination of behavioral observations with physical symptomatology such as withdrawal syndromes. Unlike DSM-III, physical tolerance and withdrawal are no longer absolutely necessary to make the diagnosis of dependence. Diagnostic criteria for substance abuse describe patterns of pathological use for at least one month, as described in the preceding outline.

The DSM-III-R then goes on to describe specifically ten different groups of psychoactive substances associated with dependence and abuse, as follows: alcohol; amphetamine or similarly acting sympathomimetics; cannabis; cocaine; hallucinogens; inhalants; nicotine; opioids; phencyclidine (PCP) or similarly acting arylcyclohexylamines; and sedative hypnotics or anxiolytics. DSM-III-R also allows for broad-spectrum categories such as polysubstance dependence, psychoactive substance dependence not otherwise specified, and psychoactive substance abuse not otherwise specified.

In addition to the diagnostic categories of abuse and dependence, DSM-III-R describes more physiologically specific diagnoses related to states of intoxication and withdrawal. This is a particularly important group of disorders as they may initially be confused with other psychiatric or physical disabilities and, in some cases, if left untreated, may have a significant morbidity and mortality. Alcohol-induced organic mental disorders include intoxication and idiosyncratic intoxication. Intoxication gives a fairly straightforward presentation, with a history of recent ingestion of alcohol, a display of behavior that shows disinhibition, and at least one of the following: slurred speech and incoordination, unsteady gait, nystagmus, and flushed face. Idiosyncratic intoxication is noteworthy for rapid onset of violent or aggressive behavior shortly after ingestion of small amounts of alcohol in a person who is not noted for this type of behavior. The withdrawal states include uncomplicated alcohol withdrawal, alcohol withdrawal delirium, and alcohol hallucinosis. These latter two diagnostic areas may

---

*May not apply to cannabis, hallucinogens, or phencyclidine (PCP).

easily be confused with other psychiatric disorders or other organic causes. DSM-III-R defines delirium as the reduced ability to maintain attention to external stimuli and to shift attention appropriately to new external stimuli. This is accompanied by disorganized thinking and at least two of the following symptoms: a reduced level of consciousness; perceptual disturbances; disturbance in sleep-wake cycle; change in the level of psychomotor activity; disorientation as to person, place, or time; or memory impairment. Delirium usually has a fluctuating course over a short period of time. There are also conditions associated with chronic use of alcohol, including alcohol amnestic disorder and dementia associated with alcoholism. Amnestic syndrome includes both short- and long-term memory impairment. Dementia includes that plus at least one other symptom, such as difficulty in abstract thinking, impaired judgment, personality change, or difficulties in higher cortical function such as aphasia, apraxia, and agnosias. DSM-III-R lists a group of sedative-, hypnotic-, or anxiolytic-induced organic mental disorders with categories somewhat similar to the alcohol states. The stimulant group of drugs, such as amphetamines, can also cause organic mental disorders that can be loosely grouped with cocaine and phencyclidine (PCP). In order to make the diagnosis of intoxication in this group, there must be a history of recent use plus maladaptive behavioral changes, such as fighting, grandiosity, hypervigilance, psychomotor agitation, impaired judgment, impaired social or occupational functioning, euphoria, belligerence, assaultiveness, impulsiveness, and unpredictability. Physical signs for cocaine and amphetamines include: tachycardia, pupillary dilation, elevated blood pressure, perspiration or chills, and nausea or vomiting. Cocaine intoxication may also include visual or tactile hallucinations. To diagnose PCP intoxication at least two of the following physical signs should be noted: vertical or horizontal nystagmus; increased blood pressure or heart rate, numbness or diminished responsiveness to pain, ataxia, dysarthria, muscle rigidity, seizures, or hyperacusis. Stimulant withdrawal states are noted to have depression, irritability, anxiety, fatigue, insomnia or hypersomnia, and psychomotor agitation. The diagnostic manual also notes that these substances may cause delirium and delusional disorder. PCP may cause organic mood disorder shortly after use.

The third major group of substances abused are the opioids. Psychiatric signs of intoxication include euphoria followed by apathy, dysphoria, psychomotor retardation, impaired judgment, and impaired social or occupational functioning. Look for pupillary constriction except in severe overdose and at least one of the following physical signs: drowsiness, slurred speech, and impairment in attention or memory. In opioid withdrawal, at least three of the following should be noted: craving for the drug, muscle aches, pupillary dilation, lacrimation or rhinorrhea, nausea or vomiting, diarrhea, insomnia, yawning or fever.

DSM-III-R also includes categories for caffeine intoxication, cannabis intoxication, and cannabis delusional disorder, as well as hallucinogen-induced hallucinosis, delusional disorder, mood disorder, and post-hallucinogen perception disorder, the so-called flashback phenomena.

The importance of recognizing these many different possibilities may not only aid in a more rapid stabilization of the patient but may also avoid unnecessary use of other psychoactive medication when the treatment of choice may be abstinence from the substance of abuse.

In summary, all physicians, including psychiatrists, family practitioners, interns, and emergency room physicians must keep a constant alert for the hidden causes of their patients' complaints. I have had many a patient who has been otherwise young and healthy report that he was evaluated for cardiac disturbance but had a negative work-up. Invariably, such patients report that they never told their physician about their cocaine use, which occurred prior to their symptomatology. Psychiatrists have long been criticized for treating alcoholics with benzodiazepines while missing the real problem. Urine and blood toxicology screens should become more routine in all physical and psychiatric work-ups. Many times, the patients will be too embarrassed or have other agendas, such as drug seeking, that will keep them from acting as good historians.

## AFFECTIVE DISORDERS

### Psychotic Illnesses

Next, we turn to the often-missed psychiatric illnesses in the identified addict or alcoholic. Conceptually speaking, the dual-diagnosis patient is usually defined as any person who simultaneously has a chemical dependency problem with a coexisting psychiatric emotional problem. The most common psychiatric diagnoses associated with substance abuse include depression, both unipolar and bipolar, [10–12] panic anxiety disorders, [13,14] attention deficit disorders [15,16] and, to a lesser degree, schizophrenia [17]. There is also a strong correlation with several of the personality disorders such as borderline and antisocial [11].

As mentioned earlier, some of the keys to making the correct psychiatric diagnosis in the chemically dependent patient is to explore the timing for the occurrence of symptoms and to wait a reasonable period of time after detox to see if the psychiatric symptoms persist or clear.

We begin with the diagnostic criteria for the affective disorders: major depression, bipolar depression, and panic/anxiety disorders.

Bipolar depression includes descriptions of manic and hypomanic behavior that, when added to depressive symptoms, distinguish it from unipolar depression.

*Mania and Hypomania* [3]
**Diagnostic Criteria**

A. A distinct period of abnormally and persistently elevated expansive or irritable mood.
B. During the period of mood disturbance, at least three of the following symptoms have persisted (four if the mood is only irritable) and had been present to a significant degree.
   1. Inflated self-esteem or grandiosity.
   2. Decreased need for sleep; e.g., feels rested after only three hours of sleep.
   3. More talkative than usual, or pressure to keep talking.
   4. Flight of ideas or subjective experience that thoughts are racing.
   5. Distractibility, i.e, attention too easily drawn to unimportant or irrelevant external stimuli.
   6. Increase in goal-directed activity (either socially, at work or school, or sexually), or psychomotor agitation.
   7. Excessive involvement in pleasurable activities which have a high potential for painful consequences, e.g., the person engages in unrestrained buying sprees, sexual indiscretions or foolish business investments.
C. This category is necessary to make the manic diagnosis. Mood disturbance is sufficiently severe to cause marked impairment in occupational functioning or in usual social activities or relationships with others, or to necessitate hospitalization to prevent harm to self or others.
D. At no time during the disturbance have there been delusions or hallucinations for as long as two weeks in the absence of prominent mood symptoms (i.e., before the mood symptoms developed or after they have remitted).
E. Not superimposed on schizophrenia, schizophreniform disorder, delusional disorder or psychotic disorder, not otherwise specified.
F. It cannot be established that an organic factor initiated and maintained the disturbance. Note: Somatic antidepressant treatment (e.g., drugs, ECT) that apparently precipitates a mood disturbance should not be considered an etiologic organic factor.

The manic syndrome may or may not have psychotic features. DSM-III-R defines delusions or hallucinations whose content is consistent with typical manic themes of inflated worth, power, knowledge, identity with, or special relationship to, a deity or famous person as mood-congruent. Persecutory delusions, thought insertion, delusions of being controlled, or catatonic symptoms indicate mood-incongruent psychotic features.

Reviewing the criteria for manic episode, one can very quickly see how alcohol or other abused substances could cover over or mimic manic symptoms. Many of these symptoms are similar to those seen in cocaine intoxication. The cocaine-intoxicated person becomes elevated and expansive and demonstrates inflated self-esteem and a decreased need to sleep. Easy distractibility and sexual indiscretions are frequent complications.

*Case History I*

Mr. T. was a 29-year-old, single, white male who came to treatment involuntarily for chemical dependency after intervention by his family. He reported abusing alcohol by the age of 13. This led to abuse of marijuana and experimentation with other drugs such as diazepam, LSD, and methaqualone. By the age of 19, he was snorting cocaine, which led to freebasing at 22 and "crack" cocaine at 26. At admission, he admitted to daily use of "crack" cocaine, daily consumption of beer, and daily use of marijuana.

The patient admitted some depression, which he related to the recent loss of his girlfriend, house, and job, along with having been in jail for some legal difficulties. He had been treated for chemical dependency on three previous occasions. Family history suggested alcoholism in his mother, bulimia in his sister, and depression in his father, paternal uncle, and grandparents. The physical work-up was unremarkable. The serum dexamethasone suppression test was normal. Neuropsychological testing revealed no significant psychopathology.

During individual sessions with us, he talked freely about his substance abuse and described himself as always having large amounts of money. He referred to himself as a supersalesman, having sold jewelry, automobiles, and furniture. Although he talked of depressing issues with other people, he denied ever being overly depressed. He admitted often being impulsive, even when it did not involve drugs. He spoke of times when he had dropped everything to go fishing. Frequently, he would get the impulse to attend Grateful Dead concerts, no matter where they were around the country. He claimed that he'd seen 167 live concerts of that musical group. He admitted that at these concerts, he would often get "stoned," intoxicated, and "high." Mental status examination, from the very beginning, revealed a hypomanic quality, with pressured, rapid speech and, at times, flight of ideas. Clinical observation over time suggested bipolar depression. He reported energy swings that occurred long before he began using drugs. His maternal grandfather had times in which he would become extremely angry and irritable, suggestive of a possible manic variant. A maternal uncle committed suicide, and his sister had similar kinds of mood and energy swings. Just prior to admission while he was in jail, he began on impulse, to bang his head against the wall, causing lacerations that required stitches. Lithobid was started, and dosage was increased gradually to 900 mg PO bid, giving a lithium level of 1.1. By the time of discharge, the patient reported feeling greater control over his energy and impulses as well as thinking in a more productive way. He was drug-free seven months post discharge, his longest drug-free period since age 13. Both the patient and his family report improvement in his emotional stability.

*Major Depressive Episodes* [3]
**Diagnostic Criteria**

A. At least five of the following symptoms have been present during the same two-week period and represent a change from previous functioning; at least one of the symptoms is either depressed mood or loss of interest or pleasure.
   1. Depressed mood (or possibly irritable mood in children and adolescents) most of the day, nearly every day, as indicated either by subjective accounts or observation by others.
   2. Markedly diminished interest or pleasure in all or almost all activities most of the day nearly every day, as indicated either by subjective account or observation of apathy most of the time.
   3. Significant weight loss or weight gain when not dieting (e.g., more than 5% of body weight in a month) or decrease or increase in appetite nearly every day. (In children, consider failure to make expected weight gain.)
   4. Insomnia or hypersomnia nearly every day.
   5. Psychomotor agitation or retardation nearly every day (observable by others rather than merely subjective feelings of restlessness or being slowed down).
   6. Fatigue or loss of energy nearly every day.
   7. Feelings of worthlessness or excessive or inappropriate guilt (which may be delusional) nearly every day (not merely self-reproach or guilt about being sick).
   8. Diminished ability to think or concentrate, or indecisiveness, nearly every day (either by subjective account or as observed by others).
   9. Recurrent thoughts of death, not just fear of dying (recurrent suicidal ideation without a suicide attempt or specific plan for committing suicide).
B. 1. It cannot be established that an organic factor initiated and maintained the disturbance.
   2. The disturbance is not a normal reaction to the death of a loved one (uncomplicated bereavement). *Note*: Morbid preoccupation with worthlessness, suicidal ideation, marked functional impairment, or psychomotor retardation for prolonged durations suggest bereavement complicated by major depression.

C.   At no time during the disturbance have there been delusions or hallucinations for as long as two weeks in the absence of prominent mood symptoms (i.e., before the mood symptoms developed or after they have remitted.)

D.   Not superimposed on schizophrenia, schizophreniform disorder, delusional disorder, or psychotic disorder not otherwise specified.

As before, psychotic features include delusions or hallucinations. If the content is consistent with typical depressive themes of personal inadequacy, guilt, disease, and death, they are mood-congruent. Mood-incongruent psychosis includes delusions (not directly related to depressive themes), thought insertion, thought broadcasting, and delusions of control. Melancholic depression is marked by lack of reactivity to usually pleasurable stimuli; depression that is regularly worse in the morning, with early morning awakening; absence of significant personality disturbance before the first major depressive episode; one or more previous major depressive episodes, followed by complete or nearly complete recovery; and previous good responses to adequate somatic antidepressant therapy, such as tricyclics, ECT, MAOI, or lithium.

The chemically dependent patient that has reached the point of coming for inpatient treatment often presents many depressive symptoms at the beginning of treatment. Many patients admit to anhedonia but attribute it to having turned all their energies to procuring their drug or maintaining their "high." Reports of significant weight loss are not unusual, especially with abuse of cocaine and stimulants. Insomnia is common in the stimulant abuser while hypersomnia is often seen in the sedative-hypnotic/alcohol abuser. In the same way, psychomotor agitation may result from stimulant use, while psychomotor retardation may come with sedative-hypnotic use. Fatigue and loss of energy occur commonly in the chemically dependent. Even stimulant users show fatigue during the recovery phase. Feelings of worthlessness and guilt are frequent, though often attributed to the problems resulting from the use of drugs. Many of the drugs of abuse diminish the ability to think or concentrate. Suicidal ideation is not uncommon during the "crash"period after cocaine or during an alcoholic blackout. Chemically dependent persons have a higher than normal rate of suicide [18].

The authors of DSM-III-R state that it cannot be established that an organic factor initiated and maintained the disturbance (see Part B in Panic Disorder outline). This is one of the greatest difficulties in sorting out the significance of depressive symptomatology. The notion of organic mood disorder may be appropriate for some patients with depression and chemical dependency, particularly if the depression clears with abstinence. We know that cocaine dependency, for example, may produce a dopamine deficiency state that may be the substrate of post-detox depression. However, these efforts to sort out diagnostic primacy can be complex and difficult, and attempts to assign primacy can lead to treatment errors. Third-party payer issues can be involved as well. As one of us has described in previous articles, there is nothing about being a chemically dependent person that protects one from having major affective illness [7]. In our experience, the most productive approach is to identify both the chemical dependency and depression (or other psychiatric problem) as coexisting, if both are present, and to treat both in an integrated program.

Once one has established the presence of either depressive symptomatology and/or mania, DSM-III-R then describes the following subcategories: bipolar disorder mixed, bipolar disorder manic, bipolar disorder depressed, cyclothymia, and bipolar disorder not otherwise specified. Cyclothymia exists when there is no evidence of major depression or focal manic episodes. Thus, it is a condition with hypomania and depressed mood not severe enough to meet the criteria for major depression. For those people presenting only depressive symptomatology, DSM-III-R lists major depressive single episode, major depression recurrent, dysthymia (or depressive neurosis), and depressive disorder not otherwise specified. We find the latter diagnosis useful since it is often impossible to rule out completely the effects of chemical dependency on the otherwise straightforward major depressive symptomatology.

*Case History II*
This was the third psychiatric admission for Mr. R., a 38-year-old father of three, who reported using opiates since his tour of duty in Vietnam at age 18. Upon returning to the United States, he was maintained on methadone through the Veterans Administration for two years. He reported taking up to 200 mg per day until 1980, when he detoxed. After one year, he began to feel better, and he stayed clean until 1984, when he required oxycodone following surgery for a ruptured disk. He reported that he began to take Percodan in steadily increasing amounts up to 20 to 30 tablets p.d. for two years. He eventually began adding Darvocet, diazepam, and marijuana, as well as about a fifth of hard liquor per day. He also admitted abusing heroin IV on a relatively frequent basis. Psychiatric history revealed an episode of depression with suicidal ideation following his first divorce. Family history revealed that his mother had been depressed and that his stepfather was alcoholic, with a history of physical abuse. The patient's wife reported that he had threatened others and was considered by the VA to be "very dangerous." Mental status showed depression but was otherwise normal. Laboratory and physical work-ups were unremarkable except for hepatitis B in the recovery phase and a positive seven-point dexamethasone suppression test. His course in the hospital went relatively smoothly. He was communicative and cooperative throughout the program, and his depression lifted with group and individual therapy.

The patient came to see us as an outpatient several months after discharge. Although he had remained clean and sober, he began to have increasing depressive symptomatology. After a trial of tricyclic antidepressant was discussed and he was put on desipramine, his depression lifted. The patient, over the last three years, has remained straight and sober, without severe depression, and is leading an active and productive life. He reported to us during one session that when he was actively using opiate, he had long ceased getting "high" but rather took it in order to maintain himself on a day-to-day basis. He admitted that taking the antidepressant gave him the same effect as taking heroin daily. He reported trying to discontinue his antidepressant several times but has always experienced a return of his depressive symptomatology.

*Case History III*
This was the first hospitalization for Mrs. Q., a white, married female about 40 years of age, who worked full time as a registered nurse. Her chief complaint at admission was: "I finally decided I had to do something for myself. I have been unable to stop drinking on my own. I want to be able to be more sociable and self-confident." The patient reported that she had experienced some level of depression for many years. However, her depressive symptoms had worsened over the past year and had become particularly severe in the six months prior to admission. Despite her low energy, anhedonia, frequent crying spells, and feelings of self-reproach and blame, she was still able to perform her job as an RN on a daily basis. She also reported difficulties with sleep, restless nights, and early morning awakening. She reported a 10-year history of continuous alcohol abuse. On an average evening, she would drink 12 shots of vodka, which would frequently lead to arguments with her husband. She reported at admission that she had attempted to stop drinking unsuccessfully on her own six months before but experienced alcohol withdrawal, including a seizure. Following this, she became frightened and began drinking again. Then she began to have suicidal ideation and had gone as far as to hide a number of pills, which she planned to use in an overdose. She had a strong, positive family history for alcoholism, with both of her parents and two brothers reportedly alcoholic. After a period of clinical observation and a positive DST, she was started on tricyclic antidepressants. Her depression lifted. She did not work a strong program of recovery but, after two years, continues to report being happy and sober.

*Case History IV*
Mr. Z. was a prominent member of the health care profession who retired in his early forties because of a disability. His chief complaint was Dilaudid dependence. This was one of multiple psychiatric hospitalizations. The patient had a history of chronic flank and right-upper-quadrant pain secondary to recurrent kidney stones. The problem had begun almost 15 years before. Following various surgeries, he became addicted to analgesic medication. The patient denied any problem with substance abuse prior to the onset of his renal and pain problems. The patient reported, at the time of this admission, that he was using 60–70 mg Dilaudid daily in addition to 20–30 mg of diazepam and occasional alcohol. The

patient denied use of any street drugs. The patient was seen in consultation on several occasions for his acute episodes of severe abdominal pain. He underwent a lengthy period of detoxification from opiates, with use of methadone and clonidine and detoxification from minor tranquilizers with the use of diazepam. The patient was treated with group, individual, and family therapies, in addition to NA and AA. Because there were some underlying vegetative signs of depression and because of the possibility of helping with his chronic pain syndrome, he was started on a serotonergic antidepressant, Surmontil and, at the time of discharge, was taking 250 mg per day. Follow-up at 18 months found that he continued to be straight and sober and, although his pain syndrome continues, he is no longer allowing it to control his life.

## Anxiety Disorders

The other group of affective disorders associated with chemical dependence are the anxiety disorders.

*Panic Disorder (with and without Agoraphobia)* [3]
**Diagnostic Criteria**

A. Sometime during the disturbance, one or more panic attacks (discrete periods of intense fear or discomfort) have occurred that were:
  1. Unexpected, i.e., did not occur immediately before, or on exposure to, a situation that almost always caused anxiety.
  2. Not triggered by situations in which the person was the focus of others' attention.
B. Either four attacks, as defined in criteria A, have occurred within a four-week period, or one or more attacks have been followed by a period of at least a month of persistent fear of having another attack.
C. At least four of the following symptoms developed during at least one of the attacks:
  1. Shortness of breath or smothering sensations.
  2. Dizziness, unsteady feelings, or faintness.
  3. Palpitations or tachycardia.
  4. Trembling or shaking.
  5. Sweating.
  6. Choking.
  7. Nausea or abdominal distress.
  8. Depersonalization or derealization.
  9. Numbness or tingling sensations.
  10. Flushes or chills.
  11. Chest pain or discomfort.
  12. Fear of dying.

13.   Fear of going crazy or doing something uncontrolled.

D.   During at least some of the attacks at least four of the symptoms in
     criterion C developed suddenly and increased in intensity within 10
     minutes of the beginning of the first symptom noticed in the attack.
E.   It cannot be established that an organic factor initiated and maintained
     the disturbance, e.g., amphetamine or caffeine intoxication, hyperthy-
     roidism. Note: Mitral valve prolapse may be an associated condition
     but does not preclude a diagnosis of panic disorder.

*Generalized Anxiety Disorder* [3]

**Diagnostic Criteria**

A.   Unrealistic or excessive anxiety and worry (apprehensive expectation)
     about two or more life circumstances, e.g., worry about possible mis-
     fortune to one's child (who is in no danger) and worry about finances
     (for no good reason) for a period of six months or longer, during which
     the person has been bothered more days than not by these concerns. In
     children and adolescents, this may take the form of anxiety and worry
     about academic, athletic, and social performance.
B.   If another Axis I disorder is present, the focus of the anxiety and worry
     in A is unrelated to it, e.g., the anxiety or worry is not about having a
     panic attack (as in panic disorder), being embarrassed in public (as in
     social phobia), being contaminated (as in obsessive-compulsive disor-
     der), or gaining weight (as in anorexia nervosa).
C.   The disturbance does not occur only during the course of a mood
     disorder or psychotic disorder.
D.   At least 6 of the following 18 symptoms are often present when anxious
     (do not include symptoms present only during panic attacks):

Motor tension:
     1.   Trembling, twitching or feeling shaky.
     2.   Muscle tension, aches, or soreness.
     3.   Restlessness.
     4.   Easy fatigability

Autonomic hyperactivity:
     5.   Shortness of breath or smothering sensations.
     6.   Palpitations or accelerated heart rate.
     7.   Sweating or cold, clammy hands.
     8.   Dry mouth.
     9.   Dizziness or light-headedness.
     10.  Nausea, diarrhea, or other abdominal distress.
     11.  Flushes or chills.

    12.   Frequent urination.

    13.   Trouble swallowing or lump in throat.

Vigilance or scanning:

    14.   Feeling keyed up or on edge.

    15.   Exaggerated startle response.

    16.   Difficulty concentrating or "mind going blank" because of anxiety.

    17.   Trouble falling asleep.

    18.   Irritability.

E.   It cannot be established that an organic factor initiated and maintained the disturbance, e.g., hyperthyroidism, caffeine intoxication.

Once again we can see, in cases IV and V, the overlap between symptoms of intoxication states and withdrawal states. However, we can also see how many people have turned to alcohol or "drugs" to "self-medicate," often effectively, at least in the beginning. It is well known that the benzodiazepine class is quite effective in dealing with generalized anxiety disorder over the short term. However, in those individuals who also have an addictive potential, an addiction may be set off by the treatment.

Another important aspect of this group of disorders is the propensity for the symptoms to intensify to the point of preventing the chemically dependent person from fully utilizing a 12-step recovery program. The "detoxed" addicts' anxiety may begin to rise, along with the emergence of agoraphobia and panic attacks.

*Case History V*

This was the first psychiatric hospitalization and the first treatment of any kind for Mrs. D., a married, white, Roman Catholic female in her thirties. Her chief complaint was "depression and Valium addiction." At the time of admission, she reported that she had been feeling increasingly depressed over the year prior to admission. She reported periods of crying, decrease in appetite, decreased libido, increase in anxiety, and difficulty falling asleep and staying asleep. She described feeling tired all the time, poor concentration, and feelings of helplessness, hopelessness, and anhedonia. She reported abusing Valium for over six years. She reported she had started out with 5–20 mg per day but, within the two months prior to admission, took up to 90 mg per day. She developed an explosive personality, with rage attacks at her husband. Historically, her depression first started at the age of 19 following an abortion. She also developed panic attacks, with sudden episodes of feeling frightened and feeling as if "she would be swallowed up." She would feel a knot in her stomach and begin to hyperventilate. Her mother had a history of "nervous breakdown," and alcoholism. Her father also drank heavily. Her sister had a history of mood swings and panic attacks. She had a positive DST. Endocrinology work-up confirmed polycystic ovarian disease. A cardiologist recommended low-dose Inderal for her symtomatic palpitations with tachycardia to 130, associated with a complete right bundle branch block and a myxomatous mitral valve. During the course of treatment, she became very motivated, attending NA and AA for several years. Following her detoxification, her depressive symptomatology and her symptomatology consistent with panic attacks were treated with a tricyclic antidepressant. However, excessive weight gain with the tricyclic led to switching antidepressants. During the period of changeover, she went through a very severe depression with marked panic attacks. It took a full six to eight weeks before she was restabilized on an alternative antidepressant. She has remained completely drug-free in terms of abuse or addiction for over three years.

## Schizophrenia [3]

In this section, we are going to discuss the interplay between the diagnoses of schizophrenia and chemical dependency. This is an important group, not so much because it is difficult to sort out the diagnosis of schizophrenia, which is often chronic and long-standing, but because it is so prevalent today for the young schizophrenic patient to have used and abused drugs [17]. There is also overlap in the sense that the presence of delusions and hallucinations can be found in a number of intoxication and withdrawal states. In addition, it is not uncommon to suspect that experimentation with substances can precipitate some latent underlying tendency toward schizophrenia.

### Diagnostic Criteria

A.  Presence of characteristic psychotic symptoms in the active phase, either 1, 2, or 3 (below) for at least one week (unless the symptoms are successfully treated):
   1.  Two of the following:
       a.  Delusions
       b.  Prominent hallucinations (throughout the day or for several weeks or several times a week for several weeks, each hallucinatory experience not being limited to a few brief moments).
       c.  Incoherence or marked loosening of associations.
       d.  Catatonic behavior.
       e.  Flat or grossly inappropriate affect.
   2.  Bizarre delusions (i.e., involving a phenomenon that the person's culture would regard as totally impossible, e.g., thought broadcasting, being controlled by a dead person).
   3.  Prominent hallucinations (as defined in 1b. of a voice with content having no apparent relation to depression or elation, or a voice keeping up a running commentary on the person's behavior or thought, or two or more voices conversing with each other).
B.  During the course of the disturbance, functioning in such areas as

work, social relations, and self-care is markedly below the highest level achieved before the onset of the disturbance.

C. Schizoaffective disorder and mood disorder, with psychotic features having been ruled out.

D. Continued signs of the disturbance for at least six months. The six-month period must include an active period (of at least one week or less if symptoms have been successfully treated) during which there were psychotic symptoms characteristic of schizophrenia with or without a prodromal or residual phase as defined below.

   1. Prodromal phase: A clear deterioration in functioning before the active phase of the disturbance that is not due to a disturbance in mood or to a psychoactive substance use disorder and that involves at least two of the symptoms listed below.

   2. Residual Phase: Following the active phase of the disturbance, a persistence of at least two of the symptoms noted below (these not being due to a disturbance in mood or to a psychoactive substance use disorder).

     a. Marked social isolation or withdrawal.

     b. Marked impairment in role functioning as wage earner, student, or homemaker.

     c. Markedly peculiar behavior (e.g., collecting garbage, talking to self in public, hoarding food).

     d. Marked impairment in personal hygiene and grooming.

     e. Blunted or inappropriate affect.

     f. Digressive, vague, overelaborate, circumstantial speech, or poverty of speech, or poverty of content of speech.

     g. Odd beliefs or magical thinking influencing behavior and inconsistent with cultural norms, e.g., superstitiousness and belief in clairvoyance, telepathy, sixth sense, "others can feel my feelings," overvalued ideas, ideas of reference.

     h. Unusual perceptual experiences, e.g., recurrent illusions, sensing the presence of a force or person not actually present.

     i. Marked lack of initiative, interest, or energy.

E. It cannot be established that an organic factor initiated or maintained the disturbance.

F. There is no history of autistic disorder; the additional diagnosis of schizophrenia is made only if the prominent delusions or hallucinations are also present.

Once again, we readily see the overlap of these symptoms with chemical dependency. Active addicts, often socially isolate, withdraw and develop impairment in role functioning. Peculiar behavior is common with many intoxication states. Personal hygiene and grooming often deteriorate in the alcoholic or cocaine addict on a binge. Vague circumstantial speech may accompany states of intoxication. As various addictions progress, initiative diminishes, interests wane, and energy levels fall. Unusual perceptual experiences are often noted during periods of heavy use. One of the common subtypes of schizophrenia is the paranoid. Paranoid thinking is very common during stimulant abuse, as well as chronic cannabis abuse.

### Attention-Deficit Hyperactivity Disorder [3]

Attention-deficit hyperactivity disorder should be mentioned when discussing the dual-diagnosis patient since a number of adolescents diagnosed with this disorder develop chemical dependency problems. At times, the hyperactivity carries over into adulthood. Chemical dependency treatment units need to take this into account since many of the same difficulties these young people suffered in school may be acted out in a treatment program. In our treatment program, we frequently have patients who are embarrassed and reluctant to admit their difficulties with reading or writing. Their secret often comes out only after they have been confronted for not completing assignments.

**Diagnostic Criteria**

A.  A disturbance of at least six months during which at least eight of the following are present:
    1.  Often fidgets with hands or feet and squirms in seat (in adolescents may be limited to subjective feelings of restlessness).
    2.  Has difficulty remaining seated when required to do so.
    3.  Is easily distracted by extraneous stimuli.
    4.  Has difficulty awaiting turn in games or group situations.
    5.  Often blurts answers to questions before they have been completed.
    6.  Has difficulty following through on instructions from others (not due to oppositional behavior or failure of comprehension), e.g., fails to finish chores.
    7.  Has difficulty sustaining attention in task or play activities.
    8.  Often shifts from one uncompleted activity to another.
    9.  Has difficulty playing quietly.
    10. Often talks excessively.
    11. Often disrupts or intrudes on others, e.g., butts into other's games.
    12. Often does not seem to listen to what is being said to him or her.
    13. Often loses things necessary for tasks or activities for school or at home, e.g., toys, pencils, books, assignments.

14. Often engages in physically dangerous activities without considering possible consequences (not for the purpose of thrill seeking),
e.g., runs into street without looking.
B. Onset before the age of 7.
C. Does not meet the criteria for pervasive developmental disorder.

*Conduct Disorder*

Another adolescent disorder frequently associated with chemical dependency is conduct disorder which, frequently, if left untreated, becomes antisocial personality disorder in persons 18 or older.

**Diagnostic Criteria** [3]

A. A disturbance of conduct lasting at least six months, during which at
least three of the following have been present.
1. Has stolen without confrontation of the victim on more than one
occasion (including forgery).
2. Has run away from home overnight at least twice while living in
parental or parental-surrogate home (or once without returning).
3. Often lies (other than to avoid physical or sexual abuse).
4. Has deliberately engaged in fire setting.
5. Is often truant from school (for older person, absent from work).
6. Has broken into someone else's house, building, or car.
7. Has deliberately destroyed others' property (other than by fire
setting).
8. Has been physically cruel to animals.
9. Has forced someone into sexual activity with him or her.
10. Has used a weapon in more than one fight.
11. Often initiates physical fights.
12. Has stolen with confrontation of a victim (e.g, mugging, purse
snatching, extortion, armed robbery).
13. Has been physically cruel to people.

As one examines the preceding outline, one can again see many symptoms frequently associated with substance abusers. Stealing, lying, fighting,
and school truancy are frequently seen as part of drug-seeking behavior. In
the same way, oppositional defiant disorder has a number of criteria that
might develop as a direct relationship to the beginning of the adolescent's
drug abuse.

Many of our adolescent patients have developed ongoing and increasingly
severe problems with their parents, teachers, and other figures. The more
their lives become unmanageable the further they sink into the vicious spiral
of anger, arguments, rule breaking, and isolation.

Adolescents who abuse drugs may also suffer from eating disorders, including anorexia nervosa, bulimia nervosa, and eating disorder [19] not otherwise specified. Some cocaine addicts, particularly women, begin to use cocaine in order to suppress appetite. Many chronic crack cocaine users have marked weight loss and border on malnutrition. Many recurrent addicts in our program began to eat somewhat vociferously. Interestingly, many of the eating-disorder treatment programs are modeled after the 12-step programs that started with Alcoholics Anonymous.

### Antisocial Personality Disorder

The personality disorders that become the basis for the Axis II diagnosis in the DSM-III-R are not uncommon in the chemically dependent population. In particular, antisocial and borderline personality disorders provide special challenges and management in treatment programs. The notion of the "addictive personality" is no longer accepted. The addictive life-style itself can mimic and teach dysfunctional interpersonal relations. However, some dysfunctional personality styles seem common in addicts.

**Diagnostic Criteria** [3]

A.  Current age at least 18.
B.  Evidence of conduct disorder with at least three of those symptoms before age 15.
C.  Pattern of irresponsibility and antisocial behavior since the age of 15 indicated by at least four of the following:
    1.  Is unable to sustain consistent work behavior as indicated by any of the following (including similar behavior in academic settings if the person is a student):
        a.  Significant unemployment for six months or more within five years when expected to work when work was available.
        b.  Repeated absences from work unexplained by illness in self or family.
        c.  Abandonment of several jobs without realistic plans for others.
    2.  Fails to conform to social norms with respect to lawful behavior, as indicated by repeatedly performing antisocial acts that are grounds for arrest (whether arrested or not), e.g., destroying property, harassing others, stealing, pursuing an illegal occupation.
    3.  Is irritable and aggressive, as indicated by repeated physical fights or assaults (not required by one's job or to defend someone or oneself), including spouse or child beating.
    4.  Repeatedly fails to honor financial obligations, as indicated by

defaulting on debts or failing to provide child support or support for other dependents on a regular basis.

5.  Fails to plan ahead or is impulsive, as indicated by one or both of the following:
    a.  Traveling from place to place without a prearranged job or clear goal for the period of travel or clear idea about when the travel will terminate.
    b.  Lack of a fixed address for a month or more.
6.  Has no regard for the truth, as indicated by repeated lying, use of aliases, or conning others for personal profit or pleasure.
7.  Is reckless regarding his or her own or other's personal safety, as indicated by driving while intoxicated or recurrent speeding.
8.  Parent or guardian lacks ability to function as a responsible parent, as indicated by one or more of the following:
    a.  Malnutrition of child.
    b.  Child's illness resulting from lack of minimal hygiene.
    c.  Failure to obtain medical care for a seriously ill child.
    d.  Child's dependence on neighbors or nonresident relatives for food or shelter.
    e.  Failure to arrange for a caretaker for young child when parent is away from home.
    f.  Repeated squandering on personal items of money required for household necessities.
9.  Has never sustained a totally monogamous relationship for more than one year.
10. Lacks remorse but feels justified at having hurt, mistreated, or stolen from another.

D.  Occurrence of antisocial behavior not exclusively during the course of schizophrenia or manic episodes.

As with conduct disorder, again, we see a number of behaviors commonly seen in drug-addicted individuals, especially when illegal substances are the drug of choice. Although some opioid and alcohol-dependent people can maintain work over long periods of time, most eventually show significant unemployment once they reach late stages of heroin use and alcoholism. Repeated absences from work are not uncommon. Becoming involved in unlawful acts, aggressive acts, impulsive acts, and lying, manipulation, failing to plan ahead, or acting impulsively are extremely common in substance abusers. Recklessness in regard to personal safety is frequent. Difficulties with parenthood are one of the more tragic consequences of chemical dependence. A new, meaningful support group, Adult Children of Alcoholics (ACOA), has grown in response to that problem. Although many chemically dependent people fulfill the criteria for antisocial personality, we feel that many of the symptoms of this personality style will fade once they have achieved and maintained sobriety over time. Thus, many chemically dependent people will turn out to have antisocial traits rather than being true antisocial personality disorders.

*Borderline Personality Disorder*

Borderline personality disorder bears special mention since these patients provide such a challenge to the treating professional. A wealth of papers and studies has been written on the borderline personality disorder; however, relatively few of these studies have appeared in the more traditional substance abuse treatment literature. The borderlines' tendency to make rapid and intense attachments, the tendency toward splitting and projective identification, the self-destructive potential, and rage often make them candidates for early departure from traditional chemical dependency treatment settings. In the same way, the traditional psychiatric community often loses sight of the significance of the borderline's chemical dependency problems. The borderline patient is a good example of the addictive illness mimicking and exacerbating psychotic behavior, and the psychiatric disorder predisposing to addictive behavior and resistance to treatment. As the subject of dual diagnosis is increasingly studied, it is clear that traditional psychotherapy will not benefit borderline patients if they are relieving internal anxiety by getting "high" rather than through learning new and healthier defenses.

**Diagnostic Criteria** [3]

A. Pervasive pattern of instability of mood, interpersonal relationships, and self-image, beginning by early adulthood and present in a variety of contexts, as indicated by at least five of the following:
  1. A pattern of unstable and intense interpersonal relationships characterized by alternating between extremes of idealization and devaluation.
  2. Impulsiveness in at least two areas that are potentially self-damaging, e.g., spending, sex, substance use, shoplifting, reckless driving, binge eating. (Do not include suicidal or self-mutilizing behavior, which is covered in item 5.)
  3. Affective instability: marked shifts from baseline mood to depression, irritability, or anxiety, usually lasting a few days and only rarely more than a few days.
  4. Inappropriate intense anger or lack of control of anger, e.g., frequent displays of temper, constant anger, recurrent physical fights.
  5. Recurrent suicidal threats, gestures, or behavior, or self-mutilating behavior.

6.  Marked and persistent identity disturbance manifested by uncertainty about at least two of the following: self-image, sexual orientation, long-term goals or career choice, type of friends desired, preferred values.
7.  Chronic feelings of emptiness or boredom.
8.  Frantic efforts to avoid real or imagined abandonment.

Again, one can see the interrelationship of symptoms with the chemically dependent. However, in this type of chemically dependent person, traditional confrontational methods may only lead to impulsiveness, affective shifts, and the inappropriate anger or dangerous behavior to themselves or others. On the more positive side, borderlines are frequently struggling with an inner sense of emptiness, lack of a sense of self, and absence of identity. They frequently have an underlying low self-esteem and low self-confidence. If they can be successfully engaged in the program of NA and AA, they can often do very well with the structure provided to them by the program, as well as the identity of recovering addict/alcoholic.

## REFERENCES:

1.  Clark J. The treatment of chemical dependence. Letters. *JAMA* 1989; 261:3239.
2.  Weiss RD. The treatment of chemical dependence. In reply. Letters *JAMA*, 1989; 261:3289.
3.  American Psychiatric Association. *Diagnostic and Statistical Manual of Mental Disorders*. 3rd ed. rev. Washington: American Psychiatric Press, 1987.
4.  Schuckit M. Alcoholic patients with psychiatric depression. *Am J Psychiatr* 1983; 140:740–714.
5.  Powell BJ, Read MR, Penick EC, Miller NS, Bingham SF. Primary and secondary depression in alcoholic men: An important distinction? *J Clin Psychiat* 1987; 48:3:98–101.
6.  Schuckit M. "Time-line history" *Psychiatr News* 1989; 5/5:14–15.
7.  Extein I, Gold MS, eds. *Medical Mimics of Psychiatric Disorders*. Washington, DC: American Psychiatric Press, 1986.
8.  Extein I, Gold MS, Groggans FC. Evaluation of affective syndromes. In: *Diagnostic and Laboratory Testing in Psychiatry*. Gold MS, Pottash ALC, eds. New York: Plenum Press, 1986.
9.  Rounsaville MJ, Kranzler JR. The DSM-III-R diagnosis of alcoholism. In: *The Rev of Psychiatry*, Vol 8. Tasman A, Hale RE, Francis AJ, eds. Washington, DC: American Psychiatric Press, 1989.
10. Mirin SM, Weiss RD, Michael J. Psychopathology in substance abusers: Diagnosis and treatment. *Am J Drug Alc Abuse* 1988; 14(2):139–157.
11. Kosten TR, Rounsaville BJ, Psychopathology in opioid addicts. *Psychiatr Clin North Amer* 1986; 9:3, 515–531.

12. Nunes F.V, Quitkin FM, Klein DF. Psychiatric diagnosis in cocaine abuse. *Psychiatr Res* 1989; 28:105–114.
13. Weissman M. Anxiety and alcoholism. *J Clin Psychiatr* 1988; 49:10, (Suppl) 17–19.
14. Gold MS. *The Good News About Panic, Anxiety and Phobias.* New York: Villard Books, 1989.
15. Schuckit MA, Sweeny S, Huey L. Hyperactivity and the risk for alcoholism. *J Clin Psychiatr* 1987; 48(7):275–277.
16. Cocores JA, Davies RK, Mueller PS, Gold MS. Cocaine abuse and adult attention deficit disorder. *J Clin Psychiatr* 1987; 48:9, 376–377.
17. Dixon L, Hass GL, Weiden PJ, Sweeny JA, Frances AJ. Schizophrenia and drug abuse: Who, what, and why? Paper Session 7, No. 20, American Psychiatric Association Annual Meeting, May 1989.
18. Marzuk PM, Mann JJ. Suicide and substance abuse. *Psychiatr Annals* 1988; 18:11,639–645.
19. Jonas JM, Gold MS, Sweeny D, Pottash ALC. Eating disorders and cocaine abuse. A survey of 259 cocaine abusers. *J Clin Psychiatr* 1987; 48:2,47–50.

# 11

## Drug Use and Addiction as Self-Medication: A Psychodynamic Perspective

**Carolyn M. Bell**

*Harvard Medical School at The Cambridge Hospital, Cambridge, Massachusetts*

**Edward J. Khantzian**

*Harvard Medical School at The Cambridge Hospital, Cambridge, Massachusetts, and Danvers State Hospital, Danvers, Massachusetts*

THE ADAPTIVE CONTEXT

"It all comes, I suppose," he decided as he said good-bye to the last branch, spun around three times, and flew gracefully into a gorse bush, "it all comes of liking honey so much. Oh, help!" [1]

A. A. Milne
*Winnie-the-Pooh*

There are few who fail to be amused by the familiar predicament of Winnie-the-Pooh. Our smiles are in identification with the tricky problem of resisting the various objects of our desires, and occasionally being confronted with the embarrassing, sometimes painful, consequences of our indulgences. Why some bears like honey "so much," and why some people develop addictions involving a variety of substances and behaviors, was explained in early psychoanalytic formulations by impulses, instincts seeking gratification, and the pleasure principle [2–4]. Freud's subsequent articulation of a dual-drive theory rather neatly, if somewhat simplistically, accounted for the negative consequences of addiction as arising out of self-destructive motivations and the death instinct [5].

Departing from classical theory, and paralleling advances in psychoanalytic perspectives on human development, views of addiction have gradually
shifted away from drive-derived explanations [6]. Increasingly, the emphasis
is on problems of adaptation — how people try to manage their lives, problem-
solve, and cope with both external reality and internal feeling states. The
adaptive perspective is the core theme of the self-medication hypothesis.

Early insights into the psychological complexities of substance abuse
were offered in the 1960s and 1970s [7–11]. These studies went beyond the
pleasure principle to suggest a more sophisticated and dynamic view of
addiction. In the process of drug experimentation, the powerful discovery is
made wherein a drug, or class of drugs, serves a deeper purpose, substitut
ing for missing psychological functions [12]. People do not abuse drugs
randomly; based on the potential of the drug(s) to serve as a coping mechanism and to attenuate painful feeling states, individuals ultimately find their
"drug of choice." [7] It is the interface between the pharmacological action
of the drug and the psychological vulnerability of the individual that poten-
tiates the addictive process. This is a radical departure from the notion that
drugs are sought to get "high" or for "kicks," and invalidates the equation of
drug abuse as "suicide on the installment plan." The self-selection process
and drug-of-choice phenomenon provide an adaptive context for compre-
hending the complexities of drug abuse and addiction.

The self-medication hypothesis proposes a correspondence between the
pharmacological effects of particular drugs or classes of drugs, on the one
hand, and feeling states, or affects, on the other [12,14]. *Stimulants* (cocaine
and amphetamines) are "activators" and act as energizers, providing the
illusion of overcoming a variety of painful feelings, such as helplessness and
passivity associated with depression. *Sedative-hypnotics*, including alcohol,
are "releasing drugs," in that they seem to allow for feelings of connectedness to others, as well as a sense of inner cohesion or intactness in individuals who tend to be rigid in their defenses and walled off from soothing
object and self-representations. *Analgesic-opiates* ("controlling-stabilizing
drugs") act to mute and counter aggression, rage, and related depression,
thereby reversing regression and helping people feel more stable and secure.
The focus on narcotics contains the clearest statement refuting earlier psychoanalytic accounts of addiction. Earlier perspectives held that opiates
represented a search for pleasurably regressive states. Here it is suggested
that these drugs stabilize the ego and act "specifically (short-term) to reverse
regressive states, by attenuating and making more bearable painful drives
and affects. . . . " (Ref. 12, p. 21)

Whereas the short-term effect of drugs may be to reverse ego regression,
in the long run — with continued use and abuse — regression becomes inevita-
ble, leaving the addict feeling more and more helpless, unhappy, isolated,
and dysfunctional. The illusion of relief from life's problems is only the eye

of the storm, which intensifies as the cycle of addiction is set in motion. There is an inverse relationship between drug addiction and personal growth that is readily observable clinically. We see many people with personality traits such as self-centered entitlement, grandiosity, and a maddening capacity to feel injured and slighted who are only minimally capable of caring for themselves in an ongoing, sensible manner. These strikingly narcissistic features probably represent both the long-term, deleterious effects of drug use and developmental deficits predisposing to chemical dependency. In this way, addiction is progressive: " . . . the more individuals depend on a drug or alcohol to calm, activate, relate to others, play, etc., the less they develop capacities to achieve them normally, and more often and tragically they . . . undermine any existing capacities they might have developed" (Ref. 12, p. 22). Although drugs aid in self-regulation, they only provide a temporary and ultimately maladaptive solution — a pseudosolution — to life's problems.

## EGO-SELF DEFICITS: PROBLEMS IN SELF-REGULATION

The acrobat on the high wire maintains his stability by continual correction of his imbalance [13].

Gregory Bateson
*Mind and Nature*

Life can seem extremely precarious for people who lack the internal psychological resources necessary for self-regulation. Drugs can function as a kind of "prosthetic" [7] to temporarily correct these psychological impairments, or ego deficits. The preference for one drug over another is related to the particular needs that the drug effects meet or fulfill. It is this "fit" between drug and user that can become malignantly compelling and may eventually develop into an addictive relationship. Four areas of self-regulation impairment constituting psychological vulnerability that can predispose to problems with substance abuse and addiction are: (1) affects, (2) self-esteem, (3) self-other relationships, and (4) self-care [15].

### Affects

Feelings can, like every other aspect of our humanity, be corrupted from their original purpose [20].

Willard Gaylin
*Feelings*

Addicts and alcoholics seem to suffer from a variety of difficulties in relation to their feelings. These problems include a propensity to experience affects in the extreme, either as intense and overwhelming or with a sense of not feeling, i.e., emotional numbing. There is a great deal of confusion associated with feelings, including problems with recognition, identification, expression, and articulation of feelings [7–10,14–18]. Addicts are not known to be able to tolerate affect well, and it is a theme often referred to and repeated among people in AA and NA that their use of drugs and alcohol was an effort to cope with psychological suffering and distress. Certain drugs may be used to calm down, self-soothe, and reduce or obliterate intensely painful feelings; other drugs help enliven the personality, relieve depression, and offset a sense of inner emptiness.

## Self-Esteem

Self-esteem refers to a capacity consolidated over time, in which attitudes of one's value, worth, efficacy, and identity become integrated into the personality. This sense of oneself is more or less cohesive, more or less positive, and more or less stable throughout one's lifespan. A fragile and unstable sense of self tends to characterize the addict and alcoholic. Negative social attitudes toward this population further undermines self-esteem, as does the impact of accumulated negative consequences of addiction itself, including deteriorating health, disintegration of family and social relationships, loss of values and ideals. At the same time, addicts and alcoholics reveal life histories and early experiences that contribute to vulnerable self-esteem.

The sense of self is not only lacking in positive self-regard, but there is a scarcity of the inner resources we all need in order to cope with a range of stresses and life crises — ways to self-soothe, feel reassured, calm ourselves, and feel intact despite life's slings and arrows. When one cannot provide these functions, the internal response can be a form of anxiety in which the subjective feeling is fear of fragmentation or breakdown of the self. People with such narcissistic vulnerabilities may self-medicate with drugs and alcohol to shore up a depleted self and counter anxiety associated with diminished self-esteem.

## Self-Other Relationships

Satisfying relationships are extremely difficult for people who are not secure within themselves and have severe problems regulating their feelings. The need for others and longings for closeness are in conflict with fears of intimacy associated with disavowed dependency needs.

Addicts and alcoholics seem to suffer with poor boundaries, which contributes to their extreme discomfort in relationships. They tend to feel cut off and isolated, yet they fantasize union with a perfect other who will magically attend to unmet needs for nurturance and affirmation. Drugs and alcohol can allow such people to experience and express their split-off, denied longings, as well as to mollify disappointment and mute rageful reactions when such relationships founder. When feelings of loss and abandonment are overwhelming, drugs can be used to ease the pain. As we will discuss in the following sections, there may be important underlying reasons why loss and abandonment are so difficult for some people to bear, thereby setting them up to use drugs and alcohol as self-medication.

## Self-Care

Self-care depends on a number of ego functions such as judgment, self-esteem, reality testing, and regulation of affect [16]. The capacity to take care of oneself is acquired. It derives from early experiences of "good-enough mothering," [19] aspects of which the child internalizes and later can count on as reliable inner resources and guides to behavior. Some addicts and alcoholics can appear so deficient in this regard as to leave little doubt as to the veracity of the death instinct.

Defects in self-care functions betray developmental failures in that sufficient care, protection, and nurturance were not provided. At the same time, it is important to recognize that society's attitudes toward addicts and alcoholics have been ambivalent at the very least — and are very frequently uncaring, abandoning, and punitive. These social attitudes are also internalized, reinforcing the addict's already low self-esteem and undermining efforts at self-care.

The function of the affects is to serve as signals and guides to behavior [20–21]. We have seen that addicts suffer from serious impairments in the realm of feeling life. Therefore, it is not surprising that self-care poses particular challenges to this population. Nevertheless, we think it is important to appreciate drug and alcohol use as an attempt to take care of the self in meaningful ways, as has been pointed out in the foregoing discussion. Efforts to manage feelings, regulate self-esteem, and protect the self from overwhelming experiences represent adaptive strivings, not self-destructive impulses. How it is that some people seem so limited in their options and do so poorly for themselves will be explored in the following pages.

## TRAUMA REVISITED

In view of the horrendous life stories told by so many of our patients, the relative neglect by psychiatry of the issue of psychological trauma is almost as intriguing as the impact of trauma itself [22].

Bessel van der Kolk
*Psychological Trauma*

The role of trauma has been neglected and de-emphasized as a meaningful causative factor in the etiology of psychological disorders [22,23]. The psychoanalytic paradigm tends to filter out data related to actual traumatic events, dating back to Freud's renunciation of the seduction theory, when the heated issue of trauma was relegated to the back burner and rapidly cooled. Psychoanalysts became preoccupied with childhood fantasies and intrapsychic conflict rather than with the actual seduction of children [24]. There is, however, a large and growing body of research and clinical evidence suggesting that trauma does indeed play a major role in the production of mental disorders [23]. In fact, not since Freud has the issue of trauma and its relationship to mental functioning been grappled with as energetically as at present. The recent resurgence of interest surrounds the growing awareness and concern about the effects of child abuse, incest, and rape. With the inclusion of post-traumatic stress disorder (PSTD) in the DSM-III-R, psychiatry has finally come to recognize and describe the symptoms and syndrome surrounding uncontrollable and overwhelming life events.

In Freud's early writings, the nature of trauma was connected to external events such that "any experience which calls up distressing affects — such as those of fright, anxiety, shame, or physical pain — may operate as a trauma." [25] Since Freud, the concept has been revised, refined, and expanded. A number of recent theoreticians emphasize early parent-child relationships, and the needs of the developing infant for safety, protection, and loving comfort [26,27]. In addition to real losses, such as death, illness, hospitalization, and divorce, experiences of psychological separation and loss are also thought to constitute traumatization to the child. Traumatic disruptions in the affiliative bond can result from serious empathic failures on the part of the primary caretaker(s). This type of loss surrounds the inability or refusal of the parent to provide soothing comfort and loving reassurance to the helplessly dependent infant and reflects a fundamental lack of attunement to the child's primary needs. This kind of early environment can result in "insecure attachment" and be experienced as traumatic by the child [28].

The traumatic situation is thought to be connected to the overwhelming fear of loss and abandonment deriving from these early painful experiences. More damage results when the child's pain and discomfort arouse the anger, blame, and humiliation — or extreme anxiety and panic — of parent(s). When such negative parental responses are internalized, aspects of the child's inner self are perceived as dangerous and threatening and may be defended against in an effort to ward off anxiety and shame associated with basic needs and feelings. The most devastating form of trauma occurs when the trauma is actually inflicted on the child at the hands of the parents. This type of experience "is the most terrible and indescribable hell known to man" (Ref. 21, p. 145). Krystal agrees with Freud that the key issue is "the development of overwhelming affects." [21] The ego or sense of self is rendered psychologically helpless: "in the acute traumatic state one stands alone, abandoned by all sources of feelings of security" (Ref. 21, p. 168).

## TRAUMATIC ANTECEDENTS OF ADDICTION

The drug-dependent personality as such does not exist. There are a variety of factors and influences, however, which make drug use, abuse and dependence more likely . . . drugs are used to avoid impending psychic trauma in circumstances which would not be potentially traumatic to other people [10].

Krystal and Raskin
*Drug Dependence*

Whenever substance abuse enters the clinical picture, we face formidable diagnostic challenges. Symptoms may represent intoxication, withdrawal, the short- and long-term effects of addiction, as well as underlying core personality traits. Another complication surrounds the apparent contradiction of addictive behavior in that drugs not only relieve suffering—they also produce and perpetuate it. One of the present authors (E. J. Khantzian) has explored this issue in a previous report and suggests that strivings for mastery and control provide a context for us to better understand this strangely compelling paradox [29]. We will continue to elaborate on this theme with a particular focus on how drug use and addiction may be understood as self-medication of post-traumatic stress disorder. We will now consider early childhood trauma and its sequelae as constituting psychological vulnerability to addiction.

The trauma syndrome is a psychobiological phenomenon [30] and involves a biphasic response. The intrusive phase entails flooding memories and associated affects. Responses include hyperreactivity, startle reaction, flashbacks, nightmares, aggressive outbursts, and reenactments. In the numbing phase, memories and affects are blocked. Responses include emotional constriction, social isolation, anhedonia, avoidance of intimacy, and all-or-nothing affects [31].

Recent research also suggests that following trauma in early life, significant biochemical and neurophysiological alterations occur within the organism that can account for "hypersensitivity" and "overreaction." [32] Traumatic separation of infants from mothers seems to produce changes in critical neurotransmitter activities that affect heart rate, body temperature, and sleep. "These changes are not transient or mild, and their persistence suggests that long-term neurobiological alterations underlie the psychological effects of early separation" (Ref. 32, p. 43).

A significant proportion of patients in treatment for chemical dependencies and addictions reveal histories of abuse, neglect, violence, and incest and have grown up in dysfunctional and/or alcoholic families. A number of researchers find that long-term effects of childhood abuse include a psychological vulnerability and motivation to seek relief in drug and alcohol use [33]. The histories of narcotics addicts frequently reveal significant abuse and family violence, and it is important to consider that these addicts may be self-medicating painful feelings deriving from such early trauma [29].

Some of the ways in which drugs and alcohol can be used to alleviate PTSD symptoms are more obvious than others. Sleep disturbances, including nightmares, are problems with which alcohol, for instance, can temporarily help. Alcohol suppresses dreaming, as well as REM sleep [34]. Generally, the sedative-hypnotic drugs can be sought for self-medication of insomnia, anxiety, agoraphobia, and flashbacks. Stimulants can offset emotional numbing, isolation, depression, and anhedonia. Narcotics can ease physical pain associated with psychosomatic conditions, which also show up as features of PTSD.

As we consider the less obvious, more subtle, and sometimes paradoxical self-medication functions of drugs and alcohol, the centrality of affects and their vicissitudes becomes apparent. It will be useful to look beyond ego defects and consider the nature of "uncontrollable suffering," i.e., the perplexing problem of a preponderance of strong affects that exacerbate existing difficulties with self-care, self-esteem, and self-other relationships.

## TRAUMA, AFFECTS, AND ADDICTION

> The problem with people who have pent-up emotions is usually not their inability to express them, but their incredible capacity to generate them [20].

> Willard Gaylin
> *Feelings*

Recent research suggests that affects develop along a line of their own [21]. When children are not protected against overwhelming internal or external stimuli, they become seriously handicapped in their affect management and tolerance [31]. Affective responses become extreme — what we sometimes observe as the "all-or-nothing response to emotional stimulation." [31] This type of response makes it virtually impossible for affects to be used as signals or guides to behavior, their primary function. In other words, it is not only a matter of structural impairment, i.e., ego defects, but a situation in which the affects themselves become distorted and dysfunctional.

In 1970, Krystal and Raskin suggested that how a person learns to tolerate physical pain becomes a model for learning how to manage psychological pain. If these developmental tasks are poorly negotiated, the individual may become "subject to stress and trauma" and vulnerable to the effects of drugs he may seek out "for the relief from pain of physical or psychic origin, in order to be able to tolerate the stresses of everyday living" (Ref. 10, p. 167).

The concept of "everyday living," however, does not capture the psychic reality of the person who suffers with the type of "uncontrollable suffering" associated with post-traumatic stress disorder. In Krystal's recent work, he makes the point most poignantly: "One must appreciate the nature of the subjective experience of patients whose affect tolerance is impaired. They are persons who were traumatized in childhood, whose affects were allowed to flood them. Among the residues of such experiences is a lifelong dread of affects" (Ref. 21, p. 29). This profound fear, a form of annihilation anxiety, surrounds the expectation of the return of the traumatic state. If feelings represent and evoke ideas associated with trauma, they may come eventually to constitute the traumatic situation itself [21].

Ironically, addicts not only have problems with painful affects but also with "proleptic affects," i.e., those experienced in the process of expecting gratification [35]. Early trauma is implicated in such difficulties in that wishes for contact and closeness evoke painful feelings associated with separation and loss. Krystal notes that if not accompanied by "hope and confidence based on previous good experiences," pleasure can convert to discomfort and may operate as a "trauma signal," stimulating panic and other defensive maneuvers, among them the use of drugs and alcohol [21]. As we have noted above, drugs and alcohol can allow the experience of longed-for closeness while warding off the associated threat of loss and abandonment deriving from this type of early trauma.

The literature continues to support the hypothesis that early developmental issues, particularly of traumatic origin, lead to problems of "pervasive dysphoria" and a tendency to use and abuse drugs and alcohol. "The persistent difficulty with modulating the intensity of affect seems to be the reason why so many traumatized individuals medicate themselves with alcohol and drugs." [31,36]

*Case Illustration:*
Jean is a 30-year-old recovering addict and alcoholic, two and a half years clean and sober. A very bright, creative, and capable woman, she has achieved much for herself, despite a 16-year history of using and abusing a variety of drugs. She enjoys a challenging, high-level job, owns two homes, and has a solid network of good friends and colleagues. She grew up in an alcoholic home, in which she assumed an overly responsible caretaking role, particularly for an alcoholic fa-

ther, helping him up when he'd stumble and fall or pass out, as he frequently would, on the front steps or in the hall. Her mother drank heavily as well, but because "she wasn't as bad as my father," and for a variety of defensive reasons, Jean denied the reality and impact of her mother's alcoholism for many years.

From the time Jean was three, until at least the age of eight or nine, she was regularly sexually abused by her older brother and occasionally by his friends. These events have haunted her all of her life and have been the core issue of her therapy.

In the early phase of her recovery, however, and during the first year of her treatment, other issues were primary and pressed for immediate attention. These issues concerned powerful daily cravings for alcohol and her extreme difficulties with her feelings. Talking at all was very hard, sometimes excruciating, for her. Jean struggled valiantly, however, coming regularly to her sessions and persevering in her efforts to find words to say what she needed to say. At the same time, her desire to drink persisted, and her anxieties seemed as relentless as her cravings.

From the first session, and for many months, Jean was very nervous, almost agitated, constantly squirming in her chair, and always watching the clock. Her mouth would become very dry, and she always brought a Coke or coffee along with her. She seemed to feel only extremes of emotion: She was either overwhelmed to the point of panic, which sometimes included physical symptoms of nausea, dizziness, and stomach cramps, or she was emotionally constricted. She had a fear of "too much all at once," which she said made her feel as if she might start to vomit and never be able to stop. Sometimes she'd go "into the fog," which was a place of nonfeeling. She'd draw a straight line through the air as across a screen to indicate the experience of going numb and inner emptiness.

The therapy task became twofold: (1) to provide a safe environment in which Jean could observe and learn to manage her feeling life, and (2) to form a relationship in which she could learn to trust someone enough to be able to speak the unspeakable. After about a year, Jean began to talk more about her history of abuse. Affect tolerance greatly improved, as she began to be able to recognize, differentiate, and articulate her feelings. Somatic symptoms became rare, and her cravings have disappeared. She is becoming self-observant, and aware of the cognitive contents of her emotions. The trauma of her childhood continues to be very difficult for her to bear, but she presses on and finds ways to talk about what happened, including how she feels about it — her rage, sadness, fear, shame, self-blame, confusion, and the many losses it represents. She no longer seems to need to externalize her control issues. In addition to AA, which has been the mainstay of her sobriety, she has started to attend Al-Anon, which has been enormously supportive of her efforts to detach from her enmeshed and very demanding family. Very importantly, she is learning how to relax and enjoy herself — learning to tolerate positive as well as painful affects.

With two and a half years of sobriety, despite over a year of cravings, she has not relapsed. Recently, she lost 80 pounds under the care of a hospital-based weight-loss program. As she separates from her family and lets go of the need to be responsible for their lives and well-being, she seems to be able to take much better care of herself. She has insight into her years of addiction as an outcome of the trauma she has endured, its functions for her in her struggle to fit in, to manage her pain, and psychologically to survive the overwhelming circumstances of her childhood. Recently she reflected, "I think about what happened to me, you know, about my brother, and all those years of drugging and drinking . . . it's hard for me to think about. It hurts. I think it's all connected, and it really affected me. I used to drink to not feel, or to feel something else. Now I have the feelings and I'm grateful for that. I can talk about it now — before, I just felt sick or nervous or crazy, or nothing at all. Sometimes, like today, when it all feels like too much and I don't even want to come here, I still know that's what I need to do. If I can say the words, it helps somehow."

This case illustrates the relationship of early childhood trauma, severe problems with affect, and the use of drugs and alcohol to self-medicate painful feelings. Jean's drugs of choice were alcohol and marijuana. It seems that each drug was able to provide specific and particular functions that connect to symptoms of PTSD. When Jean felt numb, constricted, and going "into the fog," marijuana helped her feel activated and energized (she never tried cocaine because it frightened her as did the side effects of amphetamines). Alcohol, on the other hand, acted to soothe her and as an escape from the overwhelming experience of flashbacks, intrusive memories, and associated affects of shame and helplessness. Without drugs, Jean has been finding her way back to herself by learning to recognize, talk about, and value her feelings as integral to her healing, recovery, and self-esteem.

## SELF-ESTEEM, SELF-OTHER RELATIONSHIPS, AND SELF-CARE

Recognizing the impact of early trauma deepens our appreciation of how problems in self-esteem, relationships, and self-care can develop, are intimately interrelated, and can predispose to excessive use of alcohol and drugs.

Kohut conceptualized early "traumatic disappointment" to surround the mother's failure to respond empathically to the child's basic needs for affirmation, soothing, and security. He theorized that the developmental outcome would be fragile self-esteem, impairments in the ability to maintain narcissistic equilibrium, as well as significant difficulties in the capacity for self-care [37].

As we reconsider self-care deficits in the light of recent research on the response to trauma, we come to appreciate the centrality of affects. We have already noted that the trauma response is psychobiological [32]. Both the central nervous system and the autonomic nervous system are affected such that there is an exaggerated psychophysiological response to stimuli [21,32]. Alterations in neurotransmitter systems may provide a biological basis for psychopathology of affects, including hyperarousal, lack of affect tolerance, and extremes of affect response [32]. It becomes obvious that if the reaction to relatively minor stimuli takes on a proportion and intensity appropriate to emergency situations, the capacity for self-care can be virtually nullified. Ego functions such as judgment, reality testing, anticipation, exercise of reason, and all secondary processes are disrupted. This is because the ego is once again overwhelmed by the affects, carrying with them the memory of the original trauma. This is, in theory, how retraumatization occurs. Far from constituting a wish for self-destruction, the extreme self-care deficits we see in addicts and alcoholics are more likely to be functional impairments deriving from traumatic life experiences. Although ultimately maladaptive, the motivations to use drugs and alcohol to self-medicate represent very real efforts to care for the self.

Another dimension of the self-care issue derives from separation-individuation conflicts. When the traumatic situation entails empathic failures and an early environment lacking in sufficient attunement to the child's basic needs, self-care functions are not adequately internalized. They may even become sources of conflict in that they remain reserved for the "object" (i.e., the parent or parent figure) [21]. If these functions are not integrated within the evolving self-concept, the individual cannot feel comfortable or confident in his or her assumption of self-responsibility. It can feel difficult, if not impossible, to recognize and assess one's basic needs because of this type of inhibition. When autonomous strivings arouse such anxieties, the concept of drugs used as a prosthetic gains meaning: the drug functions as an external agent of control, allowing disavowal of the wish to exercise the basic self-regulation functions essential to one's survival and well-being.

It is also possible for a compelling association to be made such that treating oneself poorly may unconsciously represent the experience of closeness or contact with the abandoning parent who, for whatever reason, was unable to respond adequately to the child's needs. Addicts have a great deal of difficulty exercising self-soothing and self-caring functions, which may be due to these internalized prohibitions. The use of drugs to perform these functions can represent a compromise in that drugs can permit some experience, however illusory, of control while reducing anxiety associated with intense conflict. The creation of a drug-induced illusion of active mastery is preferable to the sense of being out of control and prey to one's overwhelming, unpredictable, and elusive emotions. In these ways, drug use and addiction may represent "the longing to regain alienated parts of oneself," [21] as well as to seek relief from painful affects associated with these profound injuries and losses.

The nature of this compromise helps us understand the "dual aspect" of addiction: the fact that drugs not only ease pain and suffering, they also perpetuate and exacerbate distress [29]. The adaptive context, within which we recognize addiction as a behavior motivated by wishes for mastery and control, helps resolve the paradox. Looking beyond the dual aspect of addiction to the dual aspect of human motivation can help us to appreciate more fully the significance of early trauma.

The term "repetition compulsion" describes peculiar patterns of behavior involving the not infrequent human tendency to recreate situations reminiscent of earlier traumatic experiences. Children also reconstruct in play themes that connect to difficult events that they experience as overwhelming, frightening, or painful. Underlying the simple pleasures of children's play, we see valuable, even critical, opportunities to rework problems out of which a sense of control and competency develops. It is important to recognize this behavior as healthy, adaptive, and even probably essential for normal development. When childhood events are too overwhelming, however, they may not be able to be integrated and assimilated. They may remain unresolved and go underground, i.e., be repressed, later to emerge as symptoms or psychopathology. In disguised and displaced forms, these behaviors evolve as adaptive efforts to master the earlier unresolved conflicts and traumas of childhood. Such conflicts involve the clash between the motivation or unconscious wish to achieve a sense of control that struggles against the unconscious prohibition against strivings for autonomy.

*Case Illustration:*
This is the sixth session with Dan, a 40-year-old drug addict, recently admitted to a methadone clinic. He has tried to "detox" off heroin after several years in another methadone program but, within 30 days, he was back on the street shooting dope. He uses other drugs, and currently cocaine is giving him a great deal of trouble. He says if it's offered, he cannot refuse. When the therapist inquired as to how Dan feels on coke, Dan appeared perplexed, then exclaimed, "I hate cocaine! I hate everything it does to me. I feel terrible, you know, nervous, paranoid, very uncomfortable. I don't know why I do it. I really don't." Curious, the therapist encouraged the client's apparent interest in this puzzle, commenting that it seemed rather unpleasant. He described how coke brings him "to the edge," "I don't want to go that way, you know," he added. Each time he does cocaine, which he either freebases or shoots, he feels himself closer to that edge. The whole point, he explained, is to get closer and closer without going over. As he talked, he became increasingly anxious. He said it frightened him to think about it. "I've never talked about this stuff before." The therapist wondered whether there might be any sense of relief, a kind of triumph each time he "wins"—as if he's defying fate. "Oh, yeah, that's it exactly!" He looked pleased, even enthusiastic, seemingly grateful to be understood, then grew suddenly pensive, and mused, almost to himself, "I don't know why I do it, I don't want to die! I have a son. Why am I doing this?"

The therapist didn't answer, and they sat together for a couple of minutes in silence. The therapist found herself associating to the movie, *The Deer Hunter*, and the game of Russian roulette the Chris Walken character played – the scene in which DeNiro finds Walken sitting at the table with a loaded revolver aimed at his head while the crowd places bets. Walken pulls the trigger. Click. The crowd roars and money is waving in the air. When the therapist referred to this scene, Dan was quick to recognize himself in it and acknowledged that there is a gain, at least momentarily, in the sense of control he achieves when he does coke the way he does. This is what he gets out of it, even though he "hates" it.

In *The Deer Hunter*, Walken had been fighting in Vietnam and suffered prolonged torture as a POW. What is especially noteworthy is his constriction, stony countenance, walled-off quality, dissociated state, and apparent absence of any anxiety or affect. He behaves robotically, mechanically, like one already dead emotionally. His appearance and behavior suggest the numbing response to trauma.

Dan's compulsion to repeat his near-disastrous experiences with cocaine are painful and conflicted. His capacity to observe and feel anxious about it, however, is what allows him to struggle with his drug dependency. As therapy has progressed, Dan has begun to talk about how it felt for him to be a child in his family. His parents' relationship was extremely conflictual and occasionally violent. When his parents argued or discussed anything "important," they spoke in Italian, effectively shutting Dan and the other children out, and inadvertently creating an atmosphere in which a great deal of strain and worry could flourish. Dan was constantly afraid his father would harm his mother and abandon all of them. He felt helpless to protect his mother and feels guilty about this. He is beginning to realize how stressful and difficult it was for him and how helpless he, in fact, truly was to change it. He recalls that, as an adolescent, he discovered that drugs and alcohol, particularly narcotics, could help him feel calm and soothed, as well as help him forget his family problems. It is also likely that his use of drugs provided a sense of control over a world that otherwise rendered him confused and helpless.

The traumatic nature of Dan's past extends beyond his fears of violence and abandonment. Not only his fears, but all his "needy" feelings, had to be suppressed, feelings that boys were not supposed to have and certainly not to express. He came to feel shame and humiliation, as well as a great deal of rage that he was never able to convey or learn to deal with. Not insignificantly, his original preference for opiates probably derived from a need to quench his rage. There is also an important link between the need to ward off painful feelings and the maintenance of self-esteem. "In post-traumatic states, the reactions to *having* the emotion, the requirement that anxiety be absent if self-respect is to be maintained, the tendency to depression whenever everything is not well—all of these perpetuate vicious circles that prolong and deepen painful affect states" (Ref. 21, p. 70). The negative associations to experiencing one's feelings threaten self-esteem because feelings are forbidden, dangerous, and associated with loss and abandonment, i.e., the threat of the original trauma.

In adolescence, when emotional intensity tends to peak and fluctuate in normal and expectable fashion, problems with affects can interfere with phase-appropriate mourning, a necessary developmental task promoting separation-individuation and identity formation. The need to ward off such dreaded feelings "provides the motivation to maintain a manic defense against the depressive affects by chemical means if necessary" (Ref. 21, p. 70). The relationship between affects and the fear of affects produces a synergistic effect that can become malignant and overwhelming, especially when drugs enter the picture.

Dan has been able to use therapy extremely well. He has insight into how he ambivalently seeks the effects of drugs to self-medicate painful feelings but also uses them to aid in self-regulation, i.e., to effect change and a sense of some control, ephemeral and self-defeating though it may be. He is becoming aware of a crucial aspect of his use and abuse of drugs as he increases his awareness of his history, as well as his role in perpetuating his pain. He is already able to appreciate the point that ultimately drug abuse can only amount to "substituting uncontrollable suffering with controlled suffering and replacing a dysphoria which they do not understand with a drug-induced dysphoria which they do understand" (Ref. 29, p. 20).

Dan's drug dependency may also represent a variant of what has been referred to as "addiction to trauma." [30] In this connection, we finally consider the peculiar phenomenon in which both addictive behaviors and traumatic experiences may provide self-medication functions for certain individuals in reciprocal and insidious fashion. Recent research has revealed a neurochemical basis for the compulsion to repeat stressful or traumatic experiences. The phenomenon "addiction to trauma" refers to the tendency of trauma victims to reexpose themselves voluntarily to situations reminiscent of the trauma. Reexposure to severe stress seems to evoke an endogenous opioid response, identical to that of exogenous opiates [30]. This means that the psychotropic effects of exogenous narcotics can be self-induced, including tranquilization, reduction of rage and aggression, antidepressant action, and analgesia. If an individual discovers that a correlate of the experience of severe stress is relief of pain and discomfort, he or she may be motivated unconsciously to seek out and cultivate stressful or crisis situations. These findings point to the possibility that the addictive process may have an environmentally determined biochemical basis. Rather incredibly, traumatic experience may set people up not only to be vulnerable to the effects of drugs and alcohol but also to be "chemically dependent," even before the first drink or drug. The work of van der Kolk suggests that individuals who have suffered massive trauma are likely to have an overactivated endogenous opiate system. On the basis of that theory, it is not unreasonable to speculate that such individuals periodically are in the equivalent of an opiate withdrawal state. The concomitant emotional state, irritability, and other features of instability might leave them particularly vulnerable to the corrective effects of drugs and alcohol.

## COMMENTS AND CONCLUSION

Addiction is a complex process and set of behaviors with multiple determinants and multiple functions and meanings. Impairments in the areas of affects, self-esteem, self-care, and relationships make up sectors of psychological vulnerability to addiction. These structural (ego) deficits can malignantly interact with the psychoactive properties of drugs and alcohol to potentiate the addictive process. Drug and alcohol abuse is best understood to serve an adaptive purpose of providing relief from painful feelings, creating the illusion of control and mastery, and reversing regressed states.

The literature, research, and clinical evidence suggest a significant relationship between trauma and addiction. Understanding the post-traumatic syndrome and symptomatology can deepen and clarify, as well as add complexity to, the self-medication functions of substance abuse and addiction. A pervading sense of helplessness underlies the dread of affects associated with trauma; drugs can serve to shore up a depleted sense of self by providing a temporary sense of competence and efficacy. Relationships can be overwhelming for people who suffered early experiences involving real or psychological losses and abandonments; drugs may be used to mute intense affects associated with conflictual longings for closeness that are also experienced as dangerous and herald the return of the traumatic state.

Putting affect into words has been, since Anna O., the centerpiece of all psychoanalytic psychotherapy. And yet the inability to talk about one's feelings (alexithymia) accounts for a great number of treatment failures [21,38]. Addicts and alcoholics are severely impaired in the realm of their affective experience. The case of Jean illustrates the primacy of these issues for recovering people.

Trauma can lead to a range of psychological and psychobiological vulnerabilities to use and abuse drugs and alcohol in an effort to self-medicate. Treatment must address these issues, not only after a period of initial sobriety or abstinence, as is the current practice, but in the earliest phases of recovery as well. Withdrawal symptoms and cravings, for example, may be related to, and complicated by, painful memories and/or affects, which can feel overwhelming to the newly recovering person as he or she becomes aware of the early trauma.

Alcoholics Anonymous is the most reliable and successful treatment modality for alcoholism and addiction. Individual and group psychotherapy have also proved effective, once abstinence has been attained, and these approaches may be effectively combined and integrated with self-help programs [41,42]. In the present context and in consideration of the problems trauma victims suffer with, we must emphasize the efficacy of AA and recommend it as essential, if not primary, treatment. In working with trauma survivors, the group approach is considered to be a particularly useful modality. "Most people need some form of social support to overcome the effects of trauma." [39] Since addiction itself may be considered a form of trauma, [40] this is especially valid. Alcoholics Anonymous offers the kind of supportive structure recovering addicts and trauma victims require. "It is the reliving in the context of an interpersonal relationship that . . . begins the curative process." [23] Alcoholics Anonymous offers such an opportunity. For many important reasons beyond the scope of this paper, AA can be said to be a profound and sophisticated form of intensive treatment. The group provides an affirming, accepting, attuned environment and the opportunity to integrate and heal the self in the context of empathic human interaction and contact. We have described elsewhere how such group experiences also correct self-governance problems by challenging self-sufficient, narcissistic defenses, at the same time offering opportunities to listen to and tell stories that correct affect and self-care deficits [42].

Issues of dual diagnosis need to be reconsidered in the light of our understanding of trauma, PTSD, and addiction. The self-medication hypothesis can be especially useful, helping us to think through motivation and the nature of the difficulties addicts have with self-regulation. We see that early childhood trauma must be carefully considered in the etiology of both mental illness and the addictions. A very high percentage of psychiatric patients have such histories, as do addicts and alcoholics. The symptoms of PTSD can be confusing, even misleading, [23] and challenge us to refine our diagnostic skills.

For example, symptoms that represent dissociated reliving of past traumas are "potentially confusing and produce misinterpretation and clinical errors." [23] Anxiety disorders and panic states may represent symptoms of PTSD [19]. The secondary reactions to trauma can mask the underlying issue, such as emotional constriction, acting out, and drug and alcohol abuse. "These maladaptations often make it very difficult at first to establish the proper diagnosis of PTSD." [31] There is a striking overlap among borderline personality PTSD and the addictions [24]. The clinical pictures are almost identical and replicate the areas of self-regulation disturbance we find in people with addictive disorders.

To summarize, early childhood trauma can be said to powerfully potentiate vulnerability to the addictive process. Among the long-term effects of childhood abuse is a predisposition to seek relief in drugs and alcohol in an effort to control uncontrollable suffering. The adaptive context helps us resolve the apparent paradox of the dual aspect of addiction as we recognize strivings to heal, restore, and reintegrate the injured self. Within this context, we can formulate and appropriately attune treatment strategies and more empathically respond to those of our patients who suffer with these extremely difficult and resistant problems.

## REFERENCES

1.  Milne AA. *Winnie-the-Pooh*. New York: Dutton, 1926.
2.  Freud S. *Three Essays on the Theory of Sexuality, 1905*. In: *Stanford Edition*. Vol. 7. London: Hogarth, 1955.
3.  Abraham K. The psychological relation between sexuality and alcoholism. In: *Selected Papers of Karl Abraham*. New York: Basic Books, 1960.
4.  Rado S. The psychoanalysis of pharmacothymia (drug addiction). *Psychoanalyt Quart* 1933; 2:1.
5.  Freud S. *Beyond the Pleasure Principle. SE* 1920; 18:7–61.
6.  Glover E. On the etiology of drug addiction. In: *On the Early Development of the Mind*. New York: International Universities Press, 1956.
7.  Weider H, Kaplan EH. Drug use in adolescents: psychodynamic meaning and pharmacolgenic effect. *Psychoanalyt Study Child* 1969; 24:399–431.
8.  Milkman H, Frosch WA. On the preferential abuse of heroin and amphetamine. *J Nerv Ment Dis* 1973; 156:242–248.
9.  Wurmser L. Psychoanalytic considerations of the etiology of compulsive drug use. *J Am Psychoanalyt Assoc* 1974; 22:820–843.
10. Krystal H, Raskin HA. *Drug Dependence: Aspects of Ego Functions*. Detroit: Wayne State University Press, 1970.
11. Khantzian EJ, Mack JE, Schatzberg AA. Heroin use as an attempt to cope: clinical observations. *Am J Psychiatr* 1974; 131:160–164.
12. Khantzian EJ. Self selection and progression in drug dependence. *Psychiatr Digest* 1975; 10:19–22.
13. Bateson G. *Mind and Nature*. New York: Dutton, 1979.
14. Khantzian EJ. The self-medication hypothesis of addictive disorders: focus on heroin and cocaine dependence. *Am J Psychiatr* 1985; 142:1259–1264.
15. Khantzian EJ. Self-regulation and self-medication factors in alcoholism and the addictions: similarities and differences. In: *Recent Developments in Alcoholism*. Vol. 8. Galanter M, ed. New York and London: Plenum, 1990.

16. Khantzian EJ. The ego, the self and opiate addiction: theoretical and treatment considerations. *Int Rev Psychoanal* 1978; 5:189–198

17. Khantzian EJ. An ego-self theory of substance dependence. In: *Theories of Addiction*. NIDA Monograph #30. Lettieri EJ, Sayers M, Wallenstein HW, eds. Rockville, MD: National Institute of Drug Abuse, 1980.

18. Khantzian EJ, Halliday KS, McAuliffe, WE. *Addiction and the Vulnerable Self: Modified Dynamic Group Therapy for Substance Abusers.* New York: The Guilford Press, 1990.

19. Winnicott DW. Transitional objects and transitional phenomena. *Int J Psychoanal* 1953; 34:89–97.

20. Gaylin W. *Feelings: Our Vital Signs.* New York: Harper & Row, 1979.

21. Krystal H. *Integration and Self-Healing: Affect, Trauma, Alexithymia.* Hillsdale, NJ: Analytic Press, 1988.

22. van der Kolk BA. *Psychological Trauma.* Washington, DC: American Psychiatric Press, 1987.

23. Chu JA. The repetition compulsion revisited: reliving dissociated trauma. Presented at the International Conference of Multiple Personality and Dissociative States. Nov. 6, 1987.

24. Herman JL, van der Kolk BA. Traumatic antecedents of borderline personality disorder. In: *Psychological Trauma.* van der Kolk B, ed. Washington, DC: American Psychiatric Press, 1987.

25. Freud S, Breuer J. *On the Psychical Mechanism of Hysterical Phenomena: Preliminary Communication (1893).* In: *Standard Edition,* London: Hogarth, 1955; 2:1–18.

26. Lindemann E. Symptomatology and management of acute grief. *Am J Psychiatr* 1944; 101:141–148.

27. Kohut H. *The Restoration of the Self.* New York: International Universities Press, 1977.

28. Krugman S. Trauma in the family: perspectives on the intergenerational transmission of violence. In: *Psychological Trauma.* van der Kolk B, ed. Washington, DC: American Psychiatric Press, 1987.

29. Khantzian EJ. Substance dependence, repetition, and the nature of addictive suffering. Presented at the 76th Annual Meetings Amer. Psychoanalytic Association. Chicago, IL, May 9, 1987. (unpublished manuscript).

30. van der Kolk BA, Greenberg MS. The psychobiology of the trauma response: hyperarousal, constriction, and addiction to traumatic reexposure. In: *Psychological Trauma.* van der Kolk B, ed. Washington, DC: American Psychiatric Press, 1987.

31. van der Kolk BA. The psychological consequences of overwhelming life experiences. In: *Psychological Trauma.* van der Kolk B, ed. Washington, DC: American Psychiatric Press, 1987.

32. van der Kolk BA. The separation cry and the trauma response: developmental issues in the psychobiology of attachment and separation. In: *Psychological Trauma.* van der Kolk B, ed. Washington, DC: American Psychiatric Press, 1987.

33. Herman JL, Russell DE, Trocki K. Long-term effects of incestuous abuse in childhood. *Am J Psychiatr* 1986; 143:10.
34. Williams H, Salamy A. Alcohol and sleep. In: *The Biology of Alcoholism*. Vol. 2. Kissen B, Begleiter H, eds. New York: Plenum, 1973.
35. Spitz RA. Ontogenesis: the proleptic function of emotion. In: *Expression of the Emotions in Man*. Knapp PH, ed. New York: International University Press, 1963.
36. Lacoursiere R, Godfrey K, Rubey L. Traumatic neurosis in the etiology of alcoholism. *Am J Psychiatr* 1986; 137:966–968.
37. Kohut H. *The Analysis of the Self*. New York: International Universities Press, 1971.
38. Krystal H. Alexithymia and Psychotherapy. *Am J Psychother* 1979; 33(1).
39. van der Kolk BA. The role of the group in the origin and resolution of the trauma response. In: *Psychological Trauma*. van der Kolk B, ed. Washington, DC: American Psychiatric Press, 1987.
40. Bean-Bayog M. Psychopathology produced by alcoholism. In: *Psychopathology and Addictive Disorders*. Meyer RE, ed. New York and London: Guilford, 1986.
41. Khantzian EJ. The primary care therapist and patient needs in substance abuse treatment. *Am J Drug Alc Abuse* 1988; 14(2):159–167.
42. Khantzian EJ, Mack JE. Alcoholics Anonymous and contemporary psychodynamic theory. In: *Recent Developments in Alcoholism*. Vol. 7. Galanter M, ed. New York: Plenum, 1989:67–89.

# 12

## Psychopathology Resulting from Substance Abuse

### Charles A. Dackis

*Hampton Hospital, Rancocas, New Jersey*

### Mark S. Gold

*Fair Oaks Hospital, Summit, New Jersey and Delray Beach, Florida*

Psychiatrists are often asked to evaluate substance abusers and furnish much of their physician-related care. This situation would seem appropriate since psychiatric symptoms are frequently intermingled in the addict's clinical presentation. Psychiatrists are certainly most capable of recognizing and treating autonomous psychiatric disorders when necessary. On the other hand, it is important that psychiatrists exercise restraint when diagnosing and treating psychiatric syndromes that might be substance-induced. This is particularly challenging when the substance abuse is covert, as is often the case. It is nonetheless crucial to distinguish primary from secondary psychiatric illness since the treatment, prognosis, and clinical courses often differ significantly. Furthermore, unnecessary diagnoses and treatment might adversely affect recovery from addiction. This paper will outline the major types of psychiatric syndromes produced by addiction and review the diagnostic process of distinguishing these syndromes from autonomous psychiatric disorders.

## RECOGNIZING ADDICTION IN PSYCHIATRIC PATIENTS

Drug addiction has only recently been conceptualized as a separate and autonomous disorder. Corresponding expertise and training among physicians have led to refinement in our understanding of the biological basis, pathophysiology, and natural course of addiction. We now see the brain's reward center as the organ of involvement in substance abuse, much as the lung is the target organ of pneumonia.

Substance abusers are most effectively recognized, diagnosed, and treated when the crucial dynamics of addiction are understood. Drug-induced euphoria and drug craving are the major reinforcers of addiction. Euphoria resulting from the drug's pharmacological stimulation of reward centers in the brain [1] serves as a positive reinforcer, motivating repetitive drug use. The most natural behavior of addicts is to administer their drug of choice, regardless of their protest to the contrary. The reinforcing power of cocaine can be appreciated by the fact that it is repeatedly self-administered by monkeys to the point of death [2]. Over time, drug craving develops as a powerful negative reinforcer. We theorized that craving also results from the biological disruption (depletion) of reward centers by chronic drug exposure [3]. Since these reward centers are involved in natural drive states, [1] drug craving can be conceptualized as an "acquired primary drive" [4] and represents a formidable obstacle to the addict's recovery. Craving and euphoria alternate as negative and positive reinforcers to form an entrenched cycle of addiction that eventually drives itself. As the addict gradually loses control over the cycle of addiction, impairment develops in interpersonal, occupational, and medical areas. This impairment is persistently rationalized, denied, and minimized until reality intrudes and forces the addict to admit his degree of impairment.

When evaluating psychiatric symptoms, it is essential to avoid missing the diagnosis of addiction. Unlike most conditions in medicine, addiction is an affliction from which the patient initially does not want to recover. Drug addicts (including alcoholics) typically deny and minimize their impairment until irresistible family, financial, legal, or occupational pressures bear down on them. However, when seeking treatment for psychiatric or medical manifestations of addiction, the addict is often not yet ready to cease drug use and may attempt to conceal his addiction. In some cases, obfuscation is cleverly created by the patient solely to obtain a supply of addictive prescription drugs. Unfortunately, the physician must often play the role of detective to avoid misdiagnosis and inappropriate treatment of these patients.

Nearly all psychiatric syndromes can be precipitated by addiction. Depression, anxiety, psychosis, and personality disorders may all result solely from the effects of addiction, and the most difficult factor preventing the identification of addiction is often the addict's denial and dishonesty. Aside from fabrications and minimizations, there is usually a degree of defensiveness in response to questions about substance abuse. In fact, defensiveness should raise the clinician's index of suspicion for addiction. Further exploration of more objective information from the family, friends, job, or court should be pursued when addiction is suspected. Other objective measures are also more reliable than the addict, such as laboratory studies, physical examinations and past medical records.

Often, psychiatrists are tempted to view addiction as secondary to psychiatric illness and fail to appreciate the powerful biological roles of euphoria and craving. Psychiatric symptoms might even be misconceived as the cause of substance abuse when they actually result from intoxication, withdrawal, or protracted withdrawal. While self-medication of underlying psychiatric symptoms is sometimes an important dynamic in the perpetuation of addiction, it is certainly not a necessary ingredient [5] and is seldom more powerful than craving and euphoria. Furthermore, entrenched addiction will not remit solely on the basis of psychiatric stabilization but usually requires drug rehabilitation, which often differs radically from the psychiatric approach.

## MEDICAL EVALUATION

Medical evaluation of the substance abuser has been reviewed elsewhere [4] and is beyond the scope of this paper. It is emphasized now because the medical evaluation should be the starting point of any proper evaluation of the substance abusers. Aside from the obvious effects of intoxication and withdrawal, medical conditions that can mimic psychiatric illness must be ruled out before a reliable psychiatric diagnosis can be made. A full medical history and review of systems, comprehensive laboratory testing, and thorough physical examination should be obtained in *all* substance abusers prior to their psychiatric evaluation. The examining physician should be familiar with intoxication and withdrawal syndromes and with medical complications related to the route of administration and direct tissue toxicity by drugs and their adulterants. Laboratory testing should include routine blood counts, chemistries, and a properly collected and analyzed urine screen for drugs of abuse [6]. When acute intoxication or overdose is suspected, blood screens are more useful. Antibody testing for hepatitis, HTLV-III, and syphyllis is also recommended in many substance abusers. Since patients often minimize or omit crucial medical information, friend or family informants and past medical records are essential in obtaining an accurate history.

Psychiatric disorders cannot be reliably diagnosed until intoxication and withdrawal effects have resolved. After ruling out acute overdose [7–9], the most important medical issue in evaluating substance abusers is drug withdrawal. Untreated sedative-hypnotic and alcohol withdrawal can induce seizures and, as potentially fatal conditions, should never be overlooked. Polysubstance abuse with covert sedative or alcohol dependence should be suspected until information is obtained from the urine screen and other informants. Objective signs of drug withdrawal are more reliable than patient complaints. Although alcohol detoxification can usually be completed within several days, benzodiazepine and barbiturate detoxification may take several weeks, and clinicians should be familiar with appropriate detoxification protocols [10]. With mixed opiate and sedative/hypnotic dependence, sedative withdrawal is best completed before opiate detoxification [11].

## PSYCHIATRIC EVALUATION OF SUBSTANCE ABUSERS

Before reviewing specific psychiatric conditions that result from substance abuse, general principles in the overall diagnostic approach to these patients will be emphasized. Three possible diagnostic situations exist in these dually diagnosed patients. First, the psychiatric disorder may be purely secondary to the addiction, which is the focus of this paper. Examples include cocaine hallucinosis and anxiety secondary to alcohol withdrawal. These psychiatric symptoms are usually the result of intoxication, withdrawal, or protracted withdrawal syndromes. The second situation arises when substance abuse results entirely from attempts to self-medicate underlying psychiatric symptoms. Agoraphobics may overuse alcohol or benzodiazepines only for symptom relief and may not be truly addicted. It should be appreciated that self-medication may lead to entrenched addiction that does not remit with psychiatric stabilization alone. Third, addiction and psychiatric disorders may coexist, as in the case of the heroin addict with bipolar disease. It is essential to clarify which of the three diagnostic situations exists because the treatment approach will either be predominantly rehabilitative, psychiatric, or a mixture of both. In this last case, there is a significant recidivism risk since failure of either treatment generally leads to a continuation of both disorders [5]. A successful outcome depends on the skillful coordination and integration of psychiatric and rehabilitative approaches. Otherwise, these divergent therapies and their respective proponents will dictate contradictory messages to the patient.

Reliable psychiatric diagnoses in drug addicts cannot be made without some passage of time to eliminate intoxication, withdrawal, and protracted withdrawal effects. This time varies according to substances use and severity of dependence, although a two-week "washout" period after the completion of detoxification is usually sufficient. During the drug-free period, attention is directed toward any gradual diminution or spontaneous remission resolution of psychiatric symptoms.

One difficulty inherent in the psychiatric evaluation of addicts is the assurance that the patient is indeed drug-free. Serial assessments of intoxication and withdrawal for all major classes of addictive agents must be made over the course of treatment since covert drug use is common in this population. Random urine monitoring is also advisable, especially in outpatients. Pharmacological treatment of active users should be avoided since it may be unnecessary, could cause dangerous interactions with abused agents, and implies that drug abuse is medically condoned. Abstinence should be persistently encouraged, and termination of psychiatric treatment should be considered in cases of continued abuse.

Knowledge of the drug addict mentality will diminish inaccuracies in psychiatric diagnosis. These individuals are accustomed to feeling states that exceed the normal range and often have difficulty discerning more subtle feelings of anxiety, depression, or anger. Denial and minimization also distort their actual perceptions and recollections. Lying to avoid a psychiatric diagnosis, fulfill a hidden agenda, or obtain mood-altering medications may also complicate the evaluation and treatment plan. Substance abusers are unreliable historians, necessitating the use of informants and objective clinical observations.

A reliable past psychiatric history is often difficult to obtain. Psychiatric symptoms experienced during periods of active addiction are confounded by many effects of addictive agents. Attention should therefore be directed toward psychiatric symptoms that occurred during significant periods of abstinence or preceding addiction. Family reports may be helpful to verify reports of past abstinence and identity past psychiatric symptoms. If major psychiatric illness has been present prior to the onset of addiction or during significant periods of drug abstinence, an autonomous psychiatric diagnosis is more likely. A positive psychiatric family history also increases the likelihood of psychiatric illness.

In many clinical situations, hospitalization is a necessary intervention [10]. Psychiatric instability in the form of suicidality, psychosis, violence, and mania usually justifies hospitalization. Impaired judgment or reliance on self-medication of active psychiatric symptoms may interfere with outpatient rehabilitation and necessitate inpatient treatment. This is especially true when outpatient treatments have been unsuccessfully attempted. Finally, medical instability involving abstinence syndromes or active complications of addiction are more safely treated in the hospital. Intravenous use is often an indication for hospitalization due to increased severity of addiction and risks of medical complications. Hospitalization provides much more assurance that active use has ceased and allows for a more comprehensive medical and psychiatric evaluation.

## DEPRESSION

Depression is a common complaint of drug addicts and may result from primary affective illness, situational aspects of the addictive life-style, drug withdrawal, and protracted withdrawal. Protracted withdrawal has not been well researched for the various addictive agents but appears to involve neurochemical disruptions in the brain mood with the chronic use of stimulants, [3] opiates, [12] and alcohol [13]. The psychiatric evaluation should clearly distinguish patients requiring antidepressants from those likely to experience spontaneous resolution of depression with abstinence. Since the diagnosis of major depression can be made only when symptoms are not attributable to an organic cause, [14] and addiction may constitute an organic basis, past or present periods of abstinence must be scrutinized. In addition, a family history of depression raises the probability of affective illness. The self-medication of underlying depression with addictive drugs is a widely held, but probably overrated, concept [5]. For instance, while Freud first speculated that cocaine users may be self-medicating depression, [15] actual research has found that cocaine exacerbates depression [16].

Alcoholism has been associated with depression and suicidality throughout the psychiatric literature [13]. Evaluating depressive symptoms in alcoholics is difficult since many depressive symptoms, such as insomnia, anergia, decreased libido, guilt, and suicidality, are also characteristic of alcoholism. Current research suggests that alcohol-induced organic affective syndromes are common and are clinically indistinguishable from major depression on a cross-sectional basis [13]. Longitudinally, these syndromes can be easily distinguished from major depression since spontaneous remission usually occurs within a two-week period of sobriety in 80% of cases [13]. Neuroendocrine testing with the dexamethasone suppression test (DST) is a useful confirmatory test when performed after two weeks of sobriety, [17,18] but the thyrotropin-releasing hormone (TRH) test cannot distinguish depressed from nondepressed alcoholics [17].

It is imperative that the clinical implications of a severe, but rapidly resolving, affective syndrome in alcoholics be recognized. Antidepressant medications should not be prescribed for active alcoholics because the appropriate treatment is much more likely to be a period of sobriety. Clinicians should therefore be pressing for sobriety rather than prescribing medications. Furthermore, the diagnosis of major depression cannot be reliably made until two weeks of sobriety rules out the likely possibility of alcohol-induced organic affective syndrome [14]. This period should be lengthened if an improving trend is evident because protracted organic affective syndromes attributable to alcohol may occur. On the other hand, an obvious history of major depression during alcohol-free periods or persistent suicidality might justify a more rapid decision to medicate. It should be added that patients with alcohol-induced depression, unlike patients with major depression, are not subject to recurrences of depression during sobriety. Rather than drinking because they are depressed, most alcoholics appear to be depressed because they drink.

Opiate addicts have been reported by several investigators to have high rates of depression [12,18]. Prevalence rates of 17% were found for major depression in patients maintained on methadone, [18] while recently detoxified heroin- and methadone-dependent patients had rates of 25% and 60% respectively [12]. Based on these high prevalence rates, clinicians should maintain a high index of suspicion for depression in opiate addicts.

Although it has been proposed in the psychiatric literature that opiate addicts are actually medicating underlying depression, [19] we suggested that depression is often opiate-induced, based on several lines of neurochemical evidence [12]. Opiates produce a number of alterations in endogenous opoid and the intimately related hypothalamic-pituitary-adrenal (HPA) axis that are also found in major depression [20]. Neurochemical disruptions may result from the "shutdown" of beta-endorphin systems in the brain and pituitary gland by exogenous opioids [21]. Disruptions of central norepinephrine [11] may contribute to depression. In addition, the high prevalence of depression in these patients is correlated with the severity of their opiate dependence [12]. Because of high rates of recidivism with depressed opiate addicts, [18] persistent depression after the completion of detoxification should be treated aggressively. Depression in opiate addicts, even if it is a result of protracted withdrawal, does not usually resolve rapidly with abstinence, as seen in the case of alcohol. Antidepressant medications are often necessary for symptom relief and are usually effective [22]. Since opiates may induce depression, depressed individuals maintained on methadone might benefit from detoxification and antidepressant treatment. It is unfortunate that opiate addicts must often overcome the three barriers of withdrawal, craving, and depression before their recovery is on a firm foundation. Their recovery rates are enhanced if the clinician recognizes and treats associated depression.

Sedative-hypnotics are widely prescribed and frequently abused alone or in conjunction with other drugs. The most commonly prescribed agents in this class are the benzodiazepines. While these medications have been heavily marketed and widely prescribed for the treatment of anxiety [23] and even depression, their addictiveness is often unappreciated by physicians and iatrogenic benzodiazepine dependence is probably a frequent occurrence. Patients notoriously omit or minimize benzodiazepine use, perhaps in part because of their physician's nonchalant attitude toward the addictive potential. Sedative withdrawal rarely mimics depression and is much more likely to produce or exacerbate anxiety syndromes. Certain depressive target symptoms, including insomnia, irritability, and psychomotor agitation, may be due to sedative withdrawal, which should not be confused with major depression. Since sedative detoxification may require several weeks of dose reduction, and a full depressive syndrome is not characteristically induced, antidepressant treatment may be indicated before the completion of detoxication.

Central stimulants, particularly cocaine and amphetamine, produce severe withdrawal ("crash") states that share many characteristics with major depression. Anergia, psychomotor retardation, depressed mood, irritability, low self-esteem, guilt, and suicidality are often present [24]. Hyperphagia and hypersomnia are found with stimulant withdrawal, while major depression usually involves anorexia and insomnia. Crashing states generally remit within several days of abstinence after cocaine bingeing, do not include craving, and occur in the context of previous binge/crash cycles. The etiology of the stimulant crash is likely to be due to the depletion of catecholamines, dopamine, and norepinephrine [25]. Inhibition of the thyroid axis after successive stimulation effects during stimulant intoxication may also contribute to crashing symptoms [26].

The initial washout period is generally sufficient to distinguish stimulant withdrawal from a depressive episode. Crashing symptoms in "pure" cocaine abusers can usually be discerned from major depression during the first week of abstinence. However, cocaine is usually abused in conjunction with other substances. Alcohol dependence is common in cocaine abusers, and alcohol-induced mood effects may confound their evaluation. When other drugs of abuse, such as sedatives, marijuana, or opiates, are found by history or urine testing, their effects on mood should also be considered. Crashing symptoms can be reversed with the dopamine agonists bromocriptine [25,27] and amantadine [27]. In most cases, the stimulant crash remits spontaneously within several days, and dopamine agonists are used in treating craving, [28,29] which is a more important and persistent force in perpetuating stimulant addiction.

There is no proven role for neuroendocrine testing for depression in stimulant addicts. The DST has not been researched with regard to diagnostic reliability for major depression in stimulant abusers. Amphetamine releases plasma cortisol in man [30] and causes adrenocortical hypertrophy in animals, [31] suggesting that stimulant use, in and of itself, may produce cortisol hypersecretion and that the DST is therefore nonspecific for depression. The TRH test has been researched and is not specific for depression in cocaine abusers [26]. One depressive symptom, decreased libido, can result from cocaine's effect on prolactin and dopamine systems [32]. Depressive symptoms persisting beyond the cocaine crash and not attributable to other substances of abuse generally respond to standard antidepressant therapy. Since tricyclic antidepressants such as desipramine are effective treatments for depression and may also diminish stimulant craving, [33] their trial is a logical starting point.

Marijuana abuse on a regular basis produces an amotivational state that could be confused with major depression. Because of its prolonged presence in the urine, marijuana abuse is easily recognized in urine samples, and chronic use may be associated with tetrahydrocannabinol (THC) levels for several weeks [34]. Psychomotor retardation, decreased concentration, decreased libido, paranoia, and guilty ruminations may be seen during intoxication states. Decreased libido may result from the inhibition of testosterone by marijuana [35]. Marijuana intoxication is best demonstrated by plasma levels or clinical signs such as mydriasis, red conjunctivae, tachycardia, tremor, dry mouth, ataxia, and nystagmus. In our experience, marijuana-induced mood effects may continue for several days but are seldom sufficiently severe to produce a syndrome comparable to major depression.

## ANXIETY

Anxiety is the hallmark of early recovery from addiction and may help to motivate the addict. At the onset of treatment, substance abusers often face the loss of their family, job, and financial security. It is therefore understandable and appropriate that they experience anxiety commensurate with their precarious situations. The indiscriminate medicating of anxiety should be avoided, as addicts must try to tolerate unpleasant feelings without relying on drugs whenever possible. Many abstinence syndromes and intoxication states involve anxiety that should not be diagnosed as independent anxiety disorders. On the other hand, patients with anxiety disorders may become drug-dependent through self-medication, especially with sedative-hypnotics, alcohol, and opiates. The evaluation of drug addicts for anxiety should clearly distinguish drug intoxication and acute withdrawal from separate anxiety disorders that require specific pharmacotherapy.

Intoxication with cocaine, amphetamine, marijuana, hallucinogens, and phencyclidine may produce panic symptoms and anxiety and should be evaluated with plasma testing, a careful history, and physical examination. These agents produce tachycardia, hypertension, diaphoresis, hyperthermia, and mydriasis. PCP also produces characteristic salivation, muscle rigidity, myoclonus, and nystagmus, while hallucinogens cause flushing. These physical signs and those of marijuana intoxication already described should be scrutinized in anxious (and psychotic) substance abusers. A washout period corresponding to the duration of action of the drug in question is essential before anxiety disorders can be diagnosed.

Sedative, alcohol, and opiate withdrawal include anxiety and should always be recognized on clinical grounds and treated appropriately. The clinical identification of drug withdrawal and detoxification has been described elsewhere [10]. Complaints of anxiety may also be feigned to procure drugs during detoxification. Although the diagnosis of anxiety disorder should be postponed until detoxification has been completed, there are instances when anxiolytic treatment is indicated before the completion of lengthy detoxification. Patients with incapacitating anxiety may benefit from supplemental beta-blockers during detoxification from sedatives. Antidepressants may also be necessary during detoxification when severe panic attacks do not respond to detoxification alone. In these cases, a panic disorder diagnosis remains in question but is likely.

Alcoholics have a high prevalence of anxiety  due to its inclusion in alcohol withdrawal and their predisposition to underlying panic disorder and social phobia [36]. Since alcohol withdrawal usually resolves within one week of sobriety, it can generally be discerned from anxiety disorders during this time period. Covert benzodiazepine abuse often occurs with alcoholics and should be assessed with urine screening *before* starting detoxification with benzodiazepines. True panic disorder usually precedes alcohol abuse, is present during periods of sobriety, and is frequently associated with mitral valve prolapse [37]. Social phobia responds well to beta-blockers. It is especially important to ameliorate social phobia in alcoholics since it interferes with their attendance at, and participation in, AA meetings.

Sedative-dependent patients pose complex diagnostic issues with regard to anxiety. Barbiturates, benzodiazepines, glutethimide, and methaqualone may require prolonged detoxification lasting several weeks. Anxiety during this period could result from acute or protracted withdrawal. Physical signs, including hypertension, tremor, diaphoresis, tachycardia, and hyperreflexia, corroborate the presence of acute withdrawal. Protracted anxiety syndromes associated with insomnia may last for several months, with gradual and irregular remission, perhaps stemming from pharmacokinetic properties and induced neuroreceptor changes [38,39]. Efforts should be made to avoid medicating the patient experiencing protracted withdrawal, and the prescribing of addictive sedatives is obviously counterindicated once acute withdrawal has resolved.

Opiate addicts report intense panic anxiety during withdrawal. Opiate withdrawal involves the physiological activation of central norepinephrine as the nucleus locus ceruleus rebounds from chronic inhibition by exogenous opiates [11,21]. Because of its similar clinical profile, acute opiate withdrawal cannot be reliably distinguished from panic anxiety, which should be diagnosed only after the completion of detoxification. Methadone-dependent patients may experience protracted withdrawal, including anxiety, for several months after detoxification, with gradual and irregular resolution [40]. These patients may seek psychiatric care and are at risk of receiving addictive sedatives, which will usually reactivate their opiate use or serve as substitute agents of abuse. Self-medication with alcohol is also seen. Empiric pharmacotherapy with nonaddictive agents, including clonidine and beta-blockers, may be effective, although there is little research in this area. Primary anxiety disorders in opiate-dependent patients can be treated conventionally but should be diagnosed carefully and only after withdrawal effects have resolved.

If a primary anxiety disorder coexists with addictive illness, a coordinated psychiatric and rehabilitative treatment approach is imperative. Untreated panic anxiety will interfere with recovery and places the addict at risk of relapse in the pursuit of symptom relief. Self-help groups often convey the notion that panic anxiety is merely protracted withdrawal, which can make some patients very resistant to pharmacotherapy. Resistance to drug rehabilitation occurs in the sedative addict who will not admit to the enjoyment of, and desire for, sedative intoxication (craving and euphoria), and addiction will usually continue in these patients since denial has not been addressed and sedative abuse is rationalized as medicinal in nature. Benzodiazepines are widely used for anxiety disorders, [23] but they lead to recidivism in addicts and should be viewed as contraindicated in this patient group.

## PSYCHOSIS

Drug addicts with psychotic symptoms are usually evaluated in the hospital to ensure their safety and assess the etiology of their psychosis. Many of these patients have underlying psychiatric illnesses such as schizophrenia or bipolar disorder that are fairly obvious in light of extensive past histories. Psychosis may also result from drug intoxication, withdrawal, protracted withdrawal, and medical complications of addiction.

Psychotic symptoms may be found in alcohol and sedative-hypnotic withdrawal [38]. Medical detoxification must be conducted quickly and appropriately to alleviate this potentially life-threatening situation. If not presenting a danger, psychotic symptoms can be observed for spontaneous remission before neuroleptics are instituted. Alcoholics tend to recognize the unreality of their hallucinations (hallucinosis) and have a propensity for visual hallucinations. Paranoia may also be a complication of alcohol intoxication and acute withdrawal. Psychotic symptoms in alcoholics tend to wear off rapidly and can therefore be distinguished from those found in schizophrenia and mania.

Psychosis is seen during intoxication states with cocaine and amphetamine, [41,42] phencyclidine (PCP), [43] hallucinogens, [44] and marijuana [45]. Covert use of these drugs should be ruled out with blood and urine testing. Central stimulants, cocaine and amphetamine, classically produce paranoid psychoses [41]. The physical examination should focus on signs of these intoxication states already described while the results of blood or urine analysis is pending. The persistence of psychosis beyond several days of drug use generally rules out substance-induced psychosis. However, with PCP, more protracted psychosis may occur [43]. PCP levels in the urine persist for several days, and there is usually a discernible trend toward clinical improvement as the drug is metabolized and eliminated.

Certain medical complications of addiction may also produce psychosis. Temporal-lobe epilepsy (TLE) may manifest during detoxification from alcohol and sedatives or intoxication with stimulants since the seizure threshold is decreased in these conditions. Psychotic symptoms associated with TLE have been reported [46] and can be evaluated by history or electroencephalography (EEG) testing. Epilepsy may be produced by stimulants through the process of kindling [47]. A sleep-deprived EEG or 24-hour telemetry EEG provides increased sensitivity and can be performed after detoxification. Addicts also have an increased incidence of neurotoxicity from drug exposure and head trauma during intoxication. These complications are especially prevalent in alcoholics and can lead to persistent psychosis. Certain viral syndromes may produce psychosis, [48] and substance abusers are often at increased risk of exposure to hepatitis and AIDS viruses. Psychosis and dementia have been reported with AID [49]. Viral antibodies in plasma or cerebral spinal fluid can be measured when viral encephalopathy is suspected. Neuropsychological testing is helpful when brain dysfunction is suspected, and structural lesion can be identified with a CAT scan or MRI of the head.

Persistence of psychotic symptoms beyond three days of drug abstinence can seldom be attributable to intoxication (except with PCP) is more typical of schizophrenia, mania, or other psychiatric and medical causes of psychosis. Past psychotic episodes during periods of drug abstinence and family history of psychosis should be assessed. Schizophrenic patients often have comorbidity with addiction and pose a difficult treatment dilemma. They usually have great difficulty interacting in self-help groups and may even decompensate with standard rehabilitative approaches. Manic patients might appear to be substance abusers in their manic state but, unless addiction occurs during euthymic and depressed states, their diagnosis of addiction is unlikely. Treatment issues involved with these dually diagnosed patients have been reviewed elsewhere [10].

## PERSONALITY DISORDERS

Characteristic features of personality disorders are common in substance abusers during active addiction. To constitute diagnostic criteria for personality disorders, these features should precede substance abuse and not result directly from the addictive life-style. Antisocial behaviors directed toward drug procurement, impulsivity during intoxication, and lying to conceal impairment are typical of active addiction but may disappear entirely with recovery. Unless there is a compelling history for a personality disorder, diagnoses should be deferred during early recovery.

With these considerations in mind, it is also important to emphasize that individuals with personality disorders or conduct disorders may be at increased risk of drug addiction [50]. Diagnostic criteria for antisocial and borderline personality disorders even include drug abuse. In addition, individuals with avoidant personality disorders often medicate phobic anxiety with drugs or alcohol. Personality disorders may therefore precede, or result from, drug addiction, and the distinction is difficult to assess during early recovery. Personality disorders should not be the focus of treatment for addiction because the erroneous message might be conveyed that drug use results entirely from psychological conflict and will cease once conflict has resolved. This reasoning ignores the essential roles of craving and euphoria in the perpetuation of addiction. Personality disorders are of crucial importance with regard to addiction treatment when they interfere with engagement and performance in drug rehabilitation. In these cases, psychotherapy often improves the chances of recovery.

## CONCLUSION

Psychiatric symptoms are often encountered in substance abusers and present a diagnostic challenge for the practitioner. Familiarity with psychiatric manifestations of intoxication, withdrawal, and protracted withdrawal is essential to avoid inaccurate psychiatric diagnoses and unnecessary pharmacotherapy. Psychiatric complications of addiction vary with the substance in question and have characteristic periods of spontaneous remission. It is often impossible to distinguish primary from secondary psychiatric syndromes solely on the basis of current symptom profile, necessitating longitudinal observation during a controlled washout period before a reliable diagnosis can be made. In addition, the physical examination and laboratory tests provide important and reliable objective measures.

The substance abuser will often resist and interfere with the evaluation process. Denial, minimization, distortions, and outright untruths are regularly encountered in these patients. This resistance requires healthy skepticism on the part of the clinician, attentiveness to details, and use of objective information from independent sources. In addition, the patient may have a hidden agenda apart from the task of recovery. Whenever possible, psychiatric diagnoses and the use of psychotropics should be deferred to allow for the spontaneous resolution of psychiatric syndromes. This conservative strategy minimizes the unnecessary use of medications and spares the addict from having to face potential ostracism from unenlightened self-help groups. A careful diagnostic approach also permits an accurate psychiatric diagnosis of substance abusers with coexistent psychiatric illnesses. Since psychiatrists are often called upon to evaluate and treat addicts, our sophistication regarding substance-induced psychiatric syndromes will positively impact recovery rates and strengthen our credibility with the recovery community.

## REFERENCES

1. Wise RA. Catecholamine theories of reward: A critical review. *Brain Res* 1978; 152:215–247.
2. Deneau GA, Yanagita T, Seevers MH. Self-administration of psychoactive substances by the monkey. *Psychopharmacologia* 1969; 16:30–48.
3. Dackis CA, Gold MS. New concepts in cocaine addiction: The dopamine depletion hypothesis. *Neurosci Biobev Rev* 1985; 9:469–477.
4. Dackis CA, Gold MS. Psychopharmacology of cocaine. *Psych Annals* 1988; 18(9):528–530.
5. Dackis CA, Gold MS, Sweeney DR. The physiology of cocaine craving and "crashing." *Arch Gen Psychiatry* 1987; 44:297–300.
6. Gold MS, Dackis CA. Role of the laboratory in the evaluation of suspected drug abuse. *J Clin Psychiatry* 1986; 47(1):17–23.
7. Gay GR. Clinical management of acute and toxic cocaine poisoning. *Ann Emerg Med* 1982; 11:562–572.
8. Goldfrank L, Bresnitz E. Toxocologic emergencies: opioids. *Hosp Physician* 1978; 10:26.
9. Olson E, McEnrue J, Greenbaum DM. Recognition, general considerations, and techniques in the management of drug intoxication. *Heart & Lung* 1983; 12(2):110–113.
10. Dackis CA, Gold MS, Estroff TW. Inpatient treatment of addiction. In: *Treatments of Psychiatric Disorders: A Task Force Report of the American Psychiatric Association*. Vol. 3. Washington, DC: American Psychiatric Association, 1989:1359–1379.
11. Gold MS, Redmond DE, Kleber HD. Clonidine in opiate withdrawal. *Lancet* 1978; 1:929–930.

12. Dackis CA, Gold MS. Depression in Opiate Addicts. In: *Substance Abuse and Psychopathology.* Mirin, SM, ed. Washington, DC: American Psychiatric Press, 1984; 19–40.
13. Dackis CA, Pottash ALC, Gold MS, Sweeney DR. Evaluating depression in alcoholics. *Psychiatr Res* 1986; 17:105–109.
14. *Diagnostic & Statistical Manual of Mental Disorders, 3rd Ed. Rev.* (DSM-III-R). Washington: DC, American Psychiatric Association, 1987:217.
15. Byck R. *Cocaine Papers: Sigmund Freud.* New York: Stonehill Publishing 1974:64.
16. Post RM, Kotin J, Goodwin FR. The effects of cocaine of depressed patients. *Am J Psychiatry* 1974; 131:511–517.
17. Dackis CA, Bailey J, Pottash ALC, Stuckey RF, Extein IL, Gold MS. Specificity of the DST and TRH test for major depression in alcoholics. *Am J Psychiatry* 1984; 141:680–682.
18. Rounsaville BJ, Weissman MM, Crits-Christoph K et al. Diagnosis and symptoms of depression in opiate addicts. *Arch Gen Psychiatry* 1982; 39:151–156.
19. Rado S. Narcotic bondage: A general theory of the dependence on narcotic drugs. *Am J Psychiatry* 1957; 114:165–170.
20. Dackis CA, Pottash ALC, Gold MS et al. The dexamethasone suppression test for major depression in opiate addicts. *Am J Psychiatry* 1984; 141:810–811.
21. Gold MS, Dackis CA, Pottash ALC et al. Naltrexone, opiate addiction and endorphins. *Med Res Rev* 1982; 2(3):211–246.
22. Woody GE, O'Brien CP, Rickels K. Depression and anxiety in heroin addicts: A placebo controlled study of doxepin in combination with methadone. *Am J Psychiatry* 1983; 40:649–653.
23. Sheehan DV. Current views on the treatment of panic and phobic disorders. *Drug Ther* 1982; 12:74–93.
24. Gawin FH, Kleber HD. Abstinence symptomatology and psychiatric diagnosis in cocaine abusers. *Arch Gen Psychiatry* 1986; 43:107–113.
25. Dackis CA, Gold MS. Pharmacological approaches to cocaine addiction. *J Subs Abuse Treat* 1985; 2:139–145.
26. Dackis CA, Estroff TW, Sweeney DR, Pottash ALC, and Gold MS. Specificity of the TRH test for major depression in patients with serious cocaine abuse: *Am J Psychiatry* 1985; 142:1097–1099.
27. Tennant FS, Sagherian AA. Double-blind comparison of amantadine hydrochloride and bromocriptine mesylate for ambulatory withdrawal from cocaine dependence. *Arch Intern Med* 1987; 147:109–112.
28. Dacksi CA, Gold MS. Bromocriptine as a treatment of cocaine abuse. *Lancet* 1985; 1:1151–1152.
29. Dackis CA, Gold MS, Sweeney DR, Byron JP, Climko R. Single dose bromocriptine reverses cocaine craving. *Psychiatr Res* 1987; 20:261–264.
30. Sachar EJ, Asnis G, Nathan S et al. Dextroamphetamine and cortisol in depression: Morning plasma cortisol levels suppressed. *Arch Gen Psychiatry* 1980; 37:755–757.

31. Kirkby RJ, Petchkovsky L. Chronic administration of cocaine: Effects on defication and adrenal hypertrophy in the rat. *Neuropharmacology* 1973; 12:1001.
32. Corcoras JA, Dackis CA, Gold MS. Sexual dysfunction secondary to cocaine abuse in two patients. *J Clin Psychiatry* 1986; 47:384–385.
33. Gawan FH, Kleber HD. Cocaine abuse treatment; open pilot trial with desipramine and lithium carbonate. *Arch Gen Psychiatry* 1984; 41:903–909.
34. Dackis CA, Pottash ALC, Annitto W et al. Persistence of urinary marijuana levels after supervised abstinence. *Am J Psychiatry* 1984; 141:810–811.
35. Kolodny RC, Masters WH, Kolodner RM. et al. Depression of plasma testosterone levels after chronic intensive marijuana use. *NEJ Med* 1974; 290:872–874.
36. Dackis CA, Gold MS. Alcoholism. In: *Advances in Psychopharmacology*. Gold MS, Lydiard RB, Carmen JS, eds. Boca Raton, FL: CRC Press, 1984: 277–288.
37. Gorman JM, Liebowitz MR, Fyer AJ, Stein J. A neuroanatomical hypothesis for panic disorder. *Am J Psychiatry* 1989; 146:148–161.
38. MacKinnon GL, Parker WA. Benzodiazepine withdrawal syndrome: A literature review and evaluation. *Am J Drug Alc Abuse* 1982; 9:19–33.
39. Schopf J. Withdrawal phenomena after long-term administration of benzodiazepines. A review of recent investigations. *J Pharmacopsychiatria* 1983; 16:1–8.
40. Lasagna L, von Felsinger JM, Beecher HK. Drug-induced mood changes in man. *JAMA* 1955; 1006–1020.
41. Seigel RK. Cocaine hallucinations. *Am J Psychiatry* 1978; 135:309–314.
42. Post RM. Cocaine psychosis: A continuum model. *Am J Psychiatry* 1975; 132:225–231.
43. Allen RM, Young SJ. Phencyclidine-induced psychosis. *Am J Psychiatry* 1978; 135(9):1081–1083.
44. Hollister LE. Effects of hallucinogens in humans. In: *Hallucinogens: neurochemical, behavioral, and clinical perspectives*. Jacobs BL, ed. New York: Raven Press, 1984; 19–34.
45. Gold MS. *Marijuana*. New York: Plenum Press, 1989:87–88.
46. Rivinus TM. Psychiatric effects of anticonvulsant regimens. *J Clin Psychopharmacology* 1982; 2(3):165–192.
47. Post RM, Kopanda RT, Black KE. Progressive effects of cocaine on behavior and central amine metabolism in the rhesus monkey: relationship to kindling and psychosis. *Biol Psychiatry* 1976; 11:403–419.
48. Henderson DA, Shelokov A. Epidemic neuromyasthenia — Clinical syndrome? *NEJ Med* 1959; 260(16):757–764.
49. Faulstich ME. Psychiatric aspects of AIDS. *Am J Psychiatry* 1987; 144:551–556.
50. Khantzian EJ, Khantzian NJ. Cocaine Addiction: Is there a psychological predisposition? *Psycho Annals* 1984; 14(10):753–759.

# TREATMENT

# 13

## Treatment of the Dually Diagnosed Alcoholic

**Norman S. Miller**

*Cornell University Medical College, White Plains, New York*

**Mark S. Gold**

*Fair Oaks Hospital, Summit, New Jersey and Delray Beach, Florida*

### ALCOHOLISM AS A CAUSE OF PSYCHIATRIC SYNDROMES

The treatment of the psychiatric syndromes in addition to alcoholism requires a knowledge of alcoholism and other psychiatric disorders and clinical skills to apply the principles of diagnoses and treatment of these conditions. Furthermore, a clear understanding of the relationship of the psychopathology between these two broad classes of clinical conditions is mandatory before effective treatment can be administered.

Alcoholism as a clinical entity causes virtually every psychiatric syndrome. Because alcoholism may mimic other psychiatric disorders, the diagnosis of additional, coexisting or underlying disorders is not only difficult but often unnecessary. The appearance of an additional psychiatric symptom in the setting of alcoholism frequently evokes the consideration of another diagnosis if the total spectrum of psychiatric symptoms produced by alcoholism is not appreciated [1].

### Symptoms Induced by Alcohol/Alcoholism

The most common psychiatric symptoms produced by alcoholism are anxiety and depression. Pharmacological studies have clearly documented that anxiety associated with either a single administration of alcohol or especially after chronic administration is an expression of a discharging central nervous system, particularly the sympathetic nervous system. The manifestation of the entire array of the anxiety disorders may be observed as consequences of chronic alcoholism. Generalized anxiety, panic, agoraphobia, and social phobias are particularly common among alcoholics. These anxiety disorders arising from alcoholism usually abate with abstinence but may take weeks, months, and years to resolve in some particularly sensitive and chronic alcoholics [2].

The occurrence of the affective states induced by alcohol are expected clinical findings, particularly from regular use of alcohol. Major depression with mood symptoms and vegetative signs are common expression of regular and significant intake of alcohol. A depressed mood and affect with disturbances in appetite and sleep from alcohol are indistinguishable from the ideopathic "affective disorders." Suicidal thinking and actions are frequent: 25% of the total suicides are by alcoholics, and 25% of alcoholics die by suicide in the United States. Behind advancing age, alcoholism is the leading cause of suicide in the United States [3,4].

Syndromes similar to bipolar disorders, characterized by the manic syndrome, may be mimicked by alcoholism, especially if a retrospective history of behaviors is utilized in the evaluation. Alcoholism is associated with hyperactivity, elevation of mood, and changes in self-attitude, with delusions. Many of the behaviors of alcohol intoxication are indistinguishable from mania. The depressive part of bipolar disorders is a similar clinical syndrome to major depression and is commonly induced by chronic alcohol consumption [5].

Alcohol as a pharmacological agent is classified as a depressant by its action on the central nervous system. The depression is a descending pharmacological paralysis of the brain, beginning in the locations containing the most sensitive neurons in the outer, cortical layers of the cerebral hemispheres, where insight, judgment, and planning are subserved. The spread of the depression continues to the center of the hemispheres, where mood and memory are contained in the limbic system, and, in increasing doses, downward to the brainstem, where consciousness and the central neurons of the sympathetic chain are situated in the midbrain and pons [5].

Depression is an expression of the intoxicating effects of alcohol, whereas anxiety is an expression of withdrawal from alcohol. The intoxicating effects of alcohol are typically euphoria, dullness, sedation, amnesia, mood depression and dysphoria, disinhibition of drive states and behaviors ordinarily under the control of the cerebral centers. Alcohol suppresses the frontal lobe, whose function is responsible for insight, judgment, and control of emotions, violent and destructive tendencies, and improper expressions of the sexual and other drives.

The tolerance and dependence syndromes that develop from the use of alcohol produce signs and symptoms as a part of the withdrawal during abstinence. The withdrawal is a reflection of the deadaptation of the nervous system to the pharmacological effects of alcohol, whereas tolerance had been a reflection of the adaptation of the nervous system to alcohol. The abstinence withdrawal syndrome is a spectrum that is usually only partially expressed only unusually and ranges from the more common occurrence of anxiety, depression, elevated blood pressure and pulse, tremors, to seizures, delusions, hallucinations, to the full composite of delirium tremens. Many other signs and symptoms are associated with the abstinence withdrawal syndromes [5,6].

The production of hallucinations and delusions by alcoholism is less common but occurs in more chronic populations of heavy consumers of alcohol. The hallucinations may occur in a clear sensorium, as in alcoholic hallucinosis, or as a part of delirium tremens. The hallucinations may be visual or auditory and are usually frightening and disturbing to the perceiver. They typically begin with abstinence and resolve over weeks in hallucinosis and days in delirium tremens without treatment [5,6].

The production of delusions in the alcoholic is also a feature of the more chronic effects of alcohol intake. These delusions are characteristically paranoid, vague, and ill-formed. The delusions may occur independently or as a part of delirium tremens. They occur in the setting of prolonged alcohol consumption and tend to resolve over days and weeks. Both the hallucinations and delusions may be indistinguishable from schizophrenia and manic syndromes. Other stigmata of the psychotic symptoms occur but less strikingly such as the negative symptoms of impoverished affect, lack of an empathetic interpersonal relationship, and an ineffective personality [5,6].

The effect on personality is dramatic. A core personality of alcoholism has been known for years. The core personality develops as a result of alcoholism and is an acquired stereotype that is a combination of pharmacological effects of alcohol on the brain and the maladaptive life-style that results from chronic alcoholism. No predisposing personality has been established as etiologic for alcoholism. The core personality is marked by a fundamental disturbance in the interpersonal relationships of the alcoholic. The personality is characterized by antisocial, immature, histrionic, narcissistic, dependent features. These are regular derangements of the personality resulting from the addictive use of alcohol. They tend to diminish over time with sustained abstinence from alcohol and particularly with specific treatment of alcoholism [7].

The presence of alcoholism, the amelioration of the symptoms with abstinence over time, and the lack of response to medications with continued alcohol intake favor alcoholism as the etiology for all the psychiatric syndromes. Furthermore, the lessening or elimination of the signs and symptoms with specific treatment of alcoholism and addiction is confirmation that alcoholism is the predominant etiology of the associated psychiatric syndromes.

Alcoholism is a primary disorder that has specific criteria for diagnosis. As a primary disorder, it does not require an "underlying" diagnosis to define and sustain it. Alcoholism, unlike other psychiatric syndromes, is not caused by, or induced by, something else, such as another psychiatric disorder. Alcoholism is an addiction to alcohol that develops because of an interaction between alcohol and the brain. The underlying substrate for the development of alcoholism has not been definitely determined although the limbic system is a likely candidate [8].

## Alcohol Addiction

Alcoholism is an addiction to alcohol. An addiction is defined as a preoccupation with acquisition, compulsive use, and a pattern of recurrent relapse in spite of adverse consequences. The addiction is autonomous, spontaneous, and relentless, with a life of its own. Underlying the criteria is loss of control over the use of alcohol sufficient to produce the behaviors of addiction. Although tolerance and dependence are frequently associated with chronic alcohol use, they are not specific for alcoholism. Tolerance and dependence appear in the absence of addictive use of alcohol and are not always clinically evident in alcoholics, particularly younger alcoholics [9,10].

## Self-Medication

Alcoholism is considered by some to be secondary to other psychiatric syndromes as an expression of a self-medication of psychiatric symptoms. An origin of the self-medication concept is from the early psychoanalytic theory, which postulated intrapsychic causes for alcohol use. According to the psychoanalytic theory, suppression of unconscious conflict is possible by the tension-reduction effects of alcohol as it is seen as euphoric and an amnestic agent. The alcoholic is seen as having weak ego functioning, which is unable to integrate and control the powerful forces of the id and the punitive influence of the superego which has developed as a result of unconscious conflicts [11].

The major difficulty with the psychoanalytic model as an etiological explanation for alcoholism is that the clinical picture of the alcoholic does not correspond to the theory. The disintegrated ego, uncontrolled id, and unbridled superego are consequences of the addiction to alcohol and not causes. No studies have confirmed that alcoholics had this particular intrapsychic dynamic prior to the onset of alcoholism. On the other hand, many clinical studies and a consensus of clinical impressions have confirmed ego disorganization as a consequence. Furthermore, once the alcoholism is clearly established, continued alcohol use leads to worsening, whereas discontinued use often results in immediate improvement in personality variables.

The biological psychiatry model also relies on the self-medication concept in attributing addictive use of alcohol to underlying affective and psychotic states. A depression is given the antecedent position of causing addictive use of alcohol. Actual experiments performed to study the effect of depression on the drinking behavior of alcoholics and nonalcoholics did not support the hypothesis that depression is a cause of addictive drinking. Three different groups of subjects were given alcohol, and their mood and affective responses to ingested alcohol were measured. The groups were depressed alcoholics, depressed nonalcoholics, and nondepressed nonalcoholics. The depressed nonalcoholics experienced the greatest enhancement of mood and affect in response to alcohol, the nondepressed alcoholics were next, and the depressed alcoholic benefited least from alcohol. The conclusion of the study was that feeling good was not the reason alcoholics drank but that alcoholics drank in spite of feeling bad, given that alcohol consumption made them depressed. Probably the reason that the self-medication hypothesis does not fit the clinical and experimental findings of alcoholism is that most of the theoretical concepts originate from examining the responses of normal and nonalcoholic depressed drinkers [12].

A review of the psychiatric literature regarding the alcohol consumption of patients with manic-depressive disorders reveals that drinking patterns do not appear to be significantly altered by depression but are influenced by mania. When manic-depressive patients who are not alcoholics are followed over time, their alcohol consumption may decrease, remain the same, or increase during a depressive episode. There does not seem to be a correlation between the onset of the depression and the frequency and quantity of alcohol consumption in these nonalcoholic manic-depressive patients. From these studies, the onset of depression in manic-depressive patients does not seem to be a motivating force in alcohol consumption. Furthermore, anecdotal clinical experience suggests that depressed patients who are not alcoholic drink less alcohol during a depressive episode. Apparently as with anxiety, depression may even be a protective state against increased alcohol consumption, presumably because either depressed patients resist feeling better or because the dysphoric effect of alcohol worsens the existing depression [13].

On the other hand, alcohol consumption does appear to increase during a manic episode although use is not clearly addictive or alcoholic. A generalized increase in the onset and amount of drinking during mania appears to correlate with the hyperactivity and increased behaviors of many types during the manic episode.

There are many motivating reasons to drink alcohol, i.e., to feel good, to forget, but these reasons do result in addictive drinking. Once addictive alcohol consumption appears, the original antecedents to drinking are secondary to the addiction, which is preeminent. Clinically, it can be assumed that if the behaviors of addiction are identified, alcoholism is producing the psychiatric syndromes. Usually, only after abstinence from alcohol and treatment of the alcoholism is it possible to determine if other psychiatric disorders exist [13,14].

## Psychiatric Syndrome from Alcoholism

Alcoholism as an addictive disorder, has associated psychiatric symptoms that may arise during the period of abstinence, especially if specific treatment of alcoholism is not employed. The so-called dry-drunk syndrome publicized by the recovering community in Alcoholics Anonymous is a description of a major depression and several types of anxiety disorders. The dry-drunk syndrome is said to occur in an abstinent alcoholic who is not otherwise engaged in a recovery program to enhance his or her spiritual awareness and well-being by the 12 steps of AA. This syndrome is frequently the immediate antecedent of a relapse and a return to active alcoholism. Although the syndrome includes a depressed mood and effect, sometimes vegetative signs, and generalized anxiety and panic disorders, it dose not respond to traditional psychiatric medications such as antidepressants and benzodiazepines [7,8].

The dry-drunk syndrome may appear at any time in the course of abstinence, after months and years of continuous abstinence. It usually has an insidious onset over weeks and months or even years, particularly if the disengagement from a recovery program in Alcoholics Anonymous, such as discontinuing attendance at meetings, is gradual over years as it typically occurs after a period of years of active membership in AA.

The term "dry drunk" refers to the signs and symptoms of the state of intoxication that are occurring in the absence of intoxication. This state is indistinguishable from the clinical condition of major depression and anxiety disorders. The basis for these clinical expressions may be in the limbic system, where the neurological substrates for addiction and mood are located. The expression of an "untreated" addiction to alcohol may be the reappearance of the moods that were associated with chronic intoxication with alcohol during active addiction.

## COEXISTENCE OF PSYCHIATRIC DISORDERS

The occurrence of other psychiatric disorders in addition to alcoholism is not particularly common in comparison to the prevalence of psychiatric symptoms induced by alcohol and caused by alcoholism. The weight of alcohol-induced psychiatric syndromes versus ideopathic syndromes is based on the pervasive pharmacological effects of alcohol and the powerful driving force of addiction. As a rule, alcoholics appear vulnerable to developing ideopathic disorders independent of alcoholism with the same frequency as the general population [15].

Studies of the prevalence of affective disorders in alcoholics do not demonstrate an increased association between alcoholism and ideopathic affective disorders. Although affective states are commonly caused by alcoholism, these alcohol-induced states are to be distinguished from the unipolar depression and bipolar illnesses that arise as genetically independent of alcoholism. The actual prevalence of alcoholism coincidental with affective disorders is statistically calculated to be 1%. This calculation is based on the assumptions that the prevalence of alcoholism is 10% and affective disorder is 10%. Because the two are genetically independent, the two are multiplied to arrive at the prevalence of 1% for coocurrence of the disorders [16].

The prevalence of psychotic disorders, such as schizophrenia, among alcoholics is approximately 1%, as it is in the general population. The prevalence of personality disorders is also no greater among alcoholics before the onset of alcoholism than is the prevalence of personality disorders in the general population. The prevalence of anxiety disorders is not as well studied, but clinical indications are that there are no differences in prevalence rates among alcoholics before the onset of alcoholism and among the general population. The prevalence rates for psychiatric disorders not induced by alcoholism are not greater among alcoholics than the prevalence rates for psychiatric disorders in the general population [17].

## TREATMENT OF PSYCHIATRIC DISORDERS IN ALCOHOLISM

The treatment of those psychiatric syndromes induced by alcoholism is considerably different from those psychiatric disorders occurring coincidentally with alcoholism. Different clinical courses are to be expected, and different modalities of treatment are employed for each class of disorders. Beginning with the most common disorders, affective and anxiety states, and the almost equally common personality disturbances, and proceeding to the less frequent psychotic states, a systematic and rational approach will adequately and fully treat any combination of psychiatric disorders possible in the alcoholic.

Retrospective diagnosis of psychiatric disorders in alcoholic populations is fraught with difficulties. Errors in diagnosis occur in the retrospective analysis of the patient's history for a variety of reasons. The patient must use recall that is distorted by the denial associated with alcoholism. Denial is a feature of alcoholism that extends beyond the accounts of the drinking history into other aspects of the patient's mental life. The tendency is to deny that alcohol is a problem and to ascribe the consequences of alcoholism to other causes such as a coincidental or causative depression [8].

Moreover, the cognitive state of the chronic drinker is impaired sufficiently to reduce recall of the actual sequence of events associated with drinking and occurring before and during active alcoholism. There is another interesting phenomenon called "state-dependent" learning, in which the alcoholic remembers only the experience surrounding the drinking when actually in the intoxicated state. Otherwise, the recollection of factors associated with alcohol consumption, including the consequences, is missing in the abstinent state. Studies have documented this state-dependent memory and alcohol consumption [17].

Also, because of diagnostic confusion, many alcoholics who seek treatment for their depression receive a diagnosis of depression without a proper evaluation of their alcoholism and its role in the depression. Therefore, such an alcoholic has a dual diagnosis by history but, in fact, may have only alcoholism and its attendant consequences. Even obtaining old records will often not be revealing because the alcoholism is often not adequately addressed in previous evaluations.

The addiction to alcohol and its symptoms take priority in the diagnosis in most instances. Once a preoccupation with the acquisition of alcohol, compulsive use of alcohol, and a relapse into drinking alcohol are established, an addiction to alcohol exists, regardless of whether a coincidental disorder is present. The addiction to alcohol is not caused by another psychiatric condition.

## Depression and Anxiety

Although persistence of significant affective and anxiety symptoms beyond weeks may still be ascribed to alcoholism, the need for medications such as antidepressants may be indicated for a period of time. Similar guidelines to the use of antidepressants in depressed nonalcoholics may be used for depressed alcoholics. The length of treatment with antidepressants would be six months at the usual therapeutic doses. At the end of six months, the antidepressant should be tapered over two to four weeks. Doses similar to those used in the treatment of depression are sometimes necessary.

A withdrawal syndrome with the use of antidepressants is to be expected and is reduced with the gradual tapering of the antidepressant. The dependence syndrome associated with antidepressants is anxiety, depression, insomnia, tremor, malaise, and anorexia. Withdrawal may persist for weeks in some individuals but lessens in severity over time. At times, the dependence syndrome to antidepressants may be confused with the symptoms of a depression from other causes. Patient follow-up usually determines whether antidepressant withdrawal is the etiology [21].

Depression and anxiety are usually present and, at times, in sufficient severity to qualify for DSM-III-R diagnosis of affective or anxiety disorder. In most instances, a period of abstinence from alcohol results in alleviation or elimination of the symptoms of depression and anxiety, even those of the magnitude of a DSM-III-R diagnosis. The time course may be days or weeks or less commonly, months for the disappearance of a major depression or a panic disorder induced by alcoholism. No pharmacological intervention is indicated and is contraindicated at this point for most alcoholics [18–20].

The existence of a "true depressive or anxiety disorder" coincidental with alcoholism should be treated like any disorder and considered to have the same clinical course and prognosis as an independent disorder. There are some differences in the outcome expectations of treatment, in that active participation in AA may result in improved functioning and fewer signs and symptoms of depression. Moreover, the personality disturbances associated with the depressions are often treated with participation in AA. However, the usual methods of treatment of depressive disorders such as antidepressants and psychotherapy are indicated in alcoholics with coincidental depressive disorders [22].

## Psychosis

The treatment of a psychotic disorder that is coincidental with alcoholism is similar to the treatment of that disorder in the absence of alcoholism. The use of antipsychotic medication is necessary to control the hallucinations and delusions of a schizophrenic process in order to increase compliance with the treatment of alcohol addiction. A schizophrenic is more likely to be able to comply with the treatment of alcoholism if the psychotic symptoms are also under control. In this instance, the schizophrenia may trigger the onset of alcohol addiction but not cause it. Once alcoholism is reactivated by the ingestion of alcohol, the addiction resumes as the preeminent disorder in the course of the dual diagnosis.

The natural history of the schizophrenic syndrome associated with alcoholism is similar to that occurring in the absence of alcoholism. The schizophrenic disease does not appear to have different characteristics whether alcoholism exists with respect to the signs and symptoms of schizophrenia. However, as stated, the treatment of schizophrenia may be affected by the disease of alcoholism. In fact, anecdotal clinical experience suggests that active participation in AA enhances some of the personality characteristics that are troublesome to the schizophrenic [23].

It is important that the schizophrenic often has special difficulties in a group-based treatment approach. The personality limitations of the schizophrenic because of the negative symptoms of schizophrenia make interaction in a group intimidating, especially in a confrontational group. Also, the structure and discipline required of the group members are sometimes difficult for the schizophrenic to accept. The poverty of emotions and the inability to form rapport with others preclude the development of group membership and identification by the schizophrenic. Expectations may be lowered for the schizophrenic, however, and group participation may be possible. Also, the deterioration in personality may not be prohibitive for sufficient participation in the group for treatment of the addiction.

## Medications

The use of medications with the alcoholic must be handled with caution. The alcoholic population is a high-risk population for the misuse of any drug, whether it has a high or low potential for abuse and addiction. Medications of any kind carry a relative contraindication in the alcoholic population. There is a hierarchy of risk for various medications and drugs. At one end of the spectrum of risk are the highly addicting stimulants, opiates, and sedative/hypnotics (benzodiazepines), and at the other end are acetylacetic acid and acetaminophen. However, any drug including medications carries a risk for addiction, tolerance, and dependence. Antidepressants and certain antipsychotic medications are probably in the middle of the spectrum.

The major reasons for the vulnerability of the alcoholic to other medications are the following. First, the alcoholic is more likely to develop an addiction to drugs because of the already existing addiction to alcohol. Eighty percent or more alcoholics under the age of 30 are addicted to at least one other drug or medication. Marijuana is the most common, followed by cocaine, benzodiazepines, and others. Between 25% and 50% of alcoholics are addicted to benzodiazepines. Second, the drug effect of a medication is troublesome to alcoholics, rendering them more vulnerable to misuse of the medication and/or relapse to alcohol. It makes the acceptance of their alcoholism more difficult and reduces the commitment to recovery and what is necessary to establish that commitment [24].

Third, the basic defect of the alcoholic is a loss of control over alcohol, which is a drug. This loss of control extends to other populations of drugs and medications, leading to the development of abuse, addiction, tolerance, and dependence. Fourth, alcoholics have been searching for a drug solution to their problems through their use of alcohol and other drugs. The "faith in a drug or pill" to solve problems is an obsession that the alcoholic continues to pursue endlessly in spite of adverse, costly and sometimes lethal consequences. The continuation of this faith in medication will distract alcoholics from making the necessary changes in their personalities in order to recover from alcoholism.

Finally, there are no pharmacological treatments specifically for addiction. The addictive behaviors do not respond to medications. The associated consequences from alcoholism, such as depression and anxiety, do not respond to medications. The benzodiazepines may initially ameliorate the anxiety from alcoholism, but tolerance, dependence, and addiction to the benzodiazepines develop readily in alcoholics, resulting in adverse consequences from addiction to benzodiazepines similar to those from addiction to alcohol. Benzodiazepines share cross-tolerance and cross-dependence with alcohol [25].

## Personality

Beginning with the initiation of abstinence and the application of the 12-step program of Alcoholics Anonymous, the personality undergoes a profound change. The AA program is specifically for addiction. The personality undergoes a fundamental change in attitude that begins with an acceptance of the disease concept of alcoholism and the establishment of a commitment to recovery. The core personality of narcissism, antisociality, immaturity, and dependence that develops as a result of the addiction to alcoholism is gradually replaced by a more outwardly sensitive, respectful, mature, and independent personality. The basic disturbance in the interpersonal relationship is improved, with a premium placed on developing productive and harmonious or, at least, inoffensive relationships [7,8].

The use of psychotherapy to assist in this transformation of personality is legitimate, beneficial, and sometimes indispensable. The form of psychotherapy that is useful in the early stages of recovery is cognitive, "in the here and now," directive, confrontational, and supportive. Insight and long-term directed analytic psychotherapy is not useful but may be harmful in the early months of sobriety because the alcoholic is not capable of much insight and often has substantial guilt that would only be intensified. However, after a period of sobriety, especially in AA, the psychoanalytic method may be very helpful in determining and resolving long-standing conflicts that may be interfering with more contented and constructive sobriety.

## Alcoholics Anonymous

The long-range treatment of choice, for most alcoholics is involvement in Alcoholics Anonymous. Although the principles of therapy in AA are spiritual in nature, the techniques are distinctly behavioral. The approach is for the alcoholic to take actions that will eventually result in a change in mood and attitude. This method of treatment for addiction is similar to the methods employed to treat depression before the advent of antidepressants. The depressed individuals were encouraged, and in some instances pushed, to take actions that resulted in an improvement in their mood.

Recent studies in the various modalities for the treatment of depression have demonstrated that nonpharmacological therapies such as psychotherapy were as effective in alleviating the symptoms of major depression as antidepressants. Although psychotherapy alone is not sufficient to treat an addiction to alcohol, it may serve as an important adjunct to participation in AA. Furthermore, AA can be considered a form of psychotherapy, administered in a group setting.

Surveys performed by the General Service Offices of Alcoholics Anonymous have revealed that those who abstain from alcohol for one year, with regular attendance at AA meetings, have statistically an 80% chance of continuing in their recovery for an additional year. The survey further shows that, of those who have abstained through participation in AA for two years, 95% have a chance of continuing their recovery for another year. And those who are sober for five years in AA have a 98% chance of recovering for another year.

## REFERENCES

1.  Schuckit MA. Alcoholism and other psychiatric disorders. *Hosp Community Psychiatry* 1983; 34(11):1022–1027.
2.  Powell BJ, Penick EC, Othmer E, Bingham SF, Rice A. Prevalence of additional psychiatric syndromes among male alcoholics. *J Clin Psychiat* 1982; 43(10): 404–407.
3.  Martin RL, Cloninger CR, Guze SB, Clayton PJ. Mortality in a follow-up of 500 psychiatric outpatients. I. Total Mortality. *Arch Gen Psychiat* 1985; 42:47–66.
4.  Murphy GF. Suicide in alcoholics. In: Roy, A, ed. *Suicide*. Williams and Wilkins, Baltimore, 1986; 89–96.
5.  Schuckit MA. The history of psychotic symptoms in alcoholics. *J Clin Psychiat* 1982; 43(2):53–57.
6.  Adams RP, Victor M. *Principles of Neurology*. 3rd ed. New York: McGraw-Hill, 1985.
7.  Miller NS. A primer of the treatment process for alcoholism and drug addiction. *Psychiatry Letter* 1987; 5(7):30–37.
8.  Milam JR, Ketcham K. *Under the Influence*. Seattle, WA: Madrona Publishers, 1981.
9.  Jaffe JH. Drug addiction and drug abuse. In: Gilman AG, Goodman LS, Rall TW, Murad F, eds. *The Pharmacological Basis of Therapeutics*. New York: Macmillan 1985: 532–540.
10. Miller NS, Gold MS. Suggestions for changes in DSM-III-R criteria for substance use disorders. *Am J Drug Alcohol Abuse* 1989; 15(2):223–230.
11. Crowley RM. Psychoanalytic literature on drug addiction and alcoholism. *Psychoanalyt Rev* 1939; 26:39–54.

12. Mayfield DG. Alcohol and affect: Experimental studies. In: Goodwin DW, Erickson CK, eds. *Alcoholism and Affective Disorders*. New York: SP Medical and Scientific Books, 1979: 99–107.
13. Schuckit MA. Alcoholism and affective disorder: Diagnostic confusion. Goodwin DW, Erickson CK, eds. *Alcoholism and Affective Disorders*. New York: SP Medical and Scientific Books, 1979:9–19.
14. Blankfield A. Psychiatric symptoms in alcohol dependence: Diagnostic and treatment implications. *J Subst Abuse Treat* 1986; 3:275–278.
15. Helzer JE, Przybeck TR. The co-occurrence of alcoholism with other psychiatric disorders in the general population and its impact on treatment. *J Stud Alc* 1988; 49(3):219–224.
16. Schuckit MA. Genetic and clinical implications of alcoholism and affective disorder. *Am J Psychiat* 1986; 143(2):140–147.
17. Goodwin DW, Guze SB. *Psychiatric Diagnosis*. New York: Oxford University Press, 1980.
18. *Psychoactive Substance Use Disorders Diagnostic and Statistical Manual of Mental Disorders*. 3rd. ed. rev. Washington, DC: American Psychiatric Association, 1987:165–185.
19. Schuckit MA. Alcoholic patients with secondary depression. *Am J Psychiat* 1983; 140:6.
20. Schuckit MA. Dual diagnosis: Substance abuse and anxiety. *Psychiatr Times* 1987; 20–21.
21. Charney DS, Heninger GR, Sternberg DE, Landis H. Abrupt discontinuation of tricyclic antidepressant drugs: Evidence for a noradrenergic hyperactivity. *Br J Psychiat* 1982; 141:377–386.
22. Woodruff RA, Guze SB, Clayton PJ, Carr D. Alcoholism and depression. In: Goodwin DW, Erickson CK, eds. *Alcoholism and Affective Disorders*. New York: SP Medical and Scientific Books, 1979:39–47.
23. Wolf AW, Schubert DSP, Patterson MB, Grande TP, Brocco KJ, Pendleton L. Association among major psychiatric diagnoses. *J Consult Clin Psychol* 1988; 56(2):292–294.
24. Miller NS, Mirin SM. Multiple drug use in alcoholics: Practical and theoretical implications. *Psychiatr Annals* 1989; 19(5):248–255.
25. Lader M, Petursson H. Long-term effects of benzodiazepines. *Neuropharmacol* 1983; 22:527–533.

# 14

## Treatment of the Dually Diagnosed Adult Drug User

**James A. Cocores**

*Fair Oaks Hospital, Summit, New Jersey*

The effective treatment of individuals suspected of having both a drug dependence and a major psychiatric disorder usually requires specialized inpatient hospitalization. The management of dually diagnosed patients can be challenging, even for the most experienced dual-diagnosis treatment team. For example, the schizophrenic patient with a drug dependence presents one of the most trying situations facing a dual-diagnosis treatment team. The use of drugs by schizophrenic patients often exacerbates psychotic symptoms and leads to noncompliance with prescribed medications. Involvement in 12-step [1] or any other group-based drug treatment is precluded by the social impairment associated with the psychotic disturbance [2]. Unfortunately, many of these people remain chronically psychotic, actively drug-dependent, and outside the reach of the health care system. Many become part of a chronic recidivism subgroup referred to as "revolving-door" admissions in veteran, county, and state psychiatric institutions. But, because schizophrenia is such a heterogeneous disorder, it is difficult to predict which dual-diagnosis patients will tolerate and benefit from drug rehabilitation. Some schizophrenics benefit greatly from the group process and fraternity of self-help. Others decompensate and become disorganized in group settings that rely on member participation. Fortunately, most other dual-diagnosis combinations are easier to manage. Accurate identification of dual-diagnosis patient populations is best accomplished by an evaluation period of not less than two weeks. A tailored treatment plan is generated after the diagnoses have been made. Some fundamental differences exist between the treatment approaches for a particular psychiatric disorder and for a drug dependence. Major psychiatric disorders frequently are managed with medications, but there is no pharmacological treatment for drug dependence. Traditionally, each disorder has been treated on separate treatment units by a corresponding treatment staff. The following case illustration serves as an example of the problems that regularly develop when both conditions are not considered, identified, and treated simultaneously and thoroughly.

*Case History*

Mr. D, a 28-year-old, single, successful stockbroker was admitted to a substance abuse rehabilitation program following a recommendation by his employer. Mr. D's employer suspected cocaine abuse because of erratic changes in behavior at work. Previously know to peers and clients as a mild-mannered, intelligent, and even-tempered person, Mr. D. gradually became increasingly anxious, irritable, paranoid, harsh, and depressed. He had been showing poor judgment with respect to the accounts he had been handling. Mr. D, following employer confrontation, confessed to having a problem with cocaine and was admitted to a rehabilitation facility for cocaine-dependence treatment. At the facility, he dominated group time with seemingly irrelevant conversation, lacked trust, and was intimidating and grandiose toward other patients. He sought medication nightly for insomnia, was oppositional toward staff, and was discharged prior to completing the inpatient drug program because he was considered treatment-resistant. The possibility of a coexisting major psychiatric disorder was not entertained by the drug-rehabilitation staff, and no psychiatric referral was made. Mr. D relapsed and was terminated from work. Months later, he was brought to an emergency room after being assaulted one evening and was admitted to a psychiatric unit because of increased psychomotor activity, paranoia, and suicidal ideation. Mr. D responded well to treatment with lithium carbonate and continued outpatient treatment for bipolar disorder. Because cocaine-dependence treatment was not emphasized by the psychiatric treatment team or, later, by the therapist, Mr. D viewed drug addiction as an appendage or a symptom of bipolar disorder. Mr. D began using cocaine "socially" and later stopped taking lithium because of the desire to do so to feel better and because of a fear of adverse effects from the lithium-cocaine mixture. In total, Mr. D was treated at four different inpatient treatment centers, each with a 28-day minimum length of stay. One hospitalization would focus on the manic-depressive illness, and another would primarily treat his drug dependence. After five hospitalizations, he reached a dual-diagnosis treatment facility where both disorders were treated effectively, with equal importance given to them both.

This case illustrates some common problems associated with partial diagnosis and treatment. Analogous case histories regularly accompany these patients. Usually, the various etiological possibilities for each disorder are considered. One possibility is that cocaine abuse and bipolar disorder are unrelated. Another possibility is that cocaine abuse may precipitate an underlying biological predisposition to bipolar disorder. Cocaine abuse may worsen an already preexisting bipolar disorder. Cocaine abuse may induce bipolar disorder symptomatology that abates with cocaine abstinence [3]. Often, valuable evaluation time is consumed by focusing on the common "chicken or egg" dilemma. Is the bipolar disorder responsible for the drug-dependent behavior, or is the cocaine abuse creating symptoms of bipolar disorder? Unfortunately, a choice is made to treat either the psychiatric disorder or the drug dependence. Less consideration is given to the possibility that two or more disorders may be operating simultaneously and that they require simultaneous clinical management. A skilled dual-diagnosis treatment team is required when treating both disorders. An essential aspect of the dual-diagnosis evaluation is a two- to three-week drug-free evaluation period. Once the dual diagnosis is made, treatment can occur in one of many treatment settings. Selection of the appropriate treatment setting depends on the severity of the dual diagnosis. There are essential components to consider when treating the dually diagnosed patient, irrespective of the treatment framework.

## TREATMENT COMPONENTS

There are many aspects of treatment common to both psychiatric disorders and drug dependence disorders. (Table 1). But there are some approaches to the management of drug dependence that are not traditionally used in the treatment of a particular psychiatric disorder (Table 2). The reverse is also true. It is the successful dual-diagnosis treatment plan that can integrate and

**Table 1**  Clinical Components Common to the Treatment of Psychiatric and Drug-Dependence Disorders

---

Group psychotherapy
Men's and women's group therapy
Stress management/relaxation therapy
Nutrition and exercise education
Vocational Counseling
Multifamily therapy
Couples therapy
Systems therapy

---

implement a nontraditional treatment modality without minimizing the impact of traditional treatments. A particular psychiatric disorder can be managed effectively using treatments that do not rely heavily on group therapy, the 12 steps, Narcotics Anonymous, and peer-oriented aftercare; but these therapies are essential to the management of drug dependence. Individual psychotherapy and psychopharmacology may not be as essential for the treatment of drug dependence as they are for many psychiatric disorders. Fortunately, most treatment components commonly implemented in treating psychiatric patients are also useful in managing drug dependence.

Urine drug screens are essential to effective drug treatment programs because they help monitor and enforce drug abstinence. Outpatient drug treatment programs are rendered valueless without urine drug screens, and even inpatient drug abstinence is impossible to enforce without the screens. A common complaint by dual-diagnosis therapists is "How can we foster trust and a therapeutic alliance and police urine drug screens simultaneously? " But a common complaint of dually diagnosed relapsers is "The other program didn't help me because they didn't take urines," or "Everybody gets over on them." Once considered, the advantages of random supervised urine drug screens outweigh the disadvantages. If most drug-dependent persons are multisubstance abusers and if the goal of drug-dependence treatment is abstinence from all dependence-prone drugs, then comprehensive urine drug screens are an essential treatment component. The comprehensive urine drug screen should consider the patient's age and drug history, drugs common to the geographic region, and test cost. For example, cocaine, cannabis, opiates, and benzodiazepines are the minimum drugs to be tested for in the New York metropolitan area. In order to contain cost, the initial screen may be conducted using inexpensive laboratory methods such as thin-layer chromatography, [4] but positives should be confirmed by more reliable methods. Because substances like benzoylecgonine (cocaine metabolite) are undetected in urine after a few days, urine drug screens must be conducted at least biweekly. Drug-dependent persons have been known to purchase urine from nondependents, adulterate the urine (i.e., add bleach), and

**Table 2**  Dual-Diagnosis Treatment Additives

| Psychiatric | Drug Dependence |
| --- | --- |
| Individual therapy | Strong Narcotics Anonymous orientation |
| Medicines | Avoidance of dependence-prone medicines |
| Therapist-oriented follow-up | Peer-oriented follow-up |

switch urine samples. These are but a few common reasons why urine screens must be supervised by staff members.

## TREATMENT FRAMEWORKS

### Adult Inpatient Dual-Diagnosis Treatment Units

Where available, dually diagnosed patients are best treated on a separate dual-diagnosis treatment unit. Inpatient treatment of the dual-diagnosis patient is indicated when outpatient treatment has consistently failed or is likely to fail [5]. An initial thorough medical, psychiatric, and psychosocial assessment, coupled with an observation period on a neuropsychiatric evaluation unit, offers the ideal diagnostic setting. The evaluation unit provides a thorough physical examination and explores possible medical mimics to mental disorders [6]. When appropriate, medical detoxification is initiated and complete psychosocial information obtained. Family information is obtained, and other patient information resources are explored. Most important, the patient is observed drug-free for about a 14-day period in order to help predict whether the patient would best benefit from a psychiatric unit, a substance abuse unit, or a dual-diagnosis unit. Vital signs are also carefully monitored to ensure safe withdrawal from drugs during the evaluation period. Only after careful evaluation, a drug-free observation period, and a thorough history, should individuals be referred for dual-diagnosis treatment.

Drug detoxification is a function best served on the evaluation unit. The medical detoxification schedule must be tailored to each person and depends on the drug dependence(s). Although undermedication can result in withdrawal seizures (i.e., alprazolam), overmedication during detoxification should be avoided as it extends the beginning of the first drug/medicine-free day which, in turn, prolongs the drug-free time needed to evaluate dual disorders efficiently. When possible, no dependence-prone medicines should be used. For example, the detoxification of opiate addicts with clonidine [7] can offer an alternative to the use of methadone.

Anticraving agents are sometimes used with cocaine smokers during the first three weeks of evaluation. Many medications have been used for this purpose and include desipramine, [8] bromocriptine, [9] and l-dopa [10]. Selection of a particular cocaine anticraving agent may be contingent on the coexisting psychiatric disorder being considered. For example, a cocaine freebaser with severe cocaine cravings, a history of major depression, and persistent major depression symptoms without psychotic features might doubly benefit by using a tricyclic antidepressant. Whichever anticraving medication is chosen, the patient should not be given a message that drug rehabilitation consists of taking anticraving medication. Instead, the medication should be presented as a small part of a multifaceted comprehensive drug treatment program. Frequent weekly urine drug screens must be obtained when a patient is taking cocaine anticraving medications, especially when being treated on an outpatient basis, to help reduce the temptation to relapse, as well as the potentially lethal cocaine/anticraving medication interaction.

The medical detoxification and neuropsychiatric evaluation can occur on a separate evaluation unit or as part of a dual-diagnosis unit. The advantage of the latter possibility is earlier patient involvement in dual-diagnosis treatment. A disadvantage is premature involvement in dual-diagnosis treatment when the evaluation eventually might have revealed that the patient would have benefitted more by a traditional psychiatric approach. Following an appropriate evaluation, the inpatient dual-diagnosis unit functions to offer a structured comprehensive treatment for each of the respective dual-diagnosis components in a parallel manner. A multidisciplinary team, experienced in both treatment approaches, harmoniously consults and supports the treatment goals for each patient.

## Adult Inpatient Substance Abuse Units

Although most hospitals do not have a separate dual-diagnosis treatment unit, most have separate substance abuse treatment units. Dual-diagnosis patients are often conveniently referred to substance abuse units, which customarily focus on drug-dependence rehabilitation. For example, an intravenous heroin addict with persistent major depression, after two weeks of detoxification/evaluation, may be transferred to a substance abuse treatment unit. The treatment team may view the patient's depressive symptoms as a manifestation of prolonged heroin abuse and withdrawal. It is not unusual for such dual-diagnosis patients with untreated major depression to suffer multiple opiate relapses. Did the patient relapse because of resistance to following drug-rehabilitation recommendations or because of the poor quality of life associated with untreated major depression [11] and the self-medication of depression with opiates [12]? This line of thinking frequently arises when attempts are made to treat the dual-diagnosis patient on a chemical-dependency unit or when the patient is simply led to believe that they did not follow recommendations or is treatment-resistant. Unidentified dual-diagnosis is commonly associated with a history of multiple relapse and hospitalizations for drug treatment. Drug treatment units faced with dual-diagnosis patients should modify or adapt their drug treatment program to accommodate psychiatric aspects of dually diagnosed patients more effectively. A separate dual-diagnosis team can be established within the confines of the drug treatment unit. If such an arrangement is impractical, a psychopharmacologist experienced with drug-dependence treatment could serve as an inpatient liaison consultant. A consulting psychologist experienced in chemical-dependency treatment is also necessary along with the psychopharmacologist as bare minimum additions required to treat the dual-diagnosis patient effectively on a chemical-dependency unit. An estimate of utilization by a dual-diagnosis consultant may be helpful prior to deciding whether to establish a separate team or arrange consultation agreements. In either case, all staff members treating the dual-diagnosis patient should meet regularly and orchestrate treatment in such a way as to minimize undermining and to enhance one another's treatment goals for the patient.

## Psychiatric Treatment Units or Hospitals

A different but equally common possibility would include admitting an intravenous-heroin-dependent person with persistent depression and suicidal ideation to a psychiatric treatment unit. Despite adequate stabilization of the affective component with medication and therapy, continued heroin use is likely to worsen the affective disorder and foster exacerbation of both illnesses. Is the exacerbated affective disorder a product of the inefficacy of the antidepressant and therapy, or is the reemerging major depression a product of opiate-induced affective symptomatology? Such patients are prone to multiple medication trials, plus other psychiatric treatment methods common to the management of affective disorders. Often, the opiate dependence is viewed as a by-product of the affective component, with the assumption that continued opiate use will be inhibited as a result of proper treatment of the depressive disorder. Dual diagnosis should be suspected in patients who have multiple psychiatric admissions, have made multiple drug treatment attempts, and are revolving-door admissions. Patients with multiple unsuccessful treatments often are unnecessarily guilt-ridden, feel hopeless, and may feel directly responsible for past failures to respond to treatment. Staff members also feel helpless and frustrated, which contributes directly to staff burnout. Frustrating, costly, and unnecessary multiple admissions can be avoided by having assessment team staff trained in dual-diagnosis identification and treatment. Ideally, the dual-diagnosis possibility is ruled out before admission or transfer to a psychiatric treatment unit. Because this is rarely a reality, substance abuse treatment methods must be made available to the psychiatric unit in order to treat the dual-diagnosis patient effectively when a separate dual-diagnosis team or unit is impossible to establish. A certified drug counselor, experienced with inpatient psychiatric treatment, is needed as a consultant to initiate and conduct individual and group drug-rehabilitation sessions for the dually diagnosed patient hospitalized on a psychiatric unit. An added measure would be to arrange weekly transportation to local Narcotics Anonymous meetings or to arrange for Narcotics Anonymous to meet on hospital grounds.

## Intensive Outpatient Drug-Rehabilitation Programs

Intensive outpatient drug programs provide comprehensive cost-effective services to drug-abusing patients not in need of 24-hour inpatient care. These programs, like many inpatient drug treatment centers, are often based on the 12 step method of recovery, [1,13] group therapy, drug education sessions, and a strong family treatment component [14]. Progress is monitored through regular and random substance abuse urine screens. In addition to the aforementioned treatment components, outpatient day drug programs stress a vocational component. Patients usually admitted for day intensive drug treatment are typically unemployed and have a lower level of functioning than evening program participants. Day patients also have a higher incidence of concurrent psychiatric disorders, and therefore day programs require dual-diagnosis treatment capabilities. Typically, patients attend treatment sessions five days per week from 9 A.M. to 3 P.M. for about eight weeks. Patients then enter an intermediate phase of drug-dependence treatment, which meets twice a week for two weeks and then once a week for the balance of a year. As the frequency of drug-clinic attendance decreases, patient attendance at local Narcotics Anonymous groups increases. Dual-diagnosis outpatients begin visiting their outpatient psychopharmacologist and psychotherapist after the dual diagnosis is made.

A similar evening program model exists for the outpatient treatment of higher-functioning drug-dependent individuals. Intensive evening drug treatment programs typically meet four days each week from 6:30 to 10:00 P.M. for six to eight weeks. Patients attend self-help groups on the days they do not attend the outpatient clinic. As with day programs, there is an intermediate phase, which is followed by weekly relapse-prevention groups, plus weekly self-help attendance for one year. Dual-diagnosis treatment capabilities are utilized less because patients admitted to evening drug treatment programs are more frequently employed and have a higher level of functioning compared to day patients. Therefore, a separate dual-diagnosis treatment team is not often needed in an outpatient evening program, but a referral network for concurrent outpatient psychiatric treatment is required. In either case, the treatment staff must be able to identify the dual-diagnosis patient.

Because these outpatient programs are available as cost-containing options to inpatient treatment, intensive outpatient drug treatment programs are often not equipped medically to manage the dual-diagnosis patient effectively. If an outpatient dual diagnosis treatment program is not available or if a dual-diagnosis outpatient team cannot be developed, the coexisting psychiatric disorder must be addressed by referring the patient to an outpatient psychopharmacologist or therapist. In this way, dual-diagnosis patients not in need of inpatient treatment can be managed effectively through attendance at structured outpatient drug treatment and, at the same time, attention to the psychiatric illness through visits to a psychopharmacologist experienced with drug-dependence treatment. During the initial frequent drug treatment attendance, the psychopharmacologist may focus more on medication titration and maintenance. Psychotherapy sessions can increase in frequency when the patient begins attending the drug clinic less frequently.

## Partial Psychiatric Hospitalization Programs

Partial-hospitalization programs provide comprehensive cost-effective psychiatric services to psychiatric patients not in need of 24-hour treatment (Table 3). A psychiatric milieu typically provides treatment Monday through Friday from 9 A.M. to 3:30 P.M. for 4 to 12 weeks. Medical components usually include daily rounds, medical supervision, pharmacotherapy assessment, medication monitoring and maintenance, and crisis intervention. Clinical components are similar to inpatient psychiatry treatment units and consist of individual psychotherapy, group psychotherapy, men's and women's group therapy, expressive group therapy, art therapy, relaxation therapy, crafts group, vocational counseling, individual family therapy, multifamily therapy, couples therapy, and assertiveness training.

Regular and ongoing dual-diagnosis staff in-services are important for partial-hospitalization programs and inpatient psychiatric treatment units. Once dual-diagnosis patients are sought among psychiatric patients, they usually are discovered and require more than standard psychiatric treat-

**Table 3** Bases for Inpatient versus Outpatient Programs

| Inpatient | Outpatient |
| --- | --- |
| Medical detoxification | Medical clearance |
| Suicidal or homocidal | Stabilized psychiatric problems |
| Acute psychiatric problems | |
| Unable to abstain from drugs and alcohol for more than one week | Unsuccessful at individual or infrequent group therapy |
| Prior unsuccessful outpatient attempts | Unsuccessful with self-help groups alone |

ment. There are several ways to incorporate drug treatment into an already existing partial-hospitalization program. One method is to establish a separate dual-diagnosis team within the partial-hospitalization program. This approach requires hiring separate staff experienced in the treatment of dual-diagnosis patients and having consultants train existing staff. If a separate team cannot be formed or if the volume of dual-diagnosis patients identified is too small to warrant a separate team, patients can be referred for parallel concurrent treatment at an outpatient drug abuse treatment center or with a counselor. In addition, evening attendance at self-help groups such as Narcotics Anonymous can often be a useful treatment supplement for the dual-diagnosis patient in a partial-hospitalization program.

## DUAL-DIAGNOSIS TREATMENT PERSONNEL

The effective diagnosis and treatment of dually diagnosed patients requires a very experienced and flexible treatment team. The causes of psychiatric disorders are multifactorial. The causes of drug-dependence disorders are multifactorial. The treatment of dually diagnosed patients involves the blending of psychiatric and drug treatment strategies. This can be difficult because this particular treatment mix involves some different and often opposing therapeutic modalities. Each staff member may also have treatment strengths or preferences that may be opposing and different. Treatment team members should be educated and experienced in the diagnosis and treatment of both psychiatric disorders and drug dependence. Although credentials and experience are important, it is more important that the treatment team function in unison. This could be said about any treatment team, but it applies especially to dual-diagnosis treatment teams. Individuals educated, trained, and experienced in psychiatry sometimes are at odds with those educated, trained, and experienced in the diagnosis and treatment of drug abuse. The reverse is also true. Therefore, an essential and key component is open-mindedness and flexibility on the part of each team member. Effective communication and mutual respect among team members is a prerequisite to a unified treatment approach. Often, the dual-diagnosis patient's uncanny ability to detect disharmony among treatment team members and (with the help of the patient community) devastate the team with staff-splitting is underestimated. Dually diagnosed patients will often staff-split in individual therapy sessions. This is especially true of treatment-resistant, oppositional, or borderline dual-diagnosis patients. This is one more reason for frequent communication among staff members.

The dual-diagnosis team leader must be well versed in medicine, psychiatry, psychology, and sociology. It is important for the physician openly to support a philosophy of treatment that represents approaches comfortable to each team member. Team leader responsibilities include:

1. Thorough medical history and physical
2. Management/supervision of crisis intervention
3. Ongoing evaluation for psychiatric disorders
4. Medical detoxification
5. Psychopharmacology
6. Keeping current with treatment advances in psychiatric and psychoactive use disorders
7. Familiarity with self-help groups
8. Supervision of all clinical staff members
9. Treatment team burnout prevention
10. Maintaining elevated treatment team morale
11. Providing medical, psychiatric, and drug education for staff and patients
12. Community education regarding dual diagnosis

Because drug-dependent persons should not be prescribed medications with the potential for abuse, the physician must have pharmacological alternatives available for the dual-diagnosis patient with medical illnesses. (Table 4). For example, in many instances, the dually diagnosed patient has been

**Table 4** Alternatives for Some Common Medical and Psychiatric Disorders

| Medical Condition | Medicine | Alternative |
|---|---|---|
| Tendonitis | Codeine | Naproxen |
| Arthritis | Oxycodone | Indomethacin |
| Seizure disorder | Phenobarbital | Dilantin |
| Glaucoma | Tetrahydrocannabinol | Carbonic anhydrase inhibitors |
| Diarrhea | Diphenoxylate | Kaolin/pectin |
| Antitussives | Alcohol-containing | Delsym |
| Antispasmodic | Barbiturate | Clidinium bromide |
| Tooth extraction | Propoxyphene | Ibuprofen |

| Psychiatric Condition | Medicine | Alternative |
|---|---|---|
| Anxiety disorder | Alprazolam | Imipramine |
| Attention Deficit | Methylphenidate | Pemoline |
| Nicotine dependence | Scopolamine | Clonidine |
| Insomnia | Flurazepam | Doxepin |

prescribed a barbiturate containing medicine for severe migraine headaches. The physician should be aware of safer nonaddicting alternate medicines such as beta-blockers or amitriptyline. If an effective alternate medicine is not prescribed, the patient is likely to obtain the barbiturate elsewhere, or the discomfort of persistent migraine headaches may serve as an excuse to relapse. Other alternatives to some common medical and psychiatric conditions treated with dependence-prone medicines are in Table 4.

The dual-diagnosis-treating physician has an added responsibility for carefully considering the psychiatric diagnosis, the drug-dependence diagnosis, the medications currently being taken, and all the possible interactions prior to prescribing for the new condition being treated. For example, an individual with schizophreniform disorder and benzodiazepine dependence who is being treated for nicotine dependence is more likely to benefit from clonidine than scopolamine [15].

The registered nurse is an important member of the dual-diagnosis treatment team. Ideal nursing experience consists of training in emergency psychiatry, intensive care, medical detoxification, and drug rehabilitation. Nurses must be skilled in differentiating the drug-seeking behavior common to dependent patients from the necessary dispensing of medications to psychiatric or medical patients. Nurses on dual-diagnosis units frequently are also group therapy leaders or cofacilitators. The nurse's job description is therefore a more inclusive variation to traditional nursing as responsibilities encompass aspects of medicine, psychiatry, and drug rehabilitation.

Psychologists also experienced in treating drug dependence in a rehabilitation setting are most helpful in the ongoing evaluation and treatment of dually diagnosed patients. Psychological test interpretations provide rapid insight and serve as invaluable diagnostic adjuncts. This is especially true when inpatient hospital length of stay is limited, disallowing adequate observation and accurate diagnosis. In this day of third-party provided influence on length of hospital stay, the treatment team is often rushed and forced to hastily generate a diagnosis. This is a big handicap for clinicians considering dual-diagnosis. The psychologist can be most instrumental in accelerating the evaluation process. Psychologists also conduct individual therapy and address issues that may be inappropriate or difficult to discuss in a group setting. Individual therapists belonging to a dual-diagnosis team regularly reinforce the importance and goals of other treatment modalities offered by the dual-diagnosis treatment team. This helps the dual-diagnosis patient to view all treatment modalities working in unison for a common goal rather than to gravitate toward one particular aspect of treatment. The psychologist is also instrumental in presenting staff education specific to dual-diagnosis treatment, as are other members of the team.

It becomes apparent, in treating either psychiatric or drug patients, that family members also need to be involved in treatment. Family members of dual-diagnosis patients may be confused, feel helpless, and be suffering from their own psychological or substance abuse problems [16]. Social workers who are also experienced in the diagnosis and treatment of drug dependence complement the treatment team by directing the essential family component of dual-diagnosis treatment. Areas of expertise that complement the traditional training of the clinical social worker include:

1. Diagnosis and treatment of codependency [17]
2. Recognition of the adult child of alcoholic syndrome [18]
3. Diagnosis and treatment of drug dependence
4. History of, and familiarity with, self-help groups such as Nar-Anon and Families Anonymous.
5. Liaison with vocational consultant or employer

Certified drug counselors complete the core of the dual-diagnosis treatment team. Certified drug counselors experienced in treating alcohol or drug dependence are easier to acquire than those who are also experienced in treating the dual-diagnosis patient. The treatment contribution of certified drug counselors often has a strong foundation in Narcotics Anonymous and a 12-step orientation. Narcotics Anonymous has produced a subculture of recovered drug-dependent counselors who reject the view of drug dependence as a symptom of underlying psychological problems. Many drug counselors working in traditional drug rehabilitation centers believe in the spontaneous remission of psychiatric symptoms coincidental to drug abstinence. Less commonly encountered are certified drug counselors with the view needed for effective participation in a dual-diagnosis team: that although many psychiatric symptoms result from drug abuse and that the majority of psychiatric symptoms abate following drug abstinence, about 20% of drug-dependent persons also have a psychiatric disorder that may not benefit from the usual drug treatment program alone. Dual-diagnosis drug counselors, therefore, must be trained to recognize psychiatric disorders and differentiate the psychiatric symptoms from drug induced psychiatric symptoms.

It is not uncommon for members of a dual-diagnosis team to have had numerous educational experiences and credentials. For example, a team member with Ph.D. and C.A.C. (Certified Alcoholism Counselor) credentials can be an invaluable asset to the dual-diagnosis treatment team. A master's level social worker who successfully completed residential treatment for drug dependence ten years earlier can also be an added asset. Although they are not essential, recovered drug-dependent members of the dual-diagnosis treatment team can be especially valuable. Their knowledge and experience can be an asset. The biggest complement to a particular dual-diagnosis team is work with a recovered dual-diagnosis peer who was treated years earlier at the same treatment facility. Patients look up to the recovered dual-diagnosis staff members because they represent achievement and treatment success. Our experience has been good employing recovered dual-diagnosis persons who are certified drug counselors. About 40% of the more than 50 drug counselors at Fair Oaks Hospital are recovered.

The identification of adult dually diagnosed patients requires a careful and accurate drug-free diagnostic period. Once diagnosed, treatment of both disorders should occur concurrently and with equal importance in a manner similar to the way in which diabetics with asthma are treated. The dual-diagnosis treatment staff must present a unified front and function truly as a team. The effective treatment of adult dually diagnosed patients requires not only specialized treatment staff and components but also availability of numerous dual-diagnosis treatment frameworks.

## REFERENCES

1. *Alcoholics Anonymous* New York: Alcoholics Anonymous World Service Office, 1976:58.
2. Dackis CA, Gold MS. Alcoholism, In: Gold MS, Lydiard RL, Carman JS, eds. *Advances in Psychopharmacology: Predicting and Improving Treatment Response.* Boca Raton, FL: CRC Press, 1984:278.
3. Cocores JA, Patel MD, Gold MS, Pottash AC. Cocaine abuse, attention deficit disorder, and bipolar disorder. *J Nerv Ment Dis* 1987; 175(7):431.
4. Verebey K, Martin D, Gold, MS. Drug abuse: interpretation of laboratory tests. In: Gold MS, Pottash ALC, eds. *Diagnostic and Laboratory Testing in Psychiatry.* New York: Plenum Press, 1986:155.
5. Gold MS, Estroff TW. The comprehensive evaluation of cocaine and opiate abusers. In: Hall RCW, Beresford TP, eds. *Handbook of Psychiatric Diagnostic Procedures.* Jamaica, New York: Spectrum Publications, 1985:213.
6. Gross DA, Extein I, Gold MS. The psychiatrist as physician. In: Extein I, Gold MS, eds. *Medical Mimics of Psychiatric Disorders.* Washington, DC: APA Press, 1986:93.
7. Gold MS, Pottash AC, Extein I. Clonidine in acute opiate withdrawal. *NEJ Med* 1980; 302:1421.
8. Gawin FH, Kleber HD. Desipramine facilitation of initial cocaine abstinence. *Arch Gen Psychiatry* 1989; 46:117.
9. Dackis CA, Gold MS. Bromocriptine as treatment of cocaine abuse. *Lancet* 1985; 1:8438:1151.
10. Cocores JA, Gold MS. Dopaminergic treatments in cocaine withdrawal. Society for Neuroscience, 19th Annual Meeting, Phoenix, Arizona, p. 251, 1989.

11. Dackis CA, Gold MS. Opiate addiction and depression: cause or effect? *Drug Alc Depend* 1983; 11:105.
12. Khantzian EJ. Self-medication hypothesis of addictive disorders: focus on heroin and cocaine dependence. *Am J Psychiatry* 1985; 142:1259.
13. *Narcotics Anonymous.* Van Nuys, CA: World Service Office, 1984:55.
14. Cocores JA, Gold MS. Recognition and crisis intervention treatment with cocaine abusers. In: Roberts, AR, ed. *Crisis Intervention Handbook.* Pacific Grove, CA: Wadsworth, 1989:118.
15. Cocores JA, Gold MS. Transcutaneous scopolamine for nicotine dependence: use in non-addicts versus recovering addicts. Presented at 20th annual meeting of American Medical Society on Alcoholism and Other Drug Dependencies, Atlanta, GA. 1989; 8:23.
16. Cocores JA. *The 800-Cocaine Book of Drug and Alcohol Recovery.* New York: Villard Books, 1990:191.
17. Cocores JA. Co-addiction: a silent epidemic. *Fair Oaks Hospital Psychiatry Letter* 1987; 5(2):5.
18. Ceremak TL. *Diagnosing and Treating Co-Dependence.* Minneapolis, MN: Johnson Institute Books, 1986.

# 15

## Treatment of the Dually Diagnosed Adolescent

### J. Calvin Chatlos

*St. Mary Hospital, Hoboken, New Jersey*

### Judith B. Tufaro

*Fair Oaks Hospital, Summit, New Jersey*

The use of alcohol and drugs by adolescents has led to the recognition of substance abuse as "one of the most serious health hazards confronting our youth" [1]. Following the appearance and widespread use of crack cocaine in 1986, the extensive media coverage of the hazards of cocaine and other drug use, has led to a reduction in demand despite continued availability [2]. However, as stated by Johnston, [2] changing use in the already addicted population "is going to take longer and will depend heavily on our ability to provide adequate treatment capacity attract people into treatment, and offer effective treatment. The addicted are going to require the pound of cure, not the ounce of prevention."

This chapter will elaborate on the "pound of cure" required for effective treatment of adolescents. It will begin with a description of the extent of the problem and identify concerns specific to understanding adolescent chemical dependency. An emphasis on developing a comprehensive bio-psychosocial model will illustrate specific needs for assessment of adolescents. A detailed treatment model from the Adolescent Center for Chemical Education, Prevention and Treatment (ACCEPT) program, integrating the 12 steps of AA and psychiatric treatments, will be presented. The purpose of this chapter is to guide clinicians in treatment based on current research.

## EXTENT OF THE PROBLEM

Information about the extent of drug and alcohol use in young people is obtained primarily from two nationwide monitoring programs supported by the National Institute of Drug Abuse (NIDA): the *National Household Survey on Drug Abuse* (NHSDA), conducted by the Research Triangle Institute in North Carolina, and the University of Michigan research and reporting program entitled *Monitoring the Future: A Continuing Study of the Lifestyles and Values of Youth* (also referred to as the National High School Senior Survey).

The NHSDA has surveyed a random selection of household members age 12 and older every two or three years since 1971. The latest report [3] for 1988 shows significant decreases in drug use for the age group 12–17 years. Lifetime use of any illicit drug decreased from 44% in 1979 to 25% in 1988. Lifetime prevalence of marijuana use, the most widely used illicit drug, decreased from its peak of 37% in 1979 to 24% in 1985 to 17% in 1988. Lifetime prevalence of cocaine use dropped from its peak of 6.5% in 1982 to 3.4% in 1988. Current use of alcohol decreased from its peak of 37% in 1979 to 31% in 1985 and further to 25% in 1988.

The *Monitoring the Future* program has surveyed a representative sample of high school seniors annually since 1975 and has obtained follow-up surveys to include college students since 1977. It reports on the use of 11 separate classes of drugs (including alcohol and nicotine), as well as the grade level of first use, and attitudes and beliefs of peers, friends, and parents regarding drug use. Supporting data in the NHSDA, this survey [2] reported a significant decrease from peak prevalence of illicit drug use by 66% of high school seniors in 1981 and 1982 to 54% in 1988. During that time, lifetime marijuana use decreased from 59% to 47%, cocaine use decreased from 17% to 12%, alcohol use remained alarmingly steady at 93% to 92%, and cigarette use decreased from 71% to 66%. Further information shows that the decrease in use of marijuana and cocaine has mirrored an increase in perceived risk of harm in use in spite of continued or increased availability. (Figure 1).

Information about more extensive use revealed that 18% of high school seniors smoke cigarettes daily, 11% smoke half a pack or more a day, 2.7% smoke marijuana daily, and 4.2% drink alcohol daily, with 35% reporting having had five or more drinks in a row on at least one occasion during the two weeks just prior to the survey.

These surveys demonstrate the significant extent not only of adolescent drug and alcohol use but daily preoccupation and probable dependence. They also suggest the effects that education efforts and perceived harm of use can have on adolescents' use in spite of continued availability. To clini-

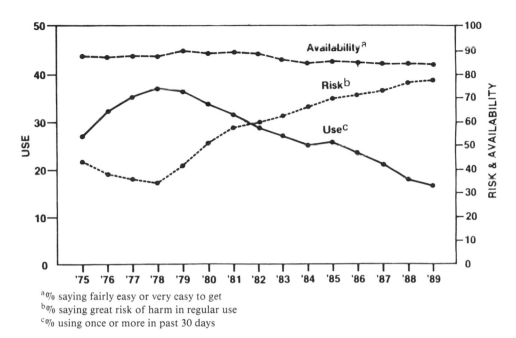

<sup>a</sup>% saying fairly easy or very easy to get
<sup>b</sup>% saying great risk of harm in regular use
<sup>c</sup>% using once or more in past 30 days

**Figure 1** Trends in marijuana availability, perceived risk of regular use, and use in past 30 days by high school seniors.

cians, they highlight the probability of 5–10% of teenagers using drugs extensively enough to require treatment.

## ADOLESCENT CHEMICAL DEPENDENCY SYNDROME

Attempts to comprehend these background data in order to make them clinically useful have led to the concept of the adolescent chemical dependency (ACD) syndrome. This concept has been developing rapidly in the past five years and has led to a comprehensive review [4]. A significant contribution to understanding the development of this concept was research demonstrating a developmental sequence, or stages, of drug use [5] as illustrated in Figure 2. Use often begins in junior high school with the chemicals socially acceptable to adults—cigarettes, beer, wine, and hard liquor. Subsequently, some users continue along an age-related progression to illicit drugs, beginning usually with marijuana and continuing to include other illicit drugs. Drugs that begin in earlier stages are continued in later stages as new drugs are added [6]. This leads to the multiple drug abuse common in

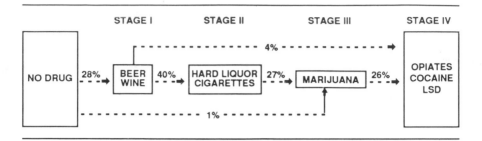

**Figure 2**   Major stages of adolescent involvement in drug use. (From Ref. 5.)

adolescents [7]. Donovan and Jessor [8] have provided support for an additional stage of "problem drinking" that occurs after marijuana use begins.

This progression is related to specific effects of the drug in inducing pleasurable affects, the role of the drug in dealing with stress, and the psychosocial setting [9]. McDonald detailed four clinical stages to the syndrome of chemical dependency: (1) learning the mood swing, (2) seeking the mood swing, (3) preoccupation with the mood swing, and (4) doing drugs to feel okay. These stages are associated with progressive drug use and dependence, and progressive use of drugs to deal with stress and problems in increasing areas of the person's life. The final stage usually involves physical deterioration and physiological dependency.

## BIOPSYCHOSOCIAL MODEL

Clinical use of these stages has guided assessment and treatment of adolescents but have not been validated by research. Attempts to understand these stages have raised many questions regarding ACD. Research has focused on antecedents, [10,11] concomitants, [12] and maintenance factors of ACD in an attempt to define the etiology of this syndrome. In recent years, as noted in a review by Bailey, [13] ACD is a condition requiring a comprehensive biopsychosocial approach.

One of the classic expressions of the biopsychosocial model described by Engel [14,15] as it relates to substance abuse was proposed by Jellinek [16] in *The Disease Concept of Alcoholism*. The specific approach to the biopsychosocial model used by the Adolescent Center for Chemical Education, Prevention and Treatment (ACCEPT) is based on the disease concept of chemical dependence (Figure 3). This particular expression of the model has been very useful for adolescents, families, and public audiences in understanding the extensive nature of ACD.

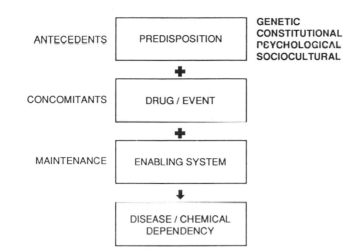

**Figure 3**   Biopsychosocial disease model.

This biopsychosocial model is divided into three parts, which correspond to research efforts on antecedents, concomitants, and maintenance factors of ACD. With adults, using alcoholism as a heuristic example, Donovan [17] divided the antecedents or predisposition into four possible sources: genetic, constitutional, psychological, and sociocultural. Family, twin, and adoption studies of adults [17–19] demonstrate evidence for a *genetic* basis that may predispose a person to alcoholism or produce a vulnerability. The 54% concordance rate for alcoholism in identical twins, and a 38% rate in paternal twins support this genetic basis. Sons of alcoholic fathers have a four times greater chance of developing alcoholism than controls. Data regarding the genetics of other drug abuse are not well defined, and the strengths that this factor contributes in ACD are yet to be determined.

Support for a *constitutional* basis again comes from adult studies showing a high heritability of alcohol-elimination rates in male twins, [20] higher levels of acetaldehyde in sons of alcoholics than in sons of nonalcoholics after an alcohol challenge, [21] and lower activity of acetaldehyde dehydrogenase in sober alcoholics than in controls [22]. Evaluation of several other markers correctly distinguished 83% of controls and 70% of sons of alcoholics [23]. The role of tetrahydroisoquinolines (THIQ) in the brain associated with alcohol administration may be related to its addictive potential [24]. As discussed by Donovan, [17] the constitutional factors may have a genetic basis or may be due to environmental influences.

*Psychological* factors have been more thoroughly studied as predisposing factors to adolescent substance abuse. These have been reviewed in Isralowitz and Singer [1] and include: negative attitude toward school and low self-esteem, low sense of psychological well-being, low self-esteem regarding school, rebelliousness, untrustworthiness, sociability and impulsive traits, tolerance of deviance, inconsistency between one's own and one's parents' opinions about drug abuse, lower academic aspirations, low school achievement, dropping out of school, mental health problems, frequent cigarette smoking, disciplinary problems in school, and delinquent and deviant behavior.

*Sociocultural* studies in adults [17,25] have demonstrated the effects of age, occupation, social class, and subcultural and religious affiliations on alcoholism. Sociocultural antecedents in adolescents have also been reviewed by Isralowitz and Singer [1] and include: parental use of hard liquor and drugs, parental divorce, parental arrest, lack of closeness between parents and children, high level of adolescent peer activity, drug use and problem behavior by close friends, broader society becoming a "drug culture," and portrayal of drugs as glamorous. Semlitz and Gold [10] also summarized additional social antecedents of chemical abuse that included the adolescent's own beliefs and values about drug use and its harmfulness, and behavior that demonstrates nonconformity, rebellion, and independence.

To all of these predisposing factors a *drug* is then introduced. Among teenagers, the major forces of introduction are peer pressure and availability [11]. Botvin [26] identifies other social, cognitive, attitudinal, personality, and developmental factors that may play a role in the initiation of substance abuse. However, once introduced, the strong positive reinforcement of the drug euphoria, the negative reinforcement of the abstinence symptoms, and genetic and biochemical effects, [11,27,28] as well as set and setting of use, [29] interact with predisposition and personality to dominate the clinical picture. Various other concomitants to drug use [12] include genetic factors associated with acute toxic reactions to drugs, vulnerability to adverse effects of toxic substances on the brain during childhood and adolescence, dislike of school, less adequate problem-solving skills, lower expectation of getting one's needs met, lower religiosity, lower cognitive development, higher life stress, frequency of school absenteeism, early premarital intercourse, running away from home, sexual promiscuity, and perceived lack of parental support.

The final factor in the biopsychosocial model equation is the *enabling system*. This is the system of people surrounding users that knowingly or unknowingly act to enable adolescents to continue use by preventing them from facing the consequences of their drug use, which leads to progression of the disease [31]. This factor has been described clinically but poorly researched. This may include promoting use without knowledge of harmful effects, modeling drug use and dependence, denial of the adolescent's use, or removal of consequences that would deter use [31]. This system may include parents, friends, teachers, therapists, physicians, judges, lawyers, law enforcement personnel, and broader aspects of a political and economic system. Singer and Anglin [32] demonstrated physician's failures to identify alcohol and drug problems in adolescents.

The interaction of the predisposition, drug effects and concomitant behaviors, and enabling system lead ACD to be a primary, progressive, chronic, and multidimensional illness [33]. According to Gitlow and Peyser, [34] primary means that "though the [alcoholic's] illness may begin from quite diverse psychological origins, once the disease of [alcoholism] has been grafted upon this personality structure, it dominates the clinical picture and eventually becomes the major determinant in both choice and efficacy of therapy." Whatever the temporal process of predisposition, drug interaction with concomitant events, and enabling system, the user eventually acquires characteristics of the ACD syndrome that are seemingly autonomous. Once alcohol or other drug abuse is grafted onto the personality, a new illness occurs that is inextricably intertwined. The intertwining develops as a result of conditioning of the body and behavior by drugs and learning effects [35,36].

This has important treatment implications since, once the drug is removed physically, the patterned behaviors—drug urges or cravings, impulsiveness, paranoia, fearfulness, and distrust—remain and are the focus of treatment. Morrison and Smith [11] have described a "biochemical-genetic" line that is crossed during addiction, after which the chemicals control the adolescent's behavior. They deemed addiction to be an "urge" that precludes logical and rational thought processes. Another way of understanding this is associated with the paradox of control, as the person becomes stimulus-responsive [37] based on interoceptive and exteroceptive stimuli that have been conditioned by drug use.

## Family Factors

The biopsychosocial model, as described, emphasizes the role of family as a maintenance factor in the enabling system part of the equation. It is important to recognize that the family is an important aspect of all three factors— the antecedent (predisposition), concomitant (drug/event), and the maintenance. An interactive/reciprocal approach is required to understand how chemical dependency affects the entire family and how the entire family affects chemical dependency [38].

Some of the antecedent factors involving the family that have been studied are birth order and sibling relationships [39]; parental mental illness, divorce and separation, and frequent geographical moves [40]; and parental substance abuse as a more important determinant of adolescent drug abuse than parental attitude toward substance abuse.

Problems often begin in early adolescence associated with new developmental issues. The onset of puberty and sexuality heralds the developmental family issues of physical changes, identity formation, autonomy, [41] and separation-individuation [42]. Dramatic physical and social changes during junior high school lead to an awareness of body function and self and experimentation of new behaviors required to adapt to these changes. Drug and alcohol use readily become part of this experimentation physically and socially as a result of strong peer pressures. As the adolescent progresses through stages of chemical dependency, the family is undergoing its own progression through stages of codependency. Kaufman [38] describes the progression of codependency that develops between adolescent and family:

> Drug-abusing adolescents generally refuse to follow parental rules for behavior at home. They associate with individuals whom their parents consider bad influences and bring them into the house. They come home just sufficiently later than curfews and without calling in a way that infuriates their parents. They drive the family car without permission and frequently get traffic citations which they can't afford to pay and which require parental court appearance. They are constantly in trouble at school, particularly through tardiness, absence, not paying attention, and unruly behavior, yet they develop a multiplicity of ways for intercepting messages from school to parents. Shoplifting as well as theft from and damage to friends' homes are also common and the adolescent may either conceal or flaunt these activities. Parents are lied to about needs for funds that are diverted to drugs and when these lies are discovered, parents are coerced into continuing to provide funds by threats of violence from debtors or of commission of crimes, and through promises of protection from incarceration. They continue to drink and to use drugs at home after they've been prohibited from doing so even with legal reinforcement. They lie about their substance abuse and destructive behavior and the lies themselves frequently become a major concern to parents. They also engage parents in frequent power struggles about whether they are high or have used drugs. This type of defiance leads many parents to feel they have totally lost control of their children.

Family members, at this point, have become preoccupied with the adolescent's behavior and their own inability to contain it, much as the teenager has become preoccupied with drugs and loss of control over use.

Some family factors that have been identified as concomitants of this progression are triangulation, [43] sibling relationships, [44] patterns of intimacy and distance, [42] inconsistency in parental rule-making and limit-setting, use of denial, covert encouragement of deviant behaviors, and impaired intergenerational mourning [45].

As the codependency progresses, families of chemically dependent children tend to be rigidly enmeshed, with blurred generational boundaries and intensely symbiotic or emotionally distant relationships [42]. The family has been described as dull and lifeless, only becoming alive when it is mobilized to deal with the crisis of drug abuse [46]. Some maintenance factors in these systems are the use of guilt by teenagers and parents; physical symptoms of depression, anxiety, or psychosomatic problems; and even parental suicide attempts blamed on the teenager [39]. Communication is most frequently negative and without praise for good behavior [46]. Levine [42] describes examples of unresolved mourning of family members maintaining substance abuse in "an ongoing deathlike process with suicidal ramifications."

All of these examples illustrate the use of the biopsychosocial model and the value of including the family in all factors of the process. This model demonstrates the complexity of the ACD syndrome and has been helpful in structuring both assessment and treatment.

## DUAL DIAGNOSIS AND BIOPSYCHOSOCIAL MODEL

As demonstrated extensively in other areas of this book, the relevance of psychiatric disorders concomitant with chemical dependency in adults is critical in assessment and treatment. Many of the same concerns occur with teenagers. However, dual diagnosis in ACD has only recently been appreciated. A review by Morrison and Smith [11] included depression, [9,47] conduct disorder, [48] attention deficit hyperactivity disorder, [49] eating disorders, [50] and borderline personality disorders [51]. A more recent review [13] includes further associations between substance abuse and depression, [52] bipolar disorder [53] antisocial behavior [7] attention deficit hyperactivity disorder, [54] borderline personality disorder, [55] and suicide [56,57].

When studies of adolescents are reviewed, the major impediment in all studies has been the lack of an adequate assessment tool for ACD. The use of DSM-III criteria was hampered by the rarity of physical signs of withdrawal occurring with ACD. The revised criteria for DSM III-R are more helpful in this regard and are more consistent with the use of a comprehensive biopsychosocial model necessary in approaching ACD. However, no specific studies validating DSM III-R criteria for substance abuse and dependence have been conducted for adolescents.

A comparison of two studies done at Fair Oaks Hospital is somewhat revealing of the situation. A retrospective study [58] of adolescents treated in 1980–1981 on an inpatient psychiatric unit assessed the presence of concomitant substance abuse using DSM III criteria. Of 41 patients in the study, 29 (71%) were abusing one or more drugs at admission. Of those 29, diagnosis was first made in 14 (48%) at admitting interview, 13 (45%) by admitting urine drug screen, and 2 (7%) at structured neuropsychiatric interview. The admitting urine drug screen was positive in 19 (65%) and negative in 10 (34%) patients with a positive clinical history of substance abuse. A subsequent study was conducted by the same author [59] at the same hospital but, in 1987, after an adolescent substance abuse inpatient unit was established. A Structured Clinical Interview for DSM III-R (SCID) of 60 consecutive adolescents admitted for substance abuse using DSM III criteria was conducted one to six weeks following admission. An SCID diagnosable Axis I illness was present in 53 (87%). The categories included conduct disorder 53 (88%), post-traumatic stress disorder 26 (42%), major depression 8 (13%), simple phobia 6 (10%), social phobia 5 (7%), agoraphobia 4 (5.7%), bulimia 3 (5%). Considering the diagnosis of post-traumatic stress disorder, it was of note that 11 (18%) had traumatic stressors precede the onset of addiction and 15 (25%) had stressors follow and were related to addiction.

In conjunction with the use of the biopsychosocial model for ACD, the psychiatric disorders are also explained using this model. For instance, a person with depression has a predisposition that includes a strong genetic component. Concordance rates for affective illness in identical twins of 67% and in paternal twins of 15%, as well as data from adoption studies, support this [60]. Supporting evidence of constitutional factors in a predisposition include neuroendocrine studies that show abnormal biogenic amines and abnormal hypothalamic-pituitary-adrenal axis [61]. Psychological and sociocultural factors continue to be relevant to understanding depression [62]. In the depression biopsychosocial model, rather than the drug serving as the event, studies have shown that life events are significantly related to the development of depression [63]. The last factor of the enabling system and maintenance factors of depression have been poorly studied, although there has been a focus on the role of support systems or intimate relationships being protective of depression. As described in further detail, [64] this model can be used in the understanding and treatment of affective disorder, post-traumatic stress disorder, conduct disorders and delinquency, sexual dependence, and personality disorders, such as narcissistic and borderline disorders, commonly found associated with chemical dependency.

## ASSESSMENT

The complexity in understanding ACD as described has made assessment difficult and poorly standardized. The role of extent of use for many years was the measure of chemical dependency. Studies began to reveal specific characteristics of the adolescent population that required a broader approach. The multiple drug use and the association with stages of a syndrome including other behaviors was described but not validated by research. Owen and Nyberg, [65] noted that adolescent chemical-dependency programs varied greatly in their assessment of ACD, with most relying on subjective judgment and on nonstandardized or adult measures. With the increasing need for treatment, the demands for accurate diagnosis have escalated.

In 1982, the Chemical Dependency Adolescent Assessment Project (CDAAP) was initiated in Minnesota. Its purpose was to develop a clinical standardized assessment battery to aid professionals in the identification, referral, and treatment of problems associated with adolescent alcohol and drug involvement. The project comprehensively reviewed efforts to date of ACD assessment [66]. These instruments are noted in Table 1. This project, supported by an NIDA initiative, [67] has been a major impetus to coordinating professional efforts at understanding and treating this problem comprehensively. It will be described in detail as part of a comprehensive evaluation of adolescents.

## NIDA ADOLESCENT ASSESSMENT-REFERRAL SYSTEM

The recognition of the need for a comprehensive biopsychosocial model in addressing adolescent issues and the importance and urgency related to the ACD syndrome has prompted a unique situation for adolescent medicine and psychiatry. The NIDA has developed a comprehensive Adolescent Assessment and Referral System program to coordinate efforts nationwide and across disciplines (Table 2).

The assessment package begins with a self-administered Problem Oriented Screening Instrument for Teenagers (POSIT) designed to identify youth in need of further assessment in 10 domains:

1. Substance use/abuse
2. Physical health status
3. Mental health status
4. Family relationships
5. Peer relations
6. Educational status
7. Vocational status
8. Social skills
9. Leisure and recreation
10. Aggressive behavior/delinquency

A Comprehensive Assessment Battery has been developed with specific instruments to further elaborate and assess any of the identified problem

**Table 1** Summary of Recently Developed or In-Progress Adolescent Chemical Involvement Assessment Tools

| Instrument Name | Source | Publication Status | Administration Format | Features |
|---|---|---|---|---|
| Adolescent Assessment and Referral System | NIDA | Unpublished | paper-and-pencil | Consists of a battery of screening measures, a diagnostic instrumentation guide, and a treatment referral guide |
| Adolescent Chemical Health Inventory | Renovex | Renovex 1988 | computer self-administered | Contains clinically oriented scales |
| Adolescent Drinking Index | Harrell and Wirtz | Psychological Assessment Resources 1989 | paper-and-pencil | Screening tool intended to measure problem drinking |
| Adolescent Drug Involvement Scale | Moberg | Unpublished | paper-and-pencil | Drug abuse screening instrument adapted from the Adolescent Alcohol Involvement Scale (Mayer and Filstead 1979) |
| Client Substance Index | Moore | Olympic Counseling Services 1983 | paper-and-pencil | Organized around Jellinek's symptoms of chemical dependency |

| Instrument | Author | Source | Format | Description |
|---|---|---|---|---|
| Drug Abuse Screening Test-Adolescent Version | Skinner | Unpublished | paper-and-pencil | Screening instrument adapted from the adult version of this test |
| Guided Rational Adolescent Substance Abuse Profile | Addiction Recovery Corporation | Addiction Recovery Corporation 1986 | semi-structured interview | Primarily organized around DSM-III criteria for substance use disorders |
| Minnesota Chemical Dependency Adolescent Assessment Package | Winters and Henly | Western Psychological Services 1988 and in press; Adolescent Assessment Project 1988 | paper-and-pencil, computer self-administered, and structured interview | Battery consists of three separate instruments: a multidimensional clinical inventory, a DSM-III-R diagnostic interview, and a problem severity screening tool |
| Perceived-Benefit of Drinking and Drug Use Scales | Petchers and Singer | Petchers and Singer 1987 | paper-and-pencil | Screening tool consisting of parallel alcohol and drug perceived-benefit items |
| Substance Involvement Instrument | Aladar | Cascade Oaks 1987 | paper-and-pencil | Organized around a rational theory concerning the progression of adolescent chemical involvement |

Winters K. The need for improved assessment of adolescent substance involvement, *J. Drug Issues* 1990; 20(3):487–502.

Table 2    Schematic Model for the Assessment-Referral System

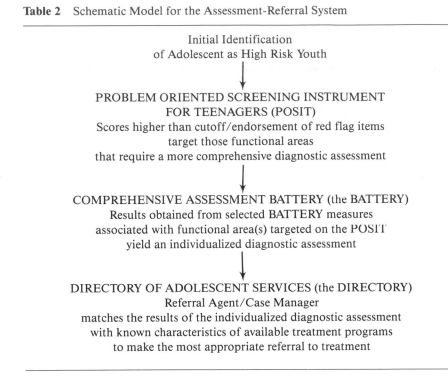

domains. The assessment of the substance use/abuse is done with the CDAAP tools to be described. The results of this extensive assessment will be used to determine referrals to appropriate treatment centers using a Directory of Adolescent Services currently being developed. It is hoped that these assessment tools and organized referral use will lead to the development of guidelines for optimal client-treatment matching as described by Hester and Miller [68].

## SUBSTANCE USE/ABUSE

Evaluation begins with a complete history. Excellent reviews on the interviewing process and guidelines for clinicians are provided by Anglin [69] and Farrow and Deisher [70]. It is recommended that information obtained by personal interview follow the domains mentioned in the NIDA Adolescent Assessment and Referral Service outline and those measured in the CDAAP assessment questionnaires. The interviewing situation may reveal unnoted areas, elaborate identified problem areas, or identify sensitive issues that are withheld on a questionnaire. Information must also be obtained from other sources such as parents, teachers, referral sources, or other agencies involved.

The CDAAP battery was developed to provide standardized measures of the ACD syndrome. It consists of three separate instruments: the Personal Experience Screen Questionnaire (PESQ), a drug abuse screening questionnaire, the Personal Experience Inventory (PEI), a multidimensional questionnaire, and the Adolescent Diagnostic Interview (ADI), a DSM-III-R-based diagnostic interview.

The Personal Experience Screen Questionnaire (PESQ) is a 38-item, self-administered 15-minute questionnaire designed to screen the severity of chemical involvement. It is useful as an initial screening tool for preassessment in deciding if a more complete assessment is warranted. School and chemical-dependency clinic norms have been collected. The design includes assessment of "faking" tendencies, and the problem severity scale is correlated highly with a similar scale on the more comprehensive Personal Experience Inventory.

The Adolescent Diagnostic Interview (ADI) is a structured diagnostic interview requiring 45–60 minutes to determine whether the client meets DSM-III-R diagnostic criteria for psychoactive substance use disorders. It begins by reviewing client and family background and also includes Axes 4 and 5, severity of psychosocial stressors and global level of functioning. It also briefly screens for six other mental disorders (affective, attention deficit, developmental, psychosis, eating, and anxiety), using approximately five screening questions for each in a yes/no format. Data demonstrate a high degree of reliability and indicate that DSM-III-R criteria for substance use disorders appear valid for adolescents.

The Personal Experience Inventory (PEI) is a 300-item, 45–60-minute self-administered questionnaire designed to evaluate comprehensively the adolescent chemical-dependency syndrome. The PEI consists of two parts: a Chemical Involvement Problem Severity Section (CIPSS) and a Psychosocial Section.

The CIPSS was developed clinically and empirically, with identification of five basic dimensions of chemical use:

1. Personal involvement with chemicals: measures global chemical use problem severity. Items focus on the specific reinforcing properties of chemicals in altering mood state and assess harmful consequences and dependency-related features.
2. Effects from use: items relate to chemical use associated with aversive psychological, physiological, and behavioral effects such as feeling out of control.

3.  Personal consequences: items relate to difficulties with friends, parents, school, and social institutions as a result of use of chemicals.
4.  Social benefits use: items reflect use associated with increased social confidence, peer acceptance, and interpersonal skills.
5.  Polydrug use: items survey use of seven drug categories (marijuana, stimulants, tranquilizers, "downers," cocaine, hallucinogens, and opioids) other than alcohol.

Findings by the CDAAP suggest that these five dimensions can adequately assess the severity of chemical use. These are correlated with the symptoms in DSM-III-R substance use disorders and reflect the multidimensional aspect of adolescent chemical dependency described previously. Using statistical analyses, questions regarding specificity of the "syndrome" concept and the ability to identify independent dimensions of ACD were evaluated. Factor analysis of the five scales demonstrated that a single factor could account for over 70% of the total variance and was unable to demonstrate independent dimensions, supporting the clinically described concept of an ACD "syndrome."

Research conducted in developing the Personal Involvement with Chemicals subscale also investigated the stagelike progression of ACD. Items included clinical signs, symptoms and behaviors based on a psychological involvement with chemicals trait continuum. Testing using this scale demonstrated the presence of stages that were identified as (1) social/recreational use, (2) mood-related use, (3) adjustment of activities to accommodate use, (4) engaging in deceptive or deviant behavior to accommodate use, and (5) use indicative of physiological adaptation [66]. These data support the concept involving stages of progression of ACD described clinically by McDonald [9]. It also indicated that the quality of progression was similar to the symptom progression often associated with adult alcoholism.

The Psychosocial Section measures aspects of psychological functioning that have been shown to be antecedent, concomitant, or maintenance factors in ACD. A Personal Risk Factor subsection includes scales of (1) negative self-image, (2) psychological disturbance, (3) social isolation, (4) uncontrolled behavior, (5) rejecting convention, (6) deviant behavior, (7) absence of goals, and (8) spiritual isolation. An Environmental Risk Factor subsection includes scales of (1) peer chemical environment, (2) sibling chemical use, (3) family pathology, and (4) family estrangement. In addition, a Specific Problem Screen questions for (1) need for psychiatric referral, (2) eating-disorder signs/symptoms, (3) sexual abuse, (4) physical abuse (intrafamilial), (5) family chemical-dependency history, and (6) suicide potential. These readily provide a screen for psychiatric problems often associated with ACD and would indicate a need for further and more extensive evaluation.

## MEDICAL

A complete medical history and physical and neurological examinations are required. These will assess antecedent medical problems that may predispose to the ACD syndrome or to problems that result from its development.

Specific aspects of the history should include prenatal risk exposure (i.e., medication, drug use, cigarette smoking, illness by mother), perinatal injury (i.e., prematurity, respiratory distress, anoxia, jaundice), developmental disability, chronic disease, allergies and accidents. The presence of chronic illness (asthma, diabetes, familial hypercholesterolemia) serves as an opportunity for further education about the effects of specific chemicals and may provide added incentive for abstinence.

Information regarding sexual development, including Tanner Stage, age of onset of puberty and relationship to peer's development, sexual activity and practices including associated use of drugs and alcohol, provides insight into aspects of self-esteem often related to drug use.

Laboratory evaluation should include CBC and a comprehensive clinical profile (SMA) to assess any medical problems that may be the result of chemical use. Medical conditions in the differential diagnosis of substance-induced organic mental disorders include temporal lobe disorder and other neurologic diseases or lesions; head trauma; toxic or metabolic disorders, including hypoglycemia, diabetic ketoacidosis, hyper- and hypothyroidism, adrenocortical disease, and vitamin deficiencies; and viral illnesses. Urine toxicology screens for chemicals of abuse should be obtained and guidelines [71,72] are helpful. Sexually active teenagers should be screened for pregnancy and for sexually transmitted diseases, including HIV. An electrocardiogram may reveal cardiac abnormalities that, with continued drug use, may be life-threatening. A sleep-deprived electroencephalogram may indicate signs of temporal lobe dysfunction or other organic mental conditions. Neuroendocrine testing, using the DST [73] or the TRH test [74] are helpful in assessing possible antidepressant responsive depressions. However, to limit the effects of prior drug use on these tests, a two- to three-week period of abstinence is suggested.

## PSYCHIATRIC EVALUATION

The assessment of psychiatric status begins with assessment of psychoactive substance–induced organic mental disorders [75] to include: intoxication, withdrawal, withdrawal delirium, hallucinosis, delusional disorder, alcohol amnestic syndrome, posthallucinogen perception disorder, and organic mood syndrome. Often the "organic" nature is determined only by resolution after two to four weeks of chemical abstinence.

Psychiatric disorders in the differential diagnosis of organic mental syndrome should include [75] schizophrenia and other nonorganic psychotic disorders, manic episode, depression, panic disorder, generalized anxiety disorder, and factitious disorder and malingering. Morrison and Smith [11] also include mental retardation, specific developmental disorders, attention deficit hyperactivity disorder, conduct disorder, oppositional disorder, and personality disorders. Assessment strategies should include questions to determine whether the onset of symptoms or behavior of the psychiatric disorder is a predisposing antecedent; a concomitant that is independent of, precipitated by, or a result of, substance abuse; and/or a maintenance factor. The Adolescent Diagnostic Interview (ADI), described as part of the CDAAP, can be instrumental in this assessment. Another evaluation tool is the Diagnostic Interview Schedule for Children (DISC), [76] which is currently being revised for DSM-III-R criteria.

## FAMILY ASSESSMENT

The family as a significant influence on predisposition and concomitant and maintenance factors has been elaborated. Family assessment is crucial both in understanding the syndrome in the specific family and in developing family as a major ally in treatment. Specific family issues to be aware of are outlined [77]. Use of the biopsychosocial model framework requires a systems theory approach to families. Obtaining a family genogram, with emphasis on chemical abuse and psychiatric disorders, opens discussion and education on the disease concept. Assessment of current family chemical use may alert staff to family denial or possible chemical dependency of family members.

A standardized questionnaire, the Family Assessment Measure (FAM), [78,79] uses a process model of family functioning and can be completed by client and parents in 30 minutes. The Family Assessment General Scale measures the health of a family along dimensions of task accomplishment, role performance, communication, affective expression, involvement, control, and values and norms. A Dyadic Relationship Scale measures the relationships between specific family member pairs on the same dimensions noted above. A Self-rating Scale measures each individual's perception of his/her own functioning in the family unit.

## PSYCHOSOCIAL ASSESSMENT

A psychosocial assessment is valuable in identifying specific psychosocial strengths that may support recovery or weaknesses and behaviors that will block recovery. An educational assessment for learning disabilities may include a WISC-R or WAIS-R and the Woodcock-Johnson Psychoeducational Battery [80]. Questions about peer relationships and involvement in risk-taking activities may reveal deviant behaviors suggesting more severe psychopathology than are assessed by structured interviews. Especially important in some regions of the country is involvement in cultlike activity that may include satanism and its cruelty to animals or people. Specific questions about aggressive behaviors, runaway behaviors, past physical and sexual abuse, promiscuity and evidence of compulsive sexual activity may alert clinicians to problems that, while initially controlled, may appear later during the stress of treatment.

## TREATMENT

The urgency and interest in treatment of teenagers with chemical dependency has paralleled the increase in extent and severity of teenagers with chemical dependency over the last 10 years. Although treatment programs have proliferated, research documenting the superiority of any single approach with adolescents has not yet occurred. The nature of ACD treatment has been based on successful treatment with adult chemical dependency developed largely by the Johnson Institute and Hazelden Foundation. This Minnesota model [81,82] is an intensive group therapy approach based on the disease concept and the 12 Steps of AA that involves chemical-dependency counselors as primary therapists. Acute care is generally followed by extended aftercare for several months to a year or more. Experience from these inpatient programs has led to development of alternative care, such as outpatient programs, as well as the use of concepts, approaches, and techniques already proven successful.

A review of the various treatment approaches [82] discusses some of the philosophic and practical dimensions regarding ACD treatment. Hoffman et al. [81] reviews multiple issues regarding evaluation of ACD programs, assessment of outcome, and the information learned from CATOR—a chemical abuse/addiction-treatment outcome registry. A major impetus in research at this time is to provide guidelines to match specific client characteristics with specific treatment approaches [68]. Since few studies have been done on adolescents, potentially predictive variables have been derived from adult literature. These include: (1) problem severity, including problem duration, severity of dependence, or consequences; (2) concomitant psychopathology; (3) social stability, including measures of family functioning and dynamics; (4) neuropsychological functioning; (5) personality characteristics; (6) cognitive style; (7) locus of control; (8) perceived choice; (9) family history; and (10) stage of change.

Treatment programs have generally been divided into outpatient, inpatient, residential, and aftercare components. In accord with most state mental health laws, treatment is to be accomplished in the "least restrictive setting." Currently, the determination of this has been poorly based on research and is usually determined by physical and economic availability [82]. The Cleveland Hospital [83] has developed criteria for determining levels of care that are currently being tested for validity. Clinically, many treatment programs determine treatment based on an assessment of the severity of the syndrome. Using descriptions of the progression of drug use from experimental to severe chemical-dependency often guides the treatment placement. This section will provide a detailed description of an inpatient treatment program specifically designed for dual-diagnosis patients to demonstrate many of the successful principles that can be modified in other settings. It will also discuss outpatient treatment as an option.

## INPATIENT TREATMENT

Some practitioners believe that the only effective treatment for adolescent chemical dependency is inpatient treatment [82]. A more usual approach is for adolescents in the later stages of daily preoccupation and severe dependency to be referred for inpatient treatment. As noted earlier, a current focus with ACD is to screen patients and match them to the specific program or aspects of the program. Because controversy is unresolved regarding the length of time after abstinence that drug effects persist, the best time to evaluate for psychiatric psychopathology, and the presence of extended denial in adolescents, ACD treatment must be approached as an extended evaluation concurrent with treatment. An approach that integrates this at the Adolescent Center for Chemical Education Prevention and Treatment (ACCEPT) is to provide a comprehensive treatment program whose structure includes an ongoing evaluation of disorders that leads to the clarification of specific needs for successful recovery. This approach is based on the Minnesota model and has been described elsewhere [64] with a case study presentation. Concepts developed by Davanloo [87] have been instrumental in the development of this model and the understanding of the biopsychosocial model presented earlier.

Certain factors define this program:

1. Use of chemical-dependency biopsychosocial disease model
2. Use of psychiatric biopsychosocial disease model
3. Treatment of the biological part of each disorder first
4. Emphasis on the "family disease" aspects of chemical dependency and psychiatric disorders
5. Focus on a commitment to abstinence
6. Therapeutic progression using the 12 steps of AA/NA
7. Structured program emphasizing "discipline" in recovery

The chemical-dependency biopsychosocial model, as presented, fosters a systemic, holistic understanding of data gathered during the evaluation and guides understanding of further information obtained by the structured treatment process. The emphasis on chemical dependency as a disease assists families and patients in working through severe guilt feelings and the sense of failure, both prominent initially in treatment. With its inclusion of "maintenance factors" and the enabling system, it fosters acceptance of responsibility in taking action to stop these behaviors and to stop the progression of the disease. This balance is often critical, as some families use their "disease" to continue defensively to deny their responsibility in the process, and others victimize and paralyze themselves by taking on full responsibility, with resulting self-pity. An attempt to have every family member understand the different factors in the equation and their role in the disease is the initial focus in treatment.

As the chemical-dependency biopsychosocial model is presented, the role of psychiatric disorders and dual or multiple diagnoses are explained. Using this model with families fosters a holistic focus on the problem rather than splitting a focus on chemical dependency and/or a focus on psychiatric disorder. Clinical experience on dual-diagnosis treatment units demonstrates how teenagers and family members can effectively use the focus on any single part of the problem (i.e., bulimia) to defensively block treatment progress. The position stated as "I'm only here for my bulimia, not my drug use!" assists continued denial.

Treatment requires a commitment to abstinence from chemical use. This is a long-term commitment that is renewed "one day at a time." Most treatment programs believe that this should be a lifelong commitment to abstinence [81]. As to whether adolescents grow out of substance abuse, [85] further research is needed.

The requirement for abstinence is based on the understanding of chemical dependency as a primary illness, as described previously. This concept actually has two different parts, which confuse clinicians because of the terminology. First, the primary intervention must be removal of the drug from the person's system in order to stop progression of the illness. Second, since a seemingly autonomous "primary" disorder has developed, once the drug is removed physically, the person will continue with many of the patterned behaviors—drug urges and cravings, impulsiveness, paranoia, fearfulness, and distrust—which are now the focus of treatment.

Traditionally, the psychotherapeutic approach to a chemically dependent person would be to attempt an understanding of how they developed psychologically. By understanding specific issues and conflicts related to past life experiences, it was believed that the end result would be abstinence from drug use (Figure 4). With addicts, knowledge and insight often does not lead

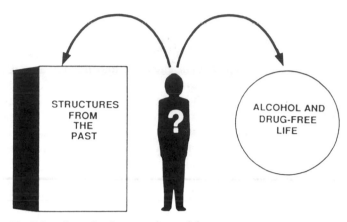

**Figure 4**   Traditional psychotherapeutic model.

to action regarding abstinence from chemical use. With addiction, a more empowering approach is to begin with a commitment to abstinence. This has been known and utilized for years by the founders of Alcoholic Anonymous: "But the actual or potential alcoholic, with hardly an exception, will be absolutely unable to stop drinking on the basis of self-knowledge." [86] The AA program begins with the commitment to abstinence.

Once detoxification is completed and evidence of any substance-induced organic syndrome is absent, beginning with the commitment to abstinence leads to predictable effects. As teenagers meaningfully verbalize this commitment, certain emotional and behavioral reactions occur. These reactions display patterns of behavior that demonstrate their specific and individual psychological history. These patterns are referred to as "structures from the past," a neutral term that allows discussion by psychoanalytic therapists, self-psychologists, developmental psychologists, behaviorists, and learning theorists (Figure 5).

These patterns or structures from the past are the result of learned coping patterns, including ego defenses, perceptual and cognitive distortions that may or may not have occurred during drug use, and urges. Urges are vague, poorly differentiated feelings that are strong motivators to specific actions, such as those for drugs, sex, binge/purge, violence, or suicide and self-mutilation. Understanding and working with urges are the key to successful transformation toward recovery. The focus on urges incorporates ideas presented earlier regarding a possible biochemical-genetic barrier, and the concept of primary illness. The presence of urges demonstrates how the addiction is grafted onto the preexisting behavior and personality structure, creating a new and seemingly autonomous entity.

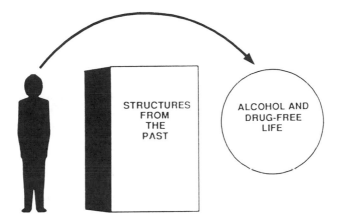

**Figure 5** Commitment to recovery.

Using the biopsychosocial model with dual-diagnosis patients requires that the commitment to abstinence be extended. As with chemical dependency, other disorders, such as depression, bulimia, post-traumatic stress disorder, sexual dependency, and attention deficit hyperactivity disorder, become primary. Whatever the temporal process of predisposition, events or drug interaction, and enabling or maintenance factors, the psychiatric disorder eventually acquires characteristics that are seemingly autonomous. Therefore, as with chemical dependency, once the biological component is addressed as with medications, a commitment to abstinence must be the beginning. Because multiple disorders are being treated, this means a commitment to no drugs, no bingeing, purging, or dieting, no sex, no depression, and no impulsive violent or suicidal behaviors.

## 12 STEPS

Because it is unrealistic to expect teenagers to be capable of making and keeping these commitments early in recovery, the 12 Steps of AA [86] are used as the foundation of the therapeutic process. In addition to using the 12 Steps as an educational tool and beginning attachment to the 12 Step fellowship in preparation for aftercare, the first five steps are used as a powerful measure of progression and an impetus for change:

Step 1.  We admitted we were powerless over [drugs and] alcohol—that our lives had become unmanageable.

Step 2.  Came to believe that a power greater than ourselves could restore us to sanity.

Step 3.   Made a decision to turn our will and our lives over to the care of God — as we understood Him.

Step 4.   Made a searching and fearless moral inventory of ourselves.

Step 5.   Admitted to God, to ourselves, and to another human being the exact nature of our wrongs.

Patients are expected to make specific commitments to completion of each step successively. Written work and behavioral assignments are provided that foster this progression. Completion occurs when a cognitive-behavioral-emotional shift is noted that is consistent with the foundation of the step, as outlined in AA [86]. In working with this model, a psychology regarding commitment to abstinence has been elaborated and is somewhat predictable within a structured setting using the 12 Steps. Within their commitment to each of the steps, specific patterns of behavior occur that block progress in recovery. What is revealed is an association of memories of events with which this pattern developed, crystallized, or was significantly attached to this person.

> A 17-year-old male patient was motivated and progressed well to completion of his step 1. Following this, his mood changed; he was not as active, was often confused, and appeared to be blocked in treatment. There was no clear explanation that could be seen until he developed complaints of pain in his leg. No physical signs of a problem were present. The patient soon after recalled an injury in which he broke a leg during a soccer game at a point in his life at which he and his father had many dreams of him becoming a professional athlete. His athletics were never as productive after this injury. The disappointment to his father and himself was not resolved and resurfaced to block his progress in treatment. The disappointment and the victimizing self-pity associated with this event were blocks to his commitment to step 2 and were part of "insane" behaviors. Once the issue was examined, he was able to continue treatment successfully.

The therapeutic work involved identifying the structures from the past, recalling the events in detail; reexperiencing the thoughts, feelings, and behaviors associated with the event; and then acting in the present to produce a different result. Therapeutic techniques include processes and understandings from short-term dynamic psychotherapy, [87] behavior and learning theory, [88] and cognitive [89] or rational-emotive [90] therapy.

An important insight into this process has come from Lane and Schwartz, [91] who approached the treatment of psychiatric disorders from a cognitive-developmental viewpoint. Five levels of emotional experience were described: (1) bodily sensations, (2) body in action, (3) individual feelings, (4) blends of feelings, and (5) blends of blends of feelings. Transformations are possible as one breaks through to experience a new level of awareness. Clinically, as teenagers progress through treatment, this process appears to occur. Typically, teenagers enter with only impulsive actions and awareness of no feelings. They progress into an awareness of single feelings, usually only anger. Further breakthroughs occur as awareness of guilt and shame appear, and they progress into further distinctions to include a full range of emotional experiences.

## THERAPEUTIC PROGRESSION

Use of this treatment model has demonstrated a predictable progression through each of the steps, highlighting specific issues associated with dual diagnosis [64]. The initial guilt and shame experienced as patients review consequences of their drug use assesses the locus of control, especially related to conduct disorders and the ability for introspection. Issues of authority and discipline highlight the cognitive distortions and paranoia that may indicate an underlying schizophrenia or schizophreniformlike disorder. The confrontational method is designed to highlight this and to distinguish it from the cognitive distortions and mistrust of the borderline disorders. Patients with these latter conditions develop more organized thought processes with confrontation. However, the borderline patients develop overwhelming urges, with acting-out behaviors—urges to use drugs, to have sex, to binge or purge, to commit suicide or self-mutilate, to be violent, or to run away. With structure, the "abandonment depression" breaks through. This loneliness and depression is common as teenagers begin to feel their life without drugs, without their drug-using friends, and without behaviors used previously to cope with feelings of loneliness and alienation. The presence of depressive symptoms must be evaluated for an underlying major depressive disorder often evident with psychomotor retardation or psychotic processes. These teenagers have responded well to antidepressant medications.

Adolescents with learning disabilities and prior social and school failure experience overwhelming feelings of failure and behaviors of giving up. When they are addressed properly with remedial support and development of alternative coping strategies, treatment becomes one of their first successes in recovery.

Step 2 begins with the reading of a comprehensive drug chart to parents, breaking through the family denial, and opening a family system to building new relationships. Understanding spirituality as the "quality of our relationships to whatever or whomever is most important in our life" [92] allows concepts of object relations theory to be applicable and fosters better understanding of this step by some professionals. The many losses of relationships, ideals, and goals, and the loss of self-esteem related to prior physical and sexual abuse, require an emphasis on unresolved grief and hopelessness. The focus on spirituality assists identification of adolescents involved in satanism and other cultlike activities. Often, these teenagers have an underlying schizotypal or schizoid personality disorder, requiring treatment. Because of the intense countertransference issues that arise in dealing with teenagers at this stage, emphasis on reality testing, projection, and projective identification is critical for success. During this step, family issues are clarified in detail. Especially important are issues of codependence and being the child of alcoholic or drug-abusing parents.

Step 3 often consolidates treatment gains. Its focus on overcoming past defensive patterns, identity changes, and adopting new behaviors is often difficult for persons with a narcissistic personality disorder. Adopted teenagers often regress as "adoption" into a recovering community is experienced through past emotional experiences of loss and abandonment related to being adopted by their family. The role of this step in the separation-individuation process of adolescence is recognized by scheduling Family Week treatment at this stage. Many teenagers are unable to complete this step without concrete experiences with family members and a direct resolution of major family conflicts.

Step 4 is designed to foster personal responsibility and growth for continued self-motivated recovery. This step aims at self-acceptance and acceptance by others to "form a true partnership with another human being." [86] The openness at this point in successful treatment allows the teenager to deal with issues of intimacy and sexuality with an emotional maturity consistent with their age. This assists the family in progressing in their own emotional development, which is necessary for continued recovery.

## FAMILY TREATMENT

The two major goals of family therapy with ACD are to: (1) Restructure the maladaptive aspects of the family system, and (2) establish an ongoing method for abstinence and recovery [38].

The confused, angry, and beleaguered families that have been part of the codependency process described previously need structure and guidance [38]. Details of the treatment program expectations are outlined below:

1. All family and household members and significant others are expected to participate.
2. A "family intervention" will occur within 72 hours of admission onto the treatment unit.
3. Family attendance at two weeknight evenings in a multifamily group.
4. Attendance at a "Family Week" (Monday through Friday) midway in treatment.
5. Attendance at Al-Anon/Families Anonymous meetings weekly.
6. Optional attendance of siblings in a siblings group once a week.

7. Abstinence from all mood-altering chemicals during the course of the treatment.
8. Commitment to the 12 Steps of Al-Anon as a process for recovery.
9. Attendance in an aftercare program following treatment that may be 6 to 12 months in duration.

The expectation of abstinence by family members can be extremely valuable. It serves several purposes:

1. Allows therapeutic work to be done without the active influence of chemical use.
2. Assists family members in empathically recognizing the difficulties that the adolescents' commitment to abstinence entails.
3. Screens for family member chemical dependence.

As with the adolescent, families are expected to make commitments to full participation in the treatment program through the first three steps of Al-Anon. In a structured program like this, any deviations assist in identifying family blocks to recovery or conflicts with other priorities. These blocks, which are similar to those experienced the adolescent treatment, are often associated with "structures from the past" or unresolved family developmental issues. Identification of these may require additional individual family sessions to foster working through and continued engagement in treatment.

A *siblings group* is for brothers and sisters of all ages. It offers an opportunity for siblings to acknowledge and express their feelings and receive support and attention. Often, this group is the only place where they can talk freely about the crisis that the family is experiencing. Siblings often develop specific roles in the family that foster inflexibility and maintenance of the family dysfunction. Some roles may be (1) the "hero" and or the student doing academically well in school, (2) "lost" or ignored by the parents, (3) victimized or scapegoated (criticized by parents and patients), or (4) also using drugs or alcohol. The group setting without parents allows a compassionate setting for their concerns to be expressed.

The *"family intervention"* occurs initially in treatment when the parents are generally overwhelmed and frightened. Parents have usually felt out of control as the child controls the family with manipulative behaviors as described. This technique was developed by the Johnson Institute and has been adapted for use with teenagers. It assists in overcoming the denial of the harmful effects of their drug use, as well as denial that the parents may still have regarding the severity of the problem. Often, teenagers become poorly engaged in treatment if they believe that a parent is not fully supportive of their treatment. This is an opportunity to dispel these illusions of "rescue" regarding the parents' commitment to treatment.

Parents are given specific instructions for the interventions. They are individually asked to list harmful situations or incidents with their teenager and the effect that it had on them personally and on relationships. The intervention is then conducted by the therapist as parents individually present this to the teenager, who is expected to make no response or comments. It is often the first opportunity for the chemically dependent teenager to hear his family members drug-free. A successful intervention assists both teenager and family members to break through the denial and begin awareness of the guilt, shame, and sense of failure that have been avoided by chemical dependence and codependent behaviors.

The *multifamily groups* are a critical element in treatment. One of these groups weekly is a "beginners" group for parents whose children have recently entered treatment. The emphasis is largely educational, preparing them for involvement in the remainder of the program. Preparation includes:

1. Introduction to the disease concept and the biopsychosocial model of chemical dependency and dual diagnosis
2. Introduction to group process
3. Identification of feelings and use of "I" statements
4. Introduction to the 12 Steps of Al-Anon
5. Introduction to concepts of enabling, codependency, detachment, defenses, spirituality, commitment

The educational preparation and the compassionate support of other parents during this crisis, and relief as they detach from their codependent reactivity to their child, provides hope and an openness to further therapeutic work. The advanced multifamily group continues with educational lectures and is more therapeutic in design. It assists parents in understanding themselves, their family of origin, and their role in the addictive process. They learn to understand the predisposing and maintenance factors, as well as the interactive effect that the chemical use of their teenager has had on them. This group is both supportive and confrontational. It also prepares families for Family Week as well as supports their involvement with Al-Anon and/or Families Anonymous.

## FAMILY WEEK

Family Week is an intensive educational-psychotherapeutic experience whose goal is to restructure family patterns to support recovery. Ideally, it occurs when the adolescent has integrated step 2 and family members have acknowledged step 1 for codependents. It takes place Monday through Thursday for six hours daily, and Friday morning is devoted to a final summary and recommendations. Three to four families participate simultaneously with two cotherapists. Specific areas that are addressed by lecture or group process include:

1. Review of the disease concept and the biopsychosocial model
2. Review of personal commitment to abstinence from mood-altering drugs
3. Setting of personal goals for the week
4. Focus on commitments and "structures from the past"
5. Group rules and the role of group process in recovery
6. Barriers to communication/defenses
7. Issues, resentments, and secrets withheld and/or unresolved
8. Family roles and family interactions, including family of origin

Family Week begins with the foundation of the program – the biopsychosocial model of the disease concept and the commitment to abstinence. These are established firmly as goals for the week are expressed. The goal setting establishes a structure for the week and alerts the therapist to participants' self-awareness, openness, and manner of communication and problem solving. As with the adolescent, the structure provided by the 12 Steps of Al-Anon is a major focus.

Clinical experience with Family Week has demonstrated the developmental progression of the group process through stages related to each of the first three steps of AA, in a manner similar to that described with the adolescents as they progress through treatment.

In an attempt to dislodge the inflexible behavior patterns that maintain the enabling family system, each individual role in the family is explored. Emphasis is on an interactive understanding between teenager, parents, and siblings and an identification of feelings beyond anger and fear. This process is facilitated as the family of origin portion of "structures from the past" is demonstrated in family interactions.

Most family interactions are done in a "fishbowl" arrangement, in which one family circles together to deal with specific issues while other participants observe. Often, therapy involves a delicate balancing between individual family work and group process. By the middle of the week, tracking of group themes becomes a powerful tool in reinforcing group process and setting the stage for future group involvements.

The concept of triangulation is presented and demonstrated within family interactions to foster each member's extrication from the inflexible system. This often leads to discussions on triangulation in the family of origin and values and behaviors that have been continued through the generations. This provides an opportunity for families to change the several generations of maintenance factors for chemical dependence.

As triangulation issues in interactions are effectively worked through, by midweek, the emphasis is on parents/couples and often requires couples' focused therapy to be done in the group. This is a critical time in the process as the level of group intimacy is tested and strengthened, depending on the degree of honesty and openness present. This is often determined by the degree to which families are shame-bound systems. In a very successful group, parents and children discuss secrets and resentments never before expressed as they develop a strong desire for further closeness. Issues regarding sexual behavior including unknown pregnancies, abortions, rape, or extrarelationship affairs are discussed. Issues of family violence and abuse often associated with other chemically dependent family members are openly worked through. Many issues related to the adult child of alcoholics syndrome occur at this point and require identification with chemical use. An emphasis on experiences of full expression and forgiveness provides further impetus for continued recovery.

The final day allows family members to evaluate themselves in terms of their original goals and personal learning experiences. Requirements for aftercare and continued recovery are reviewed as emphasis is given to the ongoing nature of recovery. Family system recommendations are also made by the therapists. This may involve recommending couples or family therapy or extended service placement for the adolescent, such as a halfway house or residential care.

Family Week can be powerfully effective not only in restructuring maladaptive aspects of the family system but also in establishing an experience of behaviors and processes required for continued abstinence and fulfilling recovery.

## OUTPATIENT TREATMENT

Clients in experimental and early abuse stages often are referred for outpatient or early intervention programs. Although most adolescents with chemical dependency are treated as outpatients, there are problems associated with this. These include [13] denial of the problem by the client and/or the family, basic adolescent mistrust of adult authority, continued association with substance-abusing peer groups, unwillingness to abstain, and lack of motivation. Some criteria have been outlined for outpatient treatment [10]. These include:

1.  Absence of acute medical and/or psychiatric problems
2.  Absence of chronic medical problems that would preclude outpatient treatment
3.  Willingness to abstain from all mood-altering chemicals and cooperation with random urine testing
4.  No prior outpatient treatment failure
5.  Extent to which the family is interested and able to become involved in treatment

6.  Motivation for treatment

Denial by teenagers or their families that a problem exists or is severe enough to warrant treatment is a significant problem in outpatient treatment. For primary intervention often done by pediatricians or family practitioners, a technique called "contracting" is useful. If a problem with chemicals is perceived by the clinician but denied by the client or family, even though use is acknowledged, the physician can contract with the client to maintain abstinence. This is often done on a four-to-six-week basis and may involve urine screening and a follow-up every two weeks, with possible phone contact during weeks without visits. Return visits assess not only abstinence but "urges" to use, refusal of opportunities to use, necessity of changing life style or social situations to avoid using, and mood upon abstinence. Adolescents that are beyond the stage of experimenting with drugs find this type of contract difficult to maintain. It is often a clear demonstration of the extent of dependency that is present.

Outpatient treatment must be intensive and extended [93] to convey the seriousness of the problem and the commitment needed for successful treatment. Filstead and Anderson [93] describe a program that is conducted four times per week for four weeks, followed by twice a week for four weeks, and then once weekly for 12 weeks. During this course of treatment, the family is expected to participate twice per week, once with the client as a total family unit and once as the parental couple. Patient and parents are expected to actively attend AA and/or NA during this course of treatment.

Filstead and Anderson describe some rules that are to be maintained and that, if violated, lead to recommendations for a more restricted treatment setting, usually an inpatient setting. The rules stated are (1) no use of alcohol or other substances for any reason, (2) no violent behavior, (3) regular attendance at therapy sessions, and (4) AA/NA meetings. If any use of chemicals is suspected, urine screens are requested.

During the initial evaluation, families are often resistant to recommendation for inpatient care because of poor understanding of chemical dependency, denial of the seriousness of the problem, poor understanding of the treatment process, or fears about inpatient settings. A trial at outpatient treatment often is used to educate families in chemical dependency. Similar to the "contracting" method noted above, it often demonstrates the teenager's inability to abstain and participate in an outpatient treatment program. This use of outpatient treatment assists families in benefitting more from the subsequent inpatient treatment referral.

The specific aspects of outpatient treatment often involve adaptation of inpatient assessment and treatment goals, depending on time allotments, staff, and economic decisions. However, the focus on peer-group therapy, family involvement, and attendance at AA/NA meetings appears common. Additional community networking, with school involvement, is becoming more important as more adolescents enter treatment and must return to school settings.

## REFERENCES

1. Isralowitz R, Singer M, eds. *Adolescent Substance Abuse: A Guide to Prevention and Treatment*. New York: Haworth, 1983.
2. Johnston LD, O'Malley PM, Bachman JG. *Drug Use, Drinking, and Smoking: National Survey Results from High School, College and Young Adult Populations 1975-1988*. Rockville, MD: NIDA, 1989.
3. National Household Survey on Drug Abuse. Rockville, MD: NIDA, 1989.
4. Rogers PD, ed. Chemical dependency. *Ped Clin N Amer* 1987; 34(2).
5. Kandel DB, Stages in adolescent involvement in drug use. *Sci* 1975; 190:912-914.
6. Kandel DB, Kessler R, Margulis R. Antecedents of adolescent initiation into stages of drug abuse. *J Youth Adolescence* 1978; 7(1):13-40.
7. Clayton RP. Multiple drug use: Epidemiology, correlates, and consequences. In: Galanter, M ed. *Recent Developments in Alcoholism*. Vol. 4. New York: Plenum, 1986:7-38.
8. Donovan JE, Jessor R. Problem drinking and the dimension of involvement with drugs: A Guttman scalogram analysis. *Am J Pub Health* 1983; 73:468-472.
9. MacDonald DI. Drugs, drinking and adolescence. *Am J Dis Child* 1984; 138:117-125.
10. Semlitz L, Gold MS. Adolescent drug abuse. *Psych Clin N Amer* 1986; 9:455-473.
11. Morrison MA, Smith QT. Psychiatric issues of adolescent chemical dependence. *Ped Clin N Amer* 1987; 34(2):461-480.
12. Norem-Hebeisen A, Hedin DP. Influences on adolescent problem behavior: Causes, connections, and contexts. In: Isralowitz R, Singer M, eds. *Adolescent Substance Abuse: A Guide to Prevention and Treatment*. New York: Haworth, 1983; 35-56.
13. Bailey GW. Current perspectives on substance abuse in youth. *J Am Acad Child Adol Psych* 1989; 28(2):151-162.
14. Engel GL. The need for a new medical model. *Sci* 1977; 196:129-136.
15. Engel GL. The clinical application of the biopsychosocial model. *Am J Psych* 1980; 137(5):535-544.
16. Jellinek EM. *The Disease Concept of Alcoholism*. New Haven, CT: Hillhouse, 1960.
17. Donovan JM. An etiological model of alcoholism. *Am J Psych* 1986; 143(1):1-11.
18. Goodwin DW. Heredity and alcoholism. *Annals of Behavioral Medicine* 1986; 8:3-6.

19. Mendelson J, Mello N, eds. *Diagnosis and Treatment of Alcoholism.* New York: McGraw-Hill, 1984.
20. Vessell ES, Page JG, Passananti GT. Genetic and environmental factors affecting ethanol metabolism in man. *Clin Pharmacol Therapeut* 1971; 12:192.
21. Schuckit M, Rayses V. Ethanol ingestion: Differences in acetaldehyde concentration in relatives of alcoholics and controls. *Sci* 1979; 203:54–55.
22. Thomas M, Halsall P, Peters TJ. Role of hepatic acetaldehyde dehydrogenase in alcoholism. *Lancet* 1982; 8307(2):1057–1059.
23. Schuckit MA, Gold EO. A simultaneous evaluation of multiple markers of ethanol/placebo challenges in sons of alcoholics and controls. *Arch Gen Psych* 1988; 45(3):211–216.
24. Myers RD. Tetrahydroisoquinolines in the brain: The basis of an animal model of alcoholism. *Alcoholism: Clin Exper Res* 1978; 2:145–154.
25. Vaillant GE. *The Natural History of Alcoholism.* Cambridge, MA: Harvard University Press, 1983.
26. Botvin GJ. Substance abuse prevention research. *J School Health* 1986; 56:369–374.
27. Carroll JF. Treating multiple substance abuse clients. In: Galanter M, ed. *Recent Developments in Alcoholism.* Vol. 4. New York: Plenum, 1986; 85–103.
28. Kauffman JF, Shaffer H, Burglass ME. The biological basics: Drugs and their effects. In: Bratter TE, and Forrest GG, eds. *Alcoholism and Substance Abuse: Strategies for Clinical Intervention.* New York: The Free Press, 1985.
29. Harford TC, Grant BF. Psychosocial factors in adolescent drinking contexts. *J Stud Alc* 1987; 48:551–557.
30. Wegscheider S. *Another Choice, Hopes and Health for the Alcoholic Family.* Palo Alto, CA: Science and Behavior Books, 1981.
31. Chatlos JC. *Crack: What You Should Know About the Cocaine Epidemic.* New York: Putnam, 1987.
32. Singer M, Anglin T. The identification of adolescent substance abuse by health care professionals. *Int J Addictions* 1986; 21(2):247–254.
33. Winters K. The need for improved assessment of adolescent substance involvement. *J Drug Issues* 1990; 20(3):487–502.
34. Gitlow SE, Peyser HS, eds. *Alcoholism: A Practical Treatment Guide.* New York: Grune and Stratton, 1980.
35. Donovan DM, Marlatt GA, eds. *Assessment of Addictive Behaviors.* New York: Guilford, 1988.
36. Ray BA, ed. *Learning Factors in Substance Abuse.* NIDA Research Monograph 84. Rockville, MD: NIDA, 1988.
37. Bickel WK, Kelly TH. The relationship of stimulus control to the treatment of substance abuse. In: Ray BA, ed. *Learning Factors in Substance Abuse.* NIDA Research Monograph 84. Rockville, MD: NIDA, 1988; 122–140.
38. Kaufman E. Adolescent substance abusers and family therapy. In: Mirkin M, Koman S, eds. *Handbook of Adolescents and Family Therapy.* New York: Gardner Press, 1985; 245–254.
39. Kaufman E. Family structures of narcotics addicts. *Int J Addictions* 1981; 16: 273–282.

40. Gibbs JT. Psychosocial factors related to substance abuse among delinquent females. *Am J Orthopsychiatry* 1982; 52(2):261-271.
41. Preto NG. Transformation of the family system in adolescence. In: Carter B, McGoldrick M, eds. *The Changing Family Life Cycle: A Framework for Family Therapy*. New York: Gardner Press, 1988; 255-283.
42. Levine BL. Adolescent substance abuse: Toward an integration of family systems and individual adaptation theories. *Am Family Ther* 1985; 13(2):3-16.
43. Schwartzman J. The addict, abstinence and the family. *Amer J Psychiatry* 1975; 132:154-157.
44. Cleveland M. Families and adolescent drug use: Structural analysis of children's roles. *Family Process* 1981; 20:295-304.
45. Reilly DM. Family therapy with adolescent drug abusers and their families: Defying gravity and achieving escape velocity. *J Drug Issues* 1984; 381-391.
46. Reilly DM. Family factors in the etiology and treatment of youthful drug abuse. *Family Ther* 1976; 2:149-171.
47. Paton S, Kessler R, Kandel D. Depressive mood and adolescent illicit drug use: A longitudinal analysis. *J Gen Psyc* 1977; 131-167.
48. Robins LN. Sturdy childhood predictors of adult antisocial behavior: Replications from longitudinal studies. *Psych Med* 1978; 8:611-622.
49. Cantwell DP. Hyperactivity and antisocial behavior. *J Am Acad Child Psych* 1978; 17:252-262.
50. Pyle RL, Mitchell JE, Eckert ED. Bulimia: A report of 34 cases. *J Clin Psychiatry* 1981; 42:60-64.
51. Masterson JF. *Treatment of the Borderline Adolescent: A Developmental Approach*. New York: Wiley Interscience, 1972.
52. Kashani JH, Keller MB, Solomon N, Reid JC, Mazzola D. Double depression in adolescent substance abusers. *J Affective Disorders* 1985; 8:153-157.
53. Famularo R, Stone K, Popper C. Pre-adolescent alcohol abuse and dependence. *Am J Psych* 1985; 140:1187-1189.
54. Gittelman R, Mannuzza S, Shenker R, Bonagura N. Hyperactive boys almost grown up. *Arch Gen Psych* 1985; 42:937-947.
55. Loranger AW, Tullis EH. Family history of alcoholism in borderline personality disorders. *Arch Gen Psychiatry* 1985; 42:153-157.
56. Fowler RC, Rich CL, Young D. San Diego suicide study II. Substance abuse in young cases. *Arch Gen Psychiatry* 1986; 43:962-965.
57. Rich CL, Fowler RL, Fogarty LA, Young D. San Diego suicide study. III. Relationships between diagnosis and stressors. *Arch Gen Psych* 1988; 45:589-592.
58. Roehrich H, Gold MS. Diagnosis of substance abuse in an adolescent psychiatric population. *Int J Psychiatry Med* 1986; 16(2):137-143.
59. Roehrich HG, Jonas JM, Gold MS. Phenomenology of adolescent drug addiction. Personal communication, 1988.
60. Gershon ES, Berrettini WH, Goldin LR. Mood disorders: Genetics. In: Kaplan VH, Sadock B, eds. *Comprehensive Textbook of Psychiatry*. Baltimore: Williams and Wilkins, 1989; 1:879-888.

61. Schildkraut JJ, Green AI, Mooney JJ. Mood disorders: Biochemical aspects. In: Kaplan VH, Sadock B, eds. *Comprehensive Textbook of Psychiatry*. Baltimore: Williams and Wilkins, 1989; 1:868–879.
62. Mollica RF. Mood disorders: Epidemiology. In: Kaplan H, Sadock B, eds. *Comprehensive Textbook of Psychiatry V*. Baltimore: Williams and Wilkins, 1989; 1:859–868.
63. Hirchfeld MA, Cross CK. Epidemiology of affective disorder: Psychosocial risk factors. *Arch Gen Psych* 1982; 39(1):35–46.
64. Chatlos J. Adolescent dual diagnosis: A 12 step transformational model. *J Psychoact Drugs* 1989; 21(2):189 210.
65. Owen PL, Nyberg LR. Assessing alcohol and drug problems among adolescents: Current practices. *J Drug Educ* 1983; 13:249–254.
66. Winters K. The need for improved assessment of adolescent substance involvement. *J of Drug Issues* 1990; 20(3):487–502.
67. Rahdert ER, Grabowski J, eds. *Adolescent Drug Abuse: Analysis of Treatment Research*. NIDA Research Monograph 77. Rockville, MD: NIDA, 1988.
68. Hester RK, Miller WR. Empirical guidelines for optimal client-treatment matching. In: Rahdert ER, Grabowski J, eds. *Adolescent Drug Abuse: Analysis of Treatment Research*. NIDA Research Monograph 77. Rockville, MD: NIDA, 1988; 27–39.
69. Anglin TA. Interviewing guidelines for the clinical evaluation of adolescent substance abuse. *Ped Clin N Amer* 1987; 34(2):381–398.
70. Farrow JA, Deisher R. A practical guide to the office assessment of adolescent substance abuse. *Ped Annals* 1988; 15:675–684.
71. Mackenzie RG, Cheng M, Haftel AJ. The clinical utility and evaluation of drug screening techniques. *Ped Clin N Amer* 1987; 34(2):423–435.
72. Gold MS, Dackis CA. Role of the laboratory in the evaluation of suspected drug use. *J Clin Psych* 1986; 47:17–23.
73. Carroll BJ. Informed use of the dexamethasone suppression test. *J Clin Psychiatry* 1986; 47(1):10–12.
74. Extein I, Gold MS. Psychiatric applications of thyroid tests. *J Clin Psychiatry* 1986; 47(1):13–16.
75. DSM-III-R. Washington, D.C.: American Psychiatric Association, 1987.
76. Costello A. Structured interviewing for the assessment of child psychopathology. In: Noshpitz J, ed. *Basic Handbook of Child Psychiatry: Advances and New Directions*. New York: Basic, 1987; 143–152.
77. Huberty DJ, Huberty CE, Hobday KF, Blackmore G. Family issues in working with chemically dependent adolescents. *Ped Clin N Amer* 1987; 34(2):507–521.
78. Skinner H. Self-report instrument for family assessment. In: Jacob T, ed. *Family Intervention and Psychopathology: Theories, Methods and Findings*. New York: Plenum, 1987.
79. Skinner H, Steinhauer P, Santa-Barbera, J. The Family Assessment Measure. *Can J Community Ment Health* 1983; 2:91–105.
80. Woodcock R. *Woodcock-Johnson Psycho-Educational Battery: Technical Report*. Boston: Teaching Resources, 1977.

81.  Hoffman NG, Sonis WA, Halikas JA. Issues in the evaluation of chemical dependency treatment programs for adolescents. *Ped Clin N Amer* 1987; 34(2): 449–459.

82.  Wheeler K, Malmquist J. Treatment approaches in adolescent chemical dependency. *Ped Clin N Amer* 1987; 34(2):437–447.

83.  *Cleveland Criteria*. Greater Cleveland Hospital Association. Cleveland, OH, 1989.

84.  Davis DM. Intensive short-term dynamic psychotherapy in the treatment of chemical dependency. Part I. *Int J Short Term Psychother* 1989; 4(1).

85.  Kandel DB, Raveis VR. Cessation of illicit drug use in young adulthood. *Arch Gen Psychiatry* 1989; 46:109–116.

86.  *Alcoholics Anonymous*. 3rd ed. New York: Alcoholics Anonymous World Services, 1984.

87.  Davanloo H. *Short-term Dynamic Psychotherapy*. New York: Jason Aronson, 1980.

88.  Ross AO. *Child Behavior Therapy*. New York: Wiley, 1981.

89.  Beck AT. *Cognitive Therapy of Depression*. New York: Guilford Press, 1978.

90.  Ellis A, Bernard ME, eds. *Clinical Applications of Rational-Emotive Therapy*. New York: Plenum, 1985.

91.  Lane RD, Schwartz GE. Levels of emotional awareness: A cognitive-developmental theory and its application to psychopathology. *Am J Psych* 1987; 144(2):133–143.

92.  Bjorklund PE. What is spirituality? Center City, Minnesota: Hazelden, 1983.

93.  Filstead, WJ, Anderson CL. Conceptual and clinical issues in the treatment of adolescent alcohol and substance misuers. In: Isralowitz R, Singer M, eds. *Adolescent Substance Abuse: A Guide to Prevention and Treatment*. New York: Haworth, 103–116, 1983.

# 16

## Treating the "High and Mighty" and the "Mighty High"

**William J. Annitto**

*Greenbrook Academy, Bound Brook, New Jersey*

**Mark S. Gold**

*Fair Oaks Hospital, Summit, New Jersey and Delray Beach, Florida*

The issue of treating the special patient remains a most difficult and vexing problem. All of us as clinicians have felt the sense of positive self-worth and the depths of self-doubt engendered in the successes or failures we might have with our patients. These vagaries of our clinical skills are augmented geometrically when we are faced with the special patient. (We define our use of "special" in the next section.)

Moreover, in substance abuse, the problems of treatment are already shrouded in the murky waters of chronic disease, recidivism, and multiple treatments. Overall, the outcome for the special patient is no better nor worse than the average outcome for the nonspecial patient. However, the stakes are frequently much higher because of the visibility of the patient and the inherent guilt or affirmation by association instilled in the institution and the clinician. This paper is written from the viewpoint of the inpatient treatment of psychiatric substance abuse problems. In the context of a highly structured, multifaceted treatment program, we view drug addiction as a chronic disease associated with progressive medical, psychiatric, and psychosocial deterioration. Psychiatrically impaired addicted patients may require hospitalization before they are capable of recovery. Their specialness does not matter in this regard. Of course, it does in the sense of their willingness to be hospitalized. We all know too well the sad stories of those "special" people who, for one reason or another, were unable to accept hospitalization, and, therefore, treatment for their problems. Various celebrities and athletes have died without hospitalization or overt interventions in recent years. The major indications for hospitalization do not differ from those of the average patient. These include; (1) severe self-destructive or suicidal features, including intravenous drug use or freebasing; (2) severe impairment of psychosocial functioning; (3) severe medical and/or other psychiatric problems; (4) concurrent physical dependence on multiple drugs of abuse including alcohol, sedatives, and opiates; (5) inability or unwillingness to discontinue drug use as an outpatient, or severe recidivism.

## DESCRIPTION OF THE SPECIAL PATIENT

The category of rich and famous has been variously defined, depending upon the preferences of the author. The Group for the Advancement of Psychiatry, in their monograph on the VIP with psychiatric impairment, noted that the phrase "very important person" was first coined by Sir Winston Churchill. This connoted a person of considerable prestige or influence, especially a high official receiving special privileges. Moreover, social, political, and economic aspects are of prime significance [1]. From our clinical experience, the rich and famous patients that we have treated include sports figures; show business celebrities or "personalities"; colleagues or professionals, such as attorneys, officers of the law, and politicians; and a final category that would include family members, especially children, of the wealthy. Whether one approaches the problem of the treatment of this patient population from the side of the psychiatric aspects of the dual diagnosis or from that of the dually diagnosed substance abuser, many of the clinical problems remain the same.

Untreated psychiatric illness is associated with morbidity and interferes with recovery from addiction. The complex interface between psychiatric and addictive illnesses can be reduced to three diagnostic situations. First, psychiatric symptoms may be entirely secondary to addiction, as in the case of cocaine-induced hallucinations [2]. Second, addiction may result entirely from the self-medication of an underlying psychiatric disorder. The third situation involves the coexistence of autonomous psychiatric and addictive illnesses.

In this formulation, we see that whether the patient is "rich and famous" or an average patient makes little difference. The differences lie in the environmental aspects of treatment. The classic descriptions in the literature regarding this treatment come from a milieu-oriented adult psychiatric perspective [3,4]. The issues raised focus exclusively on the inherent problems of "VIPs" group psychodynamics on this type of unit. Thus, issues such as splitting, countertransference, and transference are dealt with on a much more flexible, intrapsychic level than is the case on a highly structured, authoritarian rehabilitation unit. As we have noted above, our programs are highly structured and organized around the 12-step peer recovery philosophy.

Treating the rich and famous from this latter perspective can be extremely difficult, based, as 12-step programs are, on acknowledging powerlessness over drugs/alcohol. A major dilemma for addicted patients is accepting that they have indeed "hit bottom." VIPs are usually protected from a severe socioeconomic bottom by their entourage, group, professional licenses, or family. Alternatively, when the VIP patient has reached bottom—for instance, when a physician's license has been pulled or when no further Hollywood agents are willing to work with performers because of their psychiatric substance abuse problems—these patients will have less denial and hence more motivation to participate in effective treatment. Thus, Main focuses his discussions on the detailed interactions that occur between staff and patient [3]. The nuances of splitting and transferences are paramount for an understanding of treatment. Within the context of treatment for drug abuse, these dynamics are seen clearly and specifically, albeit concretely, as issues of denial of one's disease and control or of failure to accept defeat and powerlessness. Hence, strictly speaking, one's specialness does not enter into this equation. One of us (WJA) treated the dually diagnosed adult child of an underworld kingpin. At the family meeting, the gruff, somewhat uncouth parent demanded to know what the son's problem was: this, after the father had surreptitiously kidnapped the child and had him detoxified privately in a hotel suite. When conventional explanations failed, the simple statement "He's a spoiled hoodlum" won the father over to the side of treatment and began the therapeutic task of educating the father to the intricate concept of enabling.

Entitlement seems to have been the symptom of the 1980s. We have seen the essence of greed defined and then redefined as an aberrant acquisitiveness proceeded through the 1980s. This, of course, is not meant to be a psychosocial diatribe, but we must place special patients in the context of their own era. Narcissism, superficiality and, to quote Grinker, "the intense pursuit of pleasure and excitement" have essentially defined this decade [5]. We are at the point in our society where the psychopathological effects of an obvious gambling disorder in a sports celebrity remain on the front page of our newspapers for over a month, and yet the commissioner of baseball, lawyers, the judges, and the family members of this celebrity are unable to approach the problem in any clinically meaningful and thereby less self-destructive way.

The patients in this category generally are all severely characterologically impaired. Grinker [5] listed the following symptoms: chronic mild depression; emptiness; boredom; superficiality; low self-awareness; lack of empathy; intense pursuit of pleasure and excitement; the belief that they can be happy with people like themselves; lack of interest in work; superficial or absent values, goals, and ideals; and the belief that buying, spending, travel, or other use of their wealth will solve all their feelings of frustration. In short, they are not ideal patients. They do not suffer greatly and are not introspective. They see action as the main solution to whatever moods they do feel [5]. Couple with this high degree of characterological impairment the intense pressure and visibility that is brought to bear on an inpatient psychiatric or rehabilitation unit, and one no longer wonders how or why specialized treatment programs for various VIP groups have arisen during the 1980s. We know that many of these specialized facilities have had great success. We think they have had success particularly because, given their own note or level of prestige, they are somewhat immunized from the pressure or stress brought to bear on facilities during the treatment of the notorious patient. Alternatively, our programs focus on the fact that addiction is a disease that is ubiquitous and has no prejudices as to financial status, race, ethnicity, or occupation. In essence, we protect the staff and the hospital from many of the side effects of treating celebrities by focusing on the commonality of the problem versus the varied psychopathological gyrations that a celebrity can bring to bear on a treatment unit.

In our experience, the VIP has many of the same characteristics as a severe drug addict. One need only reexamine Grinker's [5] list of symptoms to see that self-destructive opiate addicts are not much different in their pursuit of narcosis from the VIP in pursuit of self-aggrandizement. During treatment, self-examination begins. Being presented with a multifaceted abstinence-oriented treatment staff, the issues of control and denial are commonly amplified in the VIP patient. Within the context of the therapeutic community, the graded status system acts as the most neutral but most forcefully plebian means of modifying behavior. Within this highly structured inpatient system, then, we attempt to isolate special patients from their power base. The entourage cannot intrude onto the treatment unit. The wealthy parents of the narcissistic impaired patient must go through the standard visiting procedures and participate in the family aspects of the program just as the average parents of the average patient do. In our career, we have met only one "special" parent who was unable to do this. This parent was emphatic about maintaining nonparticipatory status and steadfastly withheld this throughout the course of a four-month treatment. One addicted offspring of this parent is now dead, and another has been in recovery for approximately three years. The decision to encourage participation, of course, stands apart from the outcome. There are certainly other parents who have participated in family programs and who have nevertheless lost children to addiction. Within our system, however, we will not cooperate with this familial negativism. It is within the nondidactic, but equally therapeutic, communal therapies that the VIP patient and family can, in fact, utilize their status to the greatest detriment. Frequently, a sadistic and patrician family member panders to the plebian peer group by taking their side in any staff-splitting dynamic that might occur.

Physicians as a group are extremely difficult to treat in the context of a plebian psychiatric drug program. We have been trained for years to believe that we are immune to the standard levels of life's emotional slings and arrows. Our levels of denial and our need for control are vastly augmented. Physicians are notoriously poor patients. We have major access to drugs of abuse and endure extremes of stress and ego gratification. The denial of illness that surrounds the physician is both self-guided and projected by society onto the physician. The physician cannot withstand the assault on the self that this pragmatic program demands. It is a marvel of therapy the power invested in licensure. Once professionals have this leverage brought to bear on their treatment denial, intellectualization and indifference melt. A united staff, well versed in the need for structure and firmly committed to a disease model of addiction, is required in order that the therapeutic milieu may continue to function as a setting for successful treatment.

Police officers are another category of special patients that are rigidly difficult to treat. Easy generalizations are of limited value in any treatment formulation. However, common threads can be delineated that define the difficulty. Law enforcement officers, like physicians, undergo daily extremes of stress. Included for the former are: facing life-and-death situations, access to drugs and to societal corruption, (such as bribes, favors, etc.). Moreover, the mythical ethos of the "men in blue" as brave, hearty, and macho directs their behaviors as well as their stereotypical image. They cannot be depressed since this is a weakness. They do not do drugs since they are illegal! Herein lies one of the most awful conundrums of modern rehabilitation. How many recovering officers can readily be found at a Narcotics Anonymous meeting? Not too many!

Another frequently insurmountable problem in treatment of law enforcement officers is the inherent "street paranoia" of their peers on the unit: "If I talk about 'copping' in front of him [the police officer] he could call his buddies and they're busted"; that is, the other addicts—their recovery group peers are loath to interact openly with the avowed lawman/patient. In practice, this negative situation is broken down by several means. First, their peers see that the staff treats the patients uniformly, i.e., the rules are the rules. Secondly, the identified "cop," if eventually involved effectively in treatment, humanizes himself by exposing his own problems and characteristics, just as their peers have.

Frequently, in our clinical experience, the "good cop" and the "baddest" peer gravitate toward each other, thus imposing a truce on the unit so that all may reap the benefits of treatment.

For the clinician, the most difficult aspect of successfully treating law enforcement officers is the issue of legality. Current myth continues to perceive alcohol as legal, hence more acceptable to their employers, while illicit substances, most frequently cannabis and cocaine, are anathema. Thus, patients may be at greater risk of losing their jobs if they admit to illicit drug use and recovery treatment than if they do not admit it. This difficulty is overcome by strict adherence to confidentiality, as well as by convincing the officers that they need a positive report to resume work although the report can be nonspecific in terms of substances abused. To obviate intrusions into confidentiality, the more enlightened police departments utilize a confidential employee-assistance program not dissimilar from the physicians' health programs of many state medical societies.

## THE SPORTING LIFE

Perhaps the most revered patient of all is the celebrity athlete. Cultivated and courted from as early as the sixth grade, the gifted athlete can be narcissistic, grandiose, and unbounded by any reasonable sense of mere mortality. Not unlike royalty, or the successful entrepreneur, society places the gifted athlete on a pedestal. The athlete's denial can be, sadly, impervious to any interventions. Pete Rose and Lloyd Daniels are examples of the complete failure of leagues, legal systems, peers, or families to intervene effectively in the progression of the disease of addiction.

The problems inherent in treating the athlete begin within the patient. Much like physicians, athletes are loath to admit to any weaknesses, such as depression, hypomania, or out-of-control drug use. Access to drugs is excessive because of the financial rewards of sports. Moreover, athletes are profoundly involved with their own corporeal splendor—they frequently suffer a unique form of "somatic" narcissism. Thus, medication treatment becomes doubly difficult. Analgesics or performance-enhancing drugs aside, what athlete would dare take a tricyclic antidepressant at the risk of blurred vision, coordination problems, and tremor? One athlete who was treated by one of us (WJA) required very low doses of desipramine for an obvious attention deficit disorder. Neither the patient nor the team owner was agreeable to this. In fact, as the patient's treatment was deteriorating clinically because of his inability to follow unit rules, the owner, not unlike an enabling parent, refused to offer any leverage against the patient's willfulness for fear of upsetting the patient: "I can't afford to lose him." Long since that meeting, the patient/athlete has dropped from the sports page to the news section, and the owner has sold the team. A rather glum pyrrhic outcome.

## SUMMARY

Treating the VIP can be extremely gratifying. One can appreciate from afar the benefits of one's clinical skills. However, the arena is strewn with difficulties, and the "failures" are public. We have found that the most important ingredients for success are a highly structured milieu with a firm, pragmatic belief in the 12-step program of recovery. A thorough and judicious medical intervention with cautious attention to side effects of medications is required of the "VIPped" physician. It is perhaps most satisfying that successful treatment of VIPs, like "average" patients, really is based on the same fundamentals of treatment. The pitfalls lie in the levels of public pressure and exposure that surrounds treatment, as well as in the ability of both clinician and patient to suspend reality and humanize the experience. As Grinker aptly stated: "Therapeutic goals include the development of an attachment to the therapist and then separation from him and deriving pleasure from ordinary activities — in short, to have the exquisite pleasure of being human." [5]

## REFERENCES

1. Group for the Advancement of Psychiatry: *The VIP with Psychiatric Impairment.* Vol VIII. Report no. 83. January 1973.
2. Seigel RK, Cocaine hallucinations. *Am J Psychiatry* 1978; 135:309–314.
3. Main TF, The ailment. *Br J Med Psych* 1957; 30:129–145.
4. Weintraub W, "The VIP syndrome": A clinical study in hospital psychiatry. *J Nerv Ment Dis* 1964; 138:181–193.
5. Grinker RR, The poor rich: The children of the super-rich. *Am J Psychiatry* 1978; 135:8:913–916.

# 17

## Problems with Inpatient Treatment of Substance Abuse Patients with Primary Psychiatric Diagnosis

**Robert Moreines**

*Fair Oaks Hospital, Summit, New Jersey*

The problem of alcohol and drug abuse within a general psychiatric inpatient population has reached enormous proportions [1,2]. Substance abuse sustains morbidity, precipitates relapse, and disrupts behavior. It presents danger in concurrent use with medications. It is difficult to diagnose and difficult to treat unless specific efforts are developed.

The special problems that drugs pose for psychiatric patients work in two directions. The drugs themselves precipitate or worsen symptoms. Psychotic patients may suffer a first break, relapses, and intensification of hallucinations and delusions with hallucinogen, PCP, or marijuana abuse [3]. Depressed patients suffer cycles of intense hopelessness and suicidal impulses worsened by alcohol or sedative abuse [4,5]. Borderline patients and antisocial patients are more likely to make suicide attempts when using alcohol or drugs [4]. Other individuals with impulse control disorders such as explosive outbursts or self-mutilation may be disinhibited by drugs. Panic attacks and anxiety symptoms are precipitated and worsened by stimulants (cocaine, amphetamines, diet pills, caffeine) [6]. Paranoid disorders can follow cocaine and amphetamine abuse [7]. A worsening of apathy, negative symptoms of schizophrenia, and amotivational syndrome can follow chronic marijuana abuse [8].

On the other hand, psychiatric patients have an added vulnerability to substance abuse [9]. Schizotypal and psychotic patients seeking to overcome their inner emptiness, stigma, and social isolation may use drugs on the periphery of a peer group [8,10]. Depressed patients and anxious patients seek solace and escape in alcohol and sedatives [11,12]. Manic patients use drugs as a result of their impulsivity and poor judgment but may also seek to temper their hyperactivity [13]. Borderline patients turn to drugs to medicate their dissociative states, anxiety, and emptiness as well as in service of their aggressive and self-destructive impulses [14]. Many patients suffering residual attention deficit disorder with hyperactivity and brain injury lack controls over their impulses and may also seek to self medicate their inner tension or distractibility [15].

I have administered a team on the general adult psychiatry unit over the past decade at Fair Oaks Hospital. Our hospital is well known for its innovative work in the treatment of substance abuse. A comprehensive Neuropsychiatric evaluation unit exists to make a full assessment of the medical, psychiatric, and psychosocial problems for each patient and to generate the differential diagnosis. In the biological sphere, the treatment of narcotic withdrawal with clonidine, [16] the investigation of bromocriptine for use in cocaine abstinence, [17] the elucidation of the neuroendocrine profile and of affective changes in alcohol and cocaine abuse were all developed at Fair Oaks [18].

Over the past four years, as director of the unit, I have developed a subprogram for the treatment of substance abuse. It has involved many developments for the staff, including the following:

1. Encouraging individuals (both nursing staff and clinicians) with an interest or willingness to work in the area to learn about substance abuse and undergo additional training, so that they may play leading roles in coordinating the program.

2. Training the rest of the staff about the special needs and difficulties of working with patients with dual diagnosis and with their families. Clinicians, in general, had to learn to be less forgiving and more confrontive, to deal more with behavior and consequences than feelings and analysis, and to familiarize themselves with the language of enabling and codependence in working with families.

3. Integrating the progress made by patients in working through a First–Step questionnaire, participation in AA and NA discussion groups and presentation of their life stories with the rest of the program [19]. This involved giving the added requirements of the substance abuse program special importance and communicating more information between clinicians in deciding such rewards for progress as status and therapeutic pass time.

4. Maintaining an ongoing assessment and strengthening of the program to enable staff to feel credible when patients accuse staff of not being "recovering" and meetings of not being "authentic" [20]; increasing resources, such as written materials from other substance abuse programs;

building up our own speakers' bureau to include people in the community and discharged former patients who had completed our program; regular staff inservice and quality assurance monitoring, and supervision by counselors or nursing staff with certification.

I should like to describe the specific issues involved in treating substance abuse among different diagnostic groups seen commonly on a general psychiatric unit. These include psychosis (schizophrenia), explosive/impulse control disorder, problems of the elderly, and severe personality disorder. Patients with affective disorder and anxiety disorder will be discussed in other chapters of this book.

## SCHIZOPHRENIA

A confusing and potentially harmful situation arises when a patient with a psychotic disorder is treated in a traditional drug counseling program. Since even disturbed behavior may not reveal the extent of the inner psychological turmoil, confusion, and distress, the inability of these patients to participate appropriately is considered "resistance." The cognitive disorganization may be interpreted as "acting dumb," the grandiose delusions as "failure to give up control," the autistic distractions and attention to inner stimuli and auditory hallucinations as "lack of motivation," and the grossly impaired social judgment as "provocative" or "testing behavior."

Such patients may have concealed their disability and psychotic decompensation for a long time. They become isolative, with little peer interaction except as a fringe participant in social drug abuse. They avoid their parents and, when questioned, respond curtly that they're OK. If they are not pushed to describe things more fully in their own words and if their performance in school or work is not closely monitored, a profound cognitive deterioration can be hidden.

In addition to the thought disorder, such individuals often suffer dysphoric feelings. There may be some awareness of their isolation, difference from peers, and deterioration in their understanding of their surroundings. They may be scapegoated and teased by peers when they join drug parties. They may seek refuge in marijuana or hallucinogens to feel more like their friends and disguise their disability. "Social acceptance" may require only sitting around "getting high" and "being into" music. Other accompanying symptoms include lack of initiative and spontaneity, paucity of speech, little facial expression or social reactivity, lack of interest in surroundings, and anhedonia. Sometimes, when hopelessness, impaired self-esteem, guilt, sleep and eating disturbances, and sustained sadness are present, a serious depression should also be diagnosed; at other times, these dysphoric symptoms are part of the course of schizophrenia.

The relationship between schizophrenia and drug abuse has been of particular interest. Hallucinogens and stimulants can cause hallucinations and paranoid delusions; they have been studied as models for psychotic illness [3]. Some individuals suffer a prolonged psychotic episode that follows drug abuse. Actually, there has been a controversy as to whether drugs could "cause" schizophrenia. It is now generally felt that these individuals already possess the potential biological and psychological illness of schizophrenia and that the drug triggers it at that time [3].

A very serious problem is that of ongoing drug abuse following diagnosis and treatment of schizophrenia [21]. Alcohol, marijuana, hallucinogens (including PCP), and stimulants are frequent choices [10,22]. Marijuana can also precipitate and perpetuate frank delusions and hallucinations in these individuals [23,24]. Marijuana may also reinforce the negative symptoms and amotivational syndrome [23]. Hallucinogens, PCP, and stimulants are particularly dangerous in maintaining the fragmented thinking, paranoia, and hallucinations [22]. Compliance with treatment, including medications, is often adversely affected, and relapses are more frequent [25,26]. There is also an association of drug abuse with increased acting out of violent and dangerous behavior [27,28]. It has unfortunately been all too common for individuals who are attending day programs to find ongoing sources of drugs in nearby areas.

Obviously, these patients have difficulty participating in traditional AA and NA programs. As noted earlier, their psychopathology is underestimated and misinterpreted both by counselors and peers. In a program where success so clearly follows the establishment of peer bonds, the schizophrenic patient is at a serious loss.

These patients have difficulty even in dual-diagnosis drug abuse groups since the higher-functioning patients become frustrated by their lack of motivation, lack of awareness, and poor judgment [29,30]. Their social limitations, distance, and lack of relatedness make true friendships rare. Therapists must explain the disability of these patients to the group and model how to interact with them. The other patients will then follow the example and realize that they have to address schizophrenic patients in a gentle and concrete manner. Cause and effect and consequences of behavior must be clearly and specifically stated. Schizophrenic patients must be required to describe things in their own words and not be permitted simply to say yes or no to the discussions of others. Peers can help to reinforce specific behavior contracts both by being aware of the patients' responsibilities and by helping to monitor their compliance and also by supporting the reasonableness of the consequences. Schizophrenic patients benefit from additional, small, more homogeneous groups where they can get the direct attention they need and be helped to form loose, less demanding relationships.

Because of the limited benefit of peer support, the therapist must play a greater role. In groups, as noted, the patient is protected and directly addressed. More individual attention is required, and this should revolve around the behavior contract, expectations, and consequences.

Family therapy, which is a crucial component in the treatment of substance abuse, [31] also has special requirements and adaptations in these cases. Family members need to be educated about the extent of the disability which they too have often underestimated. This may have a profound effect on parents, causing depressed, guilty, and even grieving feelings as the impact of the illness is felt. Parents have to be counseled that traditional "tough love" programs and ultimatums, including forcing the schizophrenic to leave home, can be disastrous. Parents must learn to have limited and specific rules and expectations for behavior and to develop some tolerance for the residual negative symptoms.

## IMPULSE CONTROL DISORDERS

Individuals with impulse control disorders, residual attention deficit disorder, or borderline intelligence are very difficult to engage in therapy. It is even more difficult for them to make lasting changes through treatment. Depressive symptoms and antiauthority problems, impaired self-esteem, intimidating and manipulative behavior, and some cognitive impairment often complicate the clinical picture.

Some of these patients have a history of traumatic brain injury or are in other ways demonstrably impaired neurologically. They may respond to medications like beta-blockers, [32] anticonvulsants, and buspirone [33] for better control of their behavior. This is a very difficult medication problem for patients with dual diagnosis in 12-step groups because the medication appears to be more a "mind-altering chemical" than do antipsychotic or antidepressant medications for more clearly recognized illnesses.

These patients have accompanying cognitive impairments that must be considered in the treatment program. Gross has extensively described the necessary program adjustments for these patients [34]. Traditional 28-day programs are often unrealistic for these patients and demand writing and memory skills, abstract thinking, and tolerance for intense interpersonal confrontation. In addition, many of these patients have developed personality traits of rationalization and denial, emotional overreactivity, need for immediate gratification, problems not feeling in control, and difficulty recalling past events accurately.

Many of the brain-injured patients will share similar cognitive impairments. These include short attention span, distractibility, and short-term memory problems. Their problem-solving abilities suffer from lack of spontaneous cause-and-effect reasoning, concrete thinking, impulsivity and difficulty following multistep processes. Interpersonal difficulties follow from language problems with frequent tangential and circumstantial speech, impaired perception of body language, emotional insensitivity, and aloofness.

For the more disturbed brain-injured patients, the following "tips" can be helpful [34]. Their cognitive impairment requires brief and direct communication with examples. They need to learn basic problem-solving skills of a stepwise nature. Written memory aids and cues, like date books and journals, are helpful. Even the 12 steps need to be described in a simple, concrete fashion.

With brain-injured patients, obvious difficulties also result from emotional impairments of affective lability, low frustration tolerance, and catastrophic overreactions. They need to develop ways to save face, to think before acting, and to feel that it's all right to depend on someone wiser and more experienced. These patients will have greater dependency needs, which the clinician must expect and accept and not interpret in some negative fashion. Instead, they should be encouraged to draw upon others to enhance problem-solving skills. Overall, the clinicians must not take things for granted and must not assume that the patient thinks as they do.

I'd like to include several examples of the "12 Steps for Brain Injured" [34] and compare them to the classic form [19].

| *Classic* | *Revised* |
|---|---|
| We admitted we were powerless over alcohol—that our lives had become unmanageable. | You must tell yourself and others that drug use or drinking will make your life more out of control. |
| Came to believe that a Power greater than ourselves could restore us to sanity. | You must believe that someone other than yourself can and must help get your life back on track and in order. |
| Made a decision to turn our will and our lives over to the care of God *as we understand Him.* | You will allow someone other than yourself to help you. Be honest and open up. |
| Made a searching and fearless moral inventory of ourselves. | Make a list of your strengths and weaknesses, of the behaviors that are good and the behaviors that are not so good. |

I have described these issues in some detail because there are definite similarities between brain-injured/neurologically impaired and the schizophrenic populations. It is very helpful to keep their limitations in mind when dealing with them. In addition, the elderly and the older adolescent similarly require adjustments in approach.

Some of these brain-injured patients who have started out on substance abuse units have had to be transferred to the adult psychiatric unit because they cannot handle the more confrontative counseling environment. Episodes of physically losing control of their behavior, damaging physical property, threatening and even harming other patients and staff members occur. Sometimes, their cognitive and emotional impairment causes them to be scapegoated. Whether these patients complete their hospitalization on the adult unit or are transferred back to a substance abuse unit depends on the severity of their drug problem and the availability of comprehensive outpatient services.

A series of group discussions with a particular patient captures the approach most fruitfully. Although I tend to stress patient interaction rather than staff intervention, there are circumstances in which staff must model an indirect approach. In general, the patients tend to attack problems head on, which can sometimes lead to defensiveness and, in these patients, potentially harmful anger.

> The patient maintained that his current marijuana use was a reasonable way of relaxing after returning home from work. He admitted to more extensive use of other drugs in college, years before, but just felt that was irrelevant.
>
> First, in a nonjudgmental way, the true extent of current drug use had to be elicited. When he went on to describe to the group smoking marijuana every evening to relax and to heighten recreational activities, we had an opening—especially when it came out that his earlier heavy use of many drugs had been responsible for his flunking out of college. It was important to delineate the *hidden* adverse effects of his current daily marijuana abuse. It was relatively easy to demonstrate to him and to the group that his was an emotional escape from thinking about problems and that it reinforced his own distortions and interpretations, promoted social isolation, drained his energy, and led to rationalization and avoidance of problem solving and, ultimately, to his feeling depressed and suicidal. It was connected to his presenting psychiatric problems of unstable mood, distorted thinking, and impulsive and aggressive behavior.
>
> Because he was not intoxicated at work nor in jeopardy of losing his job, because his drug use did not cause the financial drain of cocaine or heroin, and because marijuana was thought to be a less potent drug and a socially acceptable way of unwinding, an obvious direct assault on the consequences of his drug abuse and "hitting bottom" was impossible. Yet, in this case, we were able to lead him and the group to appreciate how marijuana abuse maintained acceptance and perpetuation of a frustrating job situation and how greatly it contributed to pent-up hostility, feelings of victimization, and antiauthority attitudes.

## THE ELDERLY

The treatment of the elderly psychiatric patient with concurrent substance abuse presents special problems. Drugs used, misused, and abused include over-the-counter (OTC) preparations, prescribed drugs, alcohol, and illicit drugs. For many reasons, the elderly are prone to suffer adverse effects; they have insufficient contact and communication with physicians, different metabolic patterns, multiple drug use for multiple medical problems, and increased sensitivity of organ systems including brain [35–37]. In addition, their abuse is more difficult to identify in that many of the consequences (e.g., job loss, social isolation, and driving infractions) seen with younger patients are often not applicable to the aged. Some physical effects such as insomnia, decreased sexual functioning, and cognitive difficulties are also hard to distinguish from natural processes [35–37].

The elderly, perhaps even more than other population segments, minimize and conceal their drug and alcohol problems. They are embarrassed by the connotations and tend not to reveal personal matters in general. Family members and other social contacts must be interviewed and urine and blood screens utilized to avoid missing this crucial diagnosis.

In a treatment program with a mixed-age population, special attention must be given to the needs of the elderly. They may be very sensitive to abusive language and not only take offense and feel intimidated but may personalize it. They may take advantage of foul language to state that it proves that they are different from the others and don't belong in the drug abuse meetings. Their connotations of "alcoholic" or "drug addict" are of the utmost degradation and shame. Often, they are totally incapable of relating to the street activities and the illegal and violent experiences reported by younger patients and may be frightened by their acting-out behavior. This can result in resistance to feedback and advice from members of a group they can't relate to.

Some of the general problems the elderly have in therapy have a similar adverse effect on their participation in the substance abuse groups. Many of the elderly patients find it exceedingly difficult to talk about problems in their personal lives. They have a strong belief that if something can't be changed, one is not supposed to express feelings about it. They are often concrete in their thinking also and don't understand what "issues" are. Many find it difficult to listen to an analysis of a problem and seek immediately to give advice or reassure the individual. It is often very hard for them to criticize and describe shortcomings of loved ones. A deceased spouse often has become idealized and is severely missed. Adult children have often become their lifeline, and dependence on them can't be endangered by speaking badly of them. There is usually a degree of rigidity and stubbornness, perhaps a fear of not being able to change.

Many of the elderly patients who have been admitted to the hospital began using and abusing prescription drugs and alcohol because they became overwhelmed by depressive and anxious symptoms. Like the deterioration seen after a hip fracture, often the current psychiatric illness follows some physical illness or disability. Their fragile homeostasis has been threatened, their belief that they can take care of themselves is shaken, and they are overwhelmed and frightened.

Elderly patients need to be encouraged to share their lives. It must be stressed that the objective is to know them and, through understanding them, to build better coping strategies upon their strengths; it is not to find faults in them or in their families and not to create problems. The multigenerational composition of the group can be used to advantage. Older patients can share the perspective of parent and grandparent and hear from others what their own children might be feeling. A particularly important encouragement is to share their feelings and memories with their children, especially memories of a deceased spouse. The staff must counter their resistance to sharing their feelings and their belief that it will hurt their children, that they will just be a burden, and that there's no use doing so as nothing will be changed.

Family therapy is very important as both the patient and the adult children need help in coping with the present circumstances. Opening communication, sharing the expression of feelings, and more direct assertion of needs are important. A behavioral contract can maintain regular contact in a predictable way. Elderly patients must develop better problem-solving skills and need to clarify what they can do for themselves and what they need help with. Moreover, the patients should have specified tasks that they can provide for their adult children. Baby-sitting and cooking meals can be their contribution at times of being together, and such offerings provide increased self-esteem and a balance in the relationship.

For many of these patients, the following measures will be sufficient. Effective and safe pharmacotherapy will manage symptoms of depression, anxiety, and chronic pain. Coordination of treatment between all involved physicians, with one designated as primary coordinator, will help avoid dangers of polypharmacy and control abuse of medications. Establishment of a behavioral program, clear communication between family members, and reestablishment of an active social network [37] will increase coping abilities. Education about the dangers of prescription and over-the-counter drugs and reinforcing their potential for abuse will decrease misuse.

During the hospital phase of treatment, these patients must attend the AA and NA meetings and discussion groups. They work on the first step and learn about substance abuse. They should also attend meetings in the community while on therapeutic pass. However, because of the resistance noted earlier, this will typically be inadequate to get them to make a commitment to attend AA.

For the patients with a more significant alcohol problem or a pattern of medication or drug abuse, regular participation in AA and NA will be necessary after discharge. Ensuring this may require treatment on a 12-step substance abuse unit after stabilization of their other psychiatric problems on the adult unit. There they will be totally immersed in the program and helped to change their feelings of being different into identification. Moreover, they will be better able to cooperate and participate by virtue of what they have learned on the adult psychiatric unit and their greater ease and familiarity with therapy. In this way, they are similar to impulsive/brain-injured patients who need preliminary treatment desensitization and engagement before they can accept the more confrontational approach of abuse groups without overreacting defensively.

## BORDERLINE PERSONALITY DISORDER

The hospitalized patient with borderline personality disorder often has accompanying Axis I pathology, which has contributed to the need for inpatient treatment. Major depression, panic disorder, substance abuse, and psychosis may occur and, at times, are minimized by staff because of the florid character pathology. These patients are familiar both to substance abuse units and to general psychiatric units, and staff are well aware of the need for consistent limit setting. Manipulation, distortions in interpersonal interactions, emotional lability and overreactivity, and the defense of splitting characterize their behavior.

These patients form a bridge for staff members in developing and applying skills to treat substance abuse on a general psychiatric unit. The need to confront behavior, to speak in the language of consequences, to correct distortions of thinking, not to be fooled by manipulative behavior, to help develop cognitive problem-solving skills and the capacity to handle emotions, and to correct the tendency to externalize responsibility for problems and to rationalize and minimize behavior are techniques required in treating substance abuse in general as well as these patients in particular.

I should like to comment on some of the special problems posed by substance-abusing borderline patients on a general psychiatric unit. Many of them will require psychotropic medication for accompanying major depression, panic disorder, transient psychosis, and cyclothymic disorder. Because symptoms of their personality disorder can be so prominent, many counselors and other clinicians will miss the accompanying Axis I diagnosis and object to their need for medication. On the other hand, their manipulative and histrionic presentation necessitate caution in making the diagnosis, and clinicians must maintain an explicit focus on objective target symptoms.

Borderline patients can have a tremendous impact on the therapeutic milieu and can be intimidating to other patients. A special benefit of treating dual-diagnosis patients on the psychiatric unit is the presence of other patients who will be able to confront the borderline on their manipulative behavior. The similarity of the behavior of borderline patients and addicts makes this possible. Many of the psychiatric patients lack the ego strength and personality style to confront both addicts and borderline patients. An isolated borderline patient can therefore be very difficult to treat. The anti-authority attitudes of such a patient can have disastrous consequences for the lower-functioning negativistic and passive patients.

The psychodynamics of a borderline patient can seduce a therapist into a rescue fantasy. These patients have often suffered genuine emotional and even physical trauma from parents and other caretakers. They express their emotions with ease, have learned the psychological jargon, and appear to have insight. Their problem is frequently a lack of cognitive skills and adaptive defenses. They will weave a credible, distorted story, with key omissions. They will make certain staff members feel special and "confide" in them material that they misleadingly state they have never told anyone before. On the other hand, they will totally alienate other staff members and treat them according to the way they view them, which is in a distorted "all-bad" fashion.

The 12-step orientation and the slogans that form the "passed on culture" of the substance abuse programs are very helpful with these patients. They tend to devote their lives to "pseudo-self-analysis," and the slogans are very effective at penetrating distorting defenses and self-destructive behavior patterns. In fact, the slogans are very useful for *all* the psychiatric patients and capture important principles of therapy in a way that makes them usable, memorable, and understandable. The slogans provide clear guides to behavior and supplement the impaired cognitive problem-solving skills often overwhelmed by intense emotional overreactions.

"One day at a time," "K.I.S.S. (Keep it simple)," "Change people, places, and things," "If the body goes, the mind will follow," "Stick with the winners," and other classic slogans reinforce the principles that must be followed.

The borderline patients have often wreaked havoc on their external support system through their manipulative, provocative, and abusive behavior. They often reject potential supportive persons because of their interpersonal sensitivity, overreactivity, and splitting defense (viewing individuals as all bad and not being able to integrate negative and positive feelings for them). They often reject family meetings, and this is something staff must not accept. Enabling behavior of the family (today's "all-bad" mother will again be tomorrow's savior) is often prominent. Impaired communication, with frequent escalation to destructive exchanges and feelings of hatred and rejection that ensue must be repaired. A behavior contract is helpful here, too, to maintain new ways of interacting and to signal dangerous return to old maladaptive patterns.

## GROUP THERAPY

Group processes have long been recognized as fundamental to the treatment of substance abuse [29,38]. These include the AA and NA fellowships, speaker meetings, 12-step meetings, supportive/confrontational discussion groups, and life story presentations. Related problem areas have also been served well by group meetings. Al-Anon and Nar-Anon for family members provide education, emotional support, and direction in changing enabling and codependent behavior. Adult Children of Alcoholics (ACOA), for the children of recovering individuals as well as substance abusers whose parents were themselves similarly afflicted, [39] reveal self-destructive patterns. Survivors' groups help victims of sexual abuse, which is frequently seen in the dysfunctional families of substance abusers and which affects women in particular. Other family support groups, such as Tough Love and multiple family groups, help parents cope with drug-abusing youngsters.

Many of these groups must be adjusted to meet the special needs of patients with concurrent psychiatric disorders [30]. Moreover, inpatient treatment of a spectrum of psychiatric conditions benefits greatly from group therapies of various kinds: clinician-led group therapy, leaderless groups, psychodrama, social skills training, and multiple family group. I have adapted the educative model for inpatient group therapy presented by Maxmen [40,41] for my adult psychiatric unit. Not only is it effective in general, but it is particularly well suited to the treatment needs of the dual-diagnosed patient.

The name of the approach can be misleading. This is not a group that simply educates patients about their illness. It teaches patients how to think clinically and work therapeutically toward and with one another. The staff is careful not to do things for the patients but to advise, guide, and occasionally model for them how to respond to one another. I have come to value the active process by the patients as much as any specific interpretation, clarification, or piece of advice given. To appreciate the benefits of this approach, it helps to think in terms of the special needs of hospitalized patients and the specific part group therapy plays in coordination with the other components of the treatment program.

I should like to describe the technique in some detail since it works to great advantage. The group can be composed of patients with any diagnosis, level of functioning, and degree of involvement with drugs as long as they behave appropriately. The group is continuous, and patients on our psychiatric unit stay between 3 and 10 weeks. All members of the multidisciplinary clinical team attend. The group meets daily for 50 minutes. The number of patients attending is usually 12–15. The patients are oriented by their peers and staff as to their responsibilities and what to expect, and this is periodically reinforced in group sessions directly.

The group starts each day with modification of Yalom's "go-round." [42] Patients are expected to bring to the attention of the group any current issue of concern. This includes problems they are facing, issues that have arisen in the context of individual or family therapy sessions, and difficulties in interpersonal behavior in the hospital itself. Patients should also bring up concerns for other patients who have avoided taking the initiative themselves. Finally, staff bring up concerns for individual patients or the group process as a whole if no one else has. In addition, during weeks when there has been an especially high turnover of patients or a number of leaders of the group have left, everyone will introduce themselves to the group and describe the circumstances and problems that led to hospitalization and what they are currently working on so as to reestablish a common group culture and knowledge base.

These techniques for starting the group encourage more people to speak, prevent people from avoiding treatment issues, and reinforce a responsibility for both one's own and others' treatment. The members then discuss how to apportion their time; this includes grouping topics together under a common theme and rating concerns according to importance, urgency, and relevance to others. This avoids domination by a particular member and determination of the day's topic by the person who speaks first. Even if a particular issue is not discussed in that day's session, it has been brought to the group's attention and can be dealt with in a different therapeutic activity or on another day.

As Maxmen [40,41] has pointed out, inpatients can be characterized by intense dependency needs and feelings of helplessness, ineffectuality, hopelessness, and demoralization, as well as estrangement from the rest of humanity. Important therapeutic factors in group therapy include the instillation of hope, a feeling of acceptance in the group cohesiveness, and opportunity for increased self-esteem through helping others, and a sense of universality in sharing similar problems.

Of course, what is of particular importance in group therapy is its interpersonal nature. In agreement with Yalom, [42] I have found that discussions of current shared and witnessed interactions with others in the therapeutic community has the greatest emotional impact. The distortions and misperceptions, miscommunications, passivity and aggression, rigidity, and all the other maladaptive behaviors can be brought to the attention of the individual. Members of the group can then offer alternative points of view, interpretations, and behavior strategies. They can undercut defensiveness and antiauthority attitudes by learning how to be both empathic and confrontational. Members are encouraged to relate similar behaviors and to identify associated feelings. All then enter a joint task to try to reflect on and analyze the behavior, to perceive recurring patterns, and to note the self-defeating and noxious consequences. Sometimes, individuals will bring insights from their concurrent individual therapy or from prior counseling experiences; their own understanding is consolidated through applying these interpretations, and the other patients become aware of these more abstract conceptualizations. When feedback comes from peers, it has greater legitimacy and authenticity and avoids the antiauthority struggles that often ensue when staff must convey these same points.

The patients are taught to be caring detectives. Commonly, peers will accept patients' descriptions of situations at face value and sympathize with them as victims. This is an important way in which dual-diagnosis patients are different from other substance abusers; they are less suspicious of conscious manipulation and deceit. Staff must persistently reinforce the need to look for alternative explanations and focus on the patients' contribution to their problems.

Similarly, patients tend immediately to try to reassure and make each other feel better and to give advice. They need to learn to tolerate emotional distress and expression and to understand it as therapeutic (the initial goal is to describe the problem fully in all its facets and to appreciate the different points of view). Especially for patients who are abusing drugs, this is of particular relevance because they have sought to avoid emotions through drugs and have little ability to tolerate dysphoric feelings without acting out. Additionally, it is a waste of group therapy time to focus on concrete solutions. It is the emotional impediments to acting more constructively that need to be identified.

A related problem is that patients must learn to appreciate the varying needs of different patients and different disorders. While a patient with compulsive personality needs to express angry feelings, a patient with borderline or histrionic traits needs to develop more cognitive problem-solving abilities and self-control. A patient with antisocial traits must be directly and forcefully confronted, while a schizophrenic patient's limitations must be considered.

The demands on the staff of this model for group therapy require vigilance not to slip into familiar but ultimately less productive interventions. The staff must relentlessly maintain responsibility with the patients and resist the appeal of making clever interpretations. When a more subtle point needs to be made that is beyond the patients' ability to articulate, it is beneficial to have patients repeat it in their own words to make the process an active one. Staff members often find it difficult to let the patients ask the questions and make the comments. It is very easy for patients to look passively to the staff for "better" interpretations. Individual therapy provides the opportunity to follow up any of these issues in greater depth.

As these patients have primary psychiatric problems, they are being treated on a general psychiatric unit. Therefore, it is a heterogeneous community, with those suffering concurrent substance abuse mixed with those who don't. Besides providing a treatment setting that is better tolerated by the dual-diagnosis patients, the program benefits from the mix. Patients with prior or current experience in AA, NA, and substance abuse programs have learned many things about their own behavior and that of others. In particular, the slogans they use frequently capture very important therapeutic principles in a way that is directly conveyed with emotional impact and is retained. These concept are often important to all the patients' treatment and enhances a general psychiatric program (examples were given in the discussion of borderline patients).

There are many other ways in which the patient mix has special benefits. Typically, nonpsychotic substance-abusing patients are relatively more verbal and direct in expressing their own views and confronting others. This is of great importance in the treatment of borderline patients, who often dominate and intimidate others on an adult psychiatric unit. Defenses are similar to the resistant behaviors that are noted in the substance abuse groups, and interventions are applicable to many of the patients.

There are a number of obstacles that must be overcome in establishing the substance abuse treatment portion of the program. Patients have to be made to take their responsibilities seriously, and mandatory tasks must be monitored. These include writing a detailed First-Step preparation, in which the effects of drugs on all aspects of one's life are recounted. Six additional groups have been added to the schedule and are compulsory. Patients also attend AA and NA meetings in the community on therapeutic passes.

We have developed our own groups, which meet around special needs and maintain the active attitude described for group therapy. When we have speaker meetings, they often feature alumni, individuals who have previously been inpatients on the unit and, therefore, have first-hand experience with psychiatric problems.

People are encouraged to return indefinitely to some of the groups and serve as models and facilitators. Two groups per week are First-Step presentations by one patient, with extensive feedback from the group members, including a written summary evaluation. Discussion and step work are highlighted. A special weekly group run by a psychodramatist focuses on the defenses and resistance present in the group.

An important goal of treatment is establishing the foundation for ongoing participation in AA and NA after discharge. It is necessary to establish the behavior during the hospital stay, first with our own meetings and later with attendance at meetings in the communities where patients will be living after discharge. Therapeutic passes during the final phase of hospitalization include AA and NA meetings and arranging for a temporary sponsor. Spot urine and drug screens are done, and the passes make a transition to discharge, when urges will arise and will have to be dealt with.

Patients develop behavior contracts with their families as the conclusion of the family therapy experience. Meetings are held weekly to educate the family about drug abuse, identify all the drug-seeking and habit-maintaining behavior of the patient, identify the enabling behavior of the family and, in general, develop more direct and sensitive communication. In developing the behavior contract, patient and family discuss expectations and consequences of behavior. An important topic is how to handle a slip. I think it is very important to distinguish a slip from a relapse and to design appropriate actions. The factors that are pertinent include openness versus deceit, defensiveness, and remorse.

## SPECIAL PROBLEMS

A number of special problems arise in the substance abuse treatment of patients with a primary psychiatric diagnosis. They require modification of traditional approaches for each area and a novel integration of confrontational and reflective attitudes.

Complications start with the First Step: acknowledging that one is an Addict (this will be used synonomously with Alcoholic for our purposes). In fact, this is how people come to introduce themselves at AA and NA meetings. For the psychiatric patients, this presents a problem. Inclusion criteria must be broad enough to include drug usage that has been associated with adverse effects (by virtue of their psychiatric illness) even though it might be considered "recreational" or intermittent use under other circumstances. Therefore, many of the patients will not, in fact, meet criteria for being an addict. Counselors can run into problems if they persist in attacking these patients as manifesting classic denial or resistance. Patients have to accept that their prior drug usage, which typically had been associated with recurrence or worsening of symptoms (such as paranoid delusions, hallucinations, mania, suicidal or other self-inflicted injury, and impulsive and aggressive behavior, or panic anxiety), is dangerous *for them*. One can demonstrate to patients how their lives are unmanageable when intoxication exacerbates other symptoms and connect substance use to the crises that led to the current hospitalization.

A related issue is the insistence on abstinence. Because the patients often don't meet independent criteria for addiction, some of the arguments of abstinence don't apply. I insist on at least three months of total abstinence after hospitalization because of the demonstrated loss of control requiring hospitalization, and the vulnerability of, and risks to, the patient upon discharge. Although arbitrary, it coincides with the goal of 90 meetings in 90 days, which is a key focus in traditional substance abuse programs, and it falls within the six-month vulnerable period for relapse and continuation medication treatment. If patients have difficulty accepting this prescription, it only provides further evidence that drug use is a problem they can't control. It contradicts their assertion that their drug use is simply a preference and a choice.

If they observe 90 days of abstinence, the issue can be more effectively dealt with at the end of that period. By then patients should have reached a deeper understanding of the problem and a commitment to health, developed a positive therapeutic relationship and support group, and substituted alternative behavior patterns for their drug use. I also draw a distinction between an occasional alcoholic drink and all other drug use. Marijuana, hallucinogens, and stimulants are forcefully prohibited. Psychotic patients are warned of the particular dangers of those drugs. Of course, in an individual case, if a single alcoholic drink leads to behavior problems, psychiatric symptoms, or more extensive substance use and abuse, then it is totally prohibited as well. I feel that this approach also maintains credibility, as the effects of different substances of abuse vary greatly in different patients.

Obviously, interactions with psychotropic medications need to be considered [43]. I caution the reader against asserting blanket prohibition of all and any drug and alcohol use because of dire medical complications. The only exception is the MAOI class of antidepressants (phenelzine or Nardil, tranylcypromine or Parnate), where there will be a serious hypertensive reaction that could be lethal if used with stimulants like cocaine and amphetamine and certain alcoholic beverages [44]. In other cases, if a patient should "test" you and take a single drink, he will typically experience an intensification of the intoxification and expected effects. This will destroy your credibility with the patient and increase the likelihood that he will "test" other therapeutic recommendations and prohibitions. *If other circumstances permit*, many patients would be able to have a single drink of alcohol, for example, without dire circumstances of a medical, psychological, or addictive nature.

In essence, one needs to individualize the approach. Again, this is a deviation from classic substance abuse programs, but it is necessary and effective with dual-diagnosis patients who are not classically addicted. The very taking of psychotropic medications will have to be dealt with differently in these patients. Typically, all medications are suspect as mind-altering, and their use is considered a way to avoid dealing directly with emotional pain or stress. In addition, the vast majority of addicts experience symptoms of depression or anxiety during withdrawal and early abstinence; the very psychiatric diagnosis may be questioned by traditional AA and NA programs [45,46]. With increased communication between psychiatrists and counselors, improved understanding and cooperation have arisen. It is hoped that psychiatrists will not be using minor tranquilizers for symptom relief in patients with a history of substance abuse. Counselors have to accept legitimate psychiatric Axis I diagnoses and not view antipsychotic, antidepressant, and mood-stabilizing medications (lithium, Tegretol) as harmful. Patients have to be warned that they might be criticized for, or counseled against, their medication by individuals at AA or NA meetings who are well meaning but don't understand the problem.

Preparation for these meetings in the community is a crucial component of the dual-diagnosis hospital treatment [20]. Patients may not follow through and make a commitment for many reasons, such as inertia, denial, intimidation, and embarrassment. Many psychiatric patients have interpersonal difficulties due to their illness. Much attention must be given to enhancing participation; e.g., attending community meetings on therapeutic day passes and arranging for a temporary sponsor while still in the hospital. If double-trouble meetings are available in the community, they should form part of the outpatient schedule.

Drug addicts are told that they must go to meetings every day. Again, because of differences in the dual-diagnosis group, this may not apply to all our patients. Establishing a real commitment to attend three or four meetings per week is often a successful achievement.

A unique form of resistance with dual-diagnosis patients is "shifting denial." They will tell their therapist that drinking is the problem and their substance abuse counselor that their drug use is only secondary to a relapse of psychiatric symptoms. This is a rather common way to avoid facing both issues and necessitates coordination between members of the treatment team.

The treatment group must tolerate a much greater range of psychopathology and levels of ego functioning than a traditional 12-step program. Schizophrenic patients will be treated with depressive and manic depressive patients, and elements of supportive therapy may differ [20,47,48]. Dependence on others and accepting disability may be necessary. Indirect and less confrontational approaches may be crucial because of concrete and autistic thinking and extreme interpersonal sensitivity.

Furthermore, the handling of confrontation itself is complicated. Borderline and antisocial patients are often in the minority, and the other members of the group frequently lack the ego strength to respond to them directly. The therapist must take the lead and not only model this for the group but practice this task. On the other hand, the weaker patients must be protected by the therapist. Their impairments in thinking must be explained, and tendencies to stigmatize and ridicule them must be dealt with quickly and openly. The schizophrenic and depressed patients may be overwhelmed by the confrontations that they witness and which may not involve them; they may require reassurance at such times.

## CONCLUSIONS

Substance abuse is an increasingly prevalent problem for patients with other primary psychiatric disorders. It is difficult to diagnose and difficult to treat and is responsible for a worsening of symptoms and increased frequency of relapse.

It has been my experience that concurrent substance abuse can be effectively treated on a general psychiatric unit. The principles of AA and NA 12-step programs need to be thoughtfully adjusted to the special needs of psychiatric patients, and resources need to be allocated. The program enhances morale of staff participants as they seek to overcome the frustration of witnessing the relapses and revolving-door readmissions of these patients. Ultimately, the inpatient experience should lead to active participation in substance abuse groups as an outpatient and to abstinence from drugs of abuse.

## REFERENCES

1. Brown V, Ridgely M, Pepper B, Levine I, Ryglewicz, H. The dual crisis: mental illness and substance abuse. *Am Psych* 1989; 44:565–569.
2. Daley D, Moss H, Campbell F. *Dual Disorders, Counseling Clients with Chemical Dependency and Mental Illness*. Minneapolis: Hazelden, 1987.
3. Moreines R. The psychedelics. In: Giannini A, Slaby A, eds. *Drugs of Abuse*. Oradell, NJ: Medical Economics, 1989.
4. Hirschfeld R, Davidson L. Risk Factors for Suicide. In: Frances A, Hales R, eds. *Review of Psychiatry. Vol. 7*. Washington, DC: American Psychiatric Press, 1988; 307–333.
5. Schuckit M. The clinical implications of primary diagnostic groups among alcoholics. *Arch Gen Psychiatry* 1985; 42:1043–1049.
6. Shear M, Fyer M. Biological and psychopathologic findings in panic disorder. In: Frances A, Hales R, eds. *Review of Psychiatry, Vol. 7*. Washington, DC: American Psychiatric Press, 1988.
7. Miller N, Gold M. Amphetamine and its derivatives. In: Giannini A, Slaby A. *Drugs of Abuse*. Oradell, NJ: Medical Economics, 1989.

8.  Pepper B, Kirshner M, Ryglewicz H. The young adult chronic patient: overview of a population. *Hosp Community Psychiatry* 1981; 32:463–469.
9.  Rounsaville B, Weissman M, Kleber H, Wilbur C. Heterogeneity of psychiatric diagnosis in treated opiate addicts. *Arch Gen Psychiatry* 1982; 39:151–156.
10. Freed E. Alcoholism and schizophrenia: The search for perspectives. *J Stud Alcohol* 1973; 36:853–881.
11. O'Sullivan K, Depression and its treatment in alcoholics: a review. *Can J Psychiatry* 1984; 29:379–383.
12. Quitkin F, Rifkin A, Kaplan J, Klein D. Phobic anxiety syndrome complicated by drug dependence and addiction. *Arch Gen Psychiatry* 1972; 27:159–166.
13. Mayfield D, Coleman B. Alcohol use and affective disorder. *Dis Nerv Syst* 1968; 29:467–474.
14. Gunderson J. *Borderline Personality Disorder*. Washington, DC: American Psychiatric Association, 1984.
15. Weiss R, Mirin S, Michael J, Sollogub A. Psychopathology in chronic cocaine abusers. *Am J Drug Alcohol Abuse* 1986; 12:17–29.
16. Gold M, Pottash A, Extein I et al. Clonidine in acute opiate withdrawal. *NEJ Med* 1980; 302:1421–1422.
17. Dackis C, Gold M. Bromocriptine as a treatment of cocaine abuse. *Lancet* 1985; 1:1151–1152.
18. Dackis C, Bailey J, Pottash A, Stuckey R, Extein I, Gold M. Specificity of the DST and the TRH test for major depression in alcoholics. *Am J Psychiatry* 1984; 141:680–683.
19. *Twelve Steps and Twelve Traditions*. New York: Alcoholics Anonymous World Services, 1953.
20. Kofoed L, Keys A. Using group therapy to persuade dual-diagnosis patients to seek substance abuse treatment. *Hosp Community Psychiatry* 1988; 39:1209–1211.
21. Safer D. Substance abuse by young adult chronic patients. *Hosp Community Psychiatry* 1987; 38:511–514.
22. Schneier FR, Siris SG. A review of psychoactive substance use and abuse in schizophrenia. Patterns of drug choice. *J Nerv Ment Dis* 1987; 175:641–652.
23. Negrete J, Knapp W, Douglas D, Smith W. Cannabis affects the severity of schizophrenic symptoms: Results of a clinical survey. *Psychol Med* 1986; 16: 515–520.
24. Treffert D. Marijuana use in schizophrenia: A clear hazard. *Am J Psychiatry* 1978; 135:1213–1215.
25. Carpenter M, Mulligan J, Bader L, Meinzer A. Multiple admissions to an urban psychiatric center. *Hosp Community Psychiatry* 1985; 36:1305–1308.
26. Drake R, Osher F, Wallach M. Alcohol use and abuse in schizophrenia, a prospective community study. *J Nerv Ment Dis* 1989; 177:408–414.
27. McCarrick A, Manderscheid R, Bertolucci D. Correlates of acting out behaviors among young adult chronic patients. *Hosp Community Psychiatry* 1985; 36:848–853.
28. Yesavage J, Zarcone V. History of drug abuse and dangerous behavior in inpatient schizophrenics. *J Clin Psychiatry* 1983; 44:259–261.

29. Lowinson J. Group psychotherapy with substance abusers and alcoholics. In: Kaplan H, Sadock B, eds. *Comprehensive Group Psychotherapy*. Baltimore: Williams and Wilkins, 1982.

30. O'Brien C. Group psychotherapy with schizophrenia and affective disorders. In: Kaplan H, Sadock B, eds. *Comprehensive Group Psychotherapy*. Baltimore: Williams and Wilkins, 1982.

31. Kaufman E. Family systems and family therapy of substance abuse. *Int J Addictions* 1985; 20(6,7),897,916.

32. Yudofsky S, Williams D, Gorman J. Propranolol in the treatment of rage and violent behavior in patients with chronic brain syndromes. *Am J Psychiatry* 1980; 138:218-220.

33. Ratey J. Psychopharmacologic treatment of aggressive behavior. Grand Rounds, Fair Oaks Hospital, Summit, NJ, July 12, 1989.

34. Gross D. Treatment of addiction in brain damaged patients. Grand Rounds, Fair Oaks Hospital, Summit, NJ, July 31, 1989.

35. Abrams R, Alexopoulos G. Substance abuse in the elderly: over-the-counter and illegal drugs. *Hosp Community Psychiatry* 1988; 39(8):822-829.

36. Abrams R, Alexopoulos G. Substance abuse in the elderly: alcohol and prescription drugs. *Hosp Community Psychiatry* 1987; 38(12):1285-1287.

37. Gorbien M. Alcoholism in the elderly. *Ger Med Today* 1989; 8:115-118.

38. Biegel D, Yamatani H. Help-giving in self-help groups. *Hosp Community Psychiatry* 1987; 38:1195-1197.

39. Woititz J. *Adult Children of Alcoholics*. Pompano Beach, FL: Health Communications, 1983.

40. Maxmen J. An educative model for inpatient group therapy. *Int J Group Psychother* 1978; 28:321-338.

41. Maxmen J. Helping patients survive theories: the practice of an educative model. *Int J Group Psychother* 1984; 34:355-368.

42. Yalom I. *Inpatient Group Psychotherapy*. New York: Basic Books, 1983.

43. Weiss R, Mirin S. The dual diagnosis alcoholic: evaluation and treatment. *Psychiatr Annals* 1989; 19:261-265.

44. Moreines R. MAO inhibitors: predicting response/maximizing efficiency, In: Gold M, Lydiard R, Carman J, eds. *Advances in Psychopharmacology: Predicting and Improving Treatment Response*. Boca Raton, FL: CRC Press, 1984.

45. Schuckit M. Alcoholism and other psychiatric disorders. *Hosp Community Psychiatry* 1983; 34:1022-1027.

46. DeSoto C, O'Donnell W, Alfred C, Lopes C. Symptomatology in alcoholics at various stages of abstinence. *Alcoholism* 1985; 9:505-512.

47. Winston A, Pinsker H, McCullough L. A review of supportive psychotherapy. *Hosp Community Psychiatry* 1986; 37:1105-1114.

48. Kaufman E, Reoux J. Guidelines for the successful psychotherapy of substance abusers. *Am J Drug Alcohol Abuse* 1988; 14:199-209.

# 18

## Pharmacotherapy and the Dual-Diagnosis Patient

**Larry Kirstein**

*The Regent Hospital, New York, New York*

Over the past decade, there has been an increasing recognition that a significant number of psychiatric patients have coexisting substance abuse problems. The negative prognostic connotation of the latter problems, coupled
with physician ignorance and lack of interest, represent several variables that
have led competent psychiatrists to misdiagnose and mistreat psychiatric
patients with varying degrees of substance abuse. Studies of the lifetime
prevalence of substance abuse problems in a psychiatric population report
that 30% of psychiatric patients are at risk for substance abuse problems
and that 70% of substance abuse patients are at risk for major psychiatric
problems [1–3]. Since intoxication, withdrawal, and chronic use states dramatically alter cognition, mood, and performance, it is imperative that the
clinician determine if substance abuse problems exist before considering
pharmacotherapy for a psychiatric disorder.

Opiate intoxication can present as a euphoric or lethargic state, whereas
opiate withdrawal can present as an autonomic arousal state, not dissimilar
from anxiety or panic states. Chronic opiate abuse states can present as
dysphoria or an anhedonic state. Opiate intoxication tends to last hours,
and opiate withdrawal tends to improve within 24 to 72 hours from time of
last use. Chronic high-dose methadone use has been implicated in producing
a prolonged abstinence state during and following detoxification. Symptoms of mood instability, anxiety, depression, agitation, and insomnia,

coupled with muscle ache, gastrointestinal distress, and sweating are common symptoms of this condition, which improves spontaneously over time.

Alcohol intoxification tends to produce a transient euphoria and more pronounced irritability and mood lability. Alcohol withdrawal states, which can last up to two weeks, present with increasing signs of autonomic discharge and anxiety. If withdrawal is left untreated, signs of organic psychosis and full-blown delirium tremens occur. Chronic alcohol abuse produces organic brain changes and dysphoria.

CNS-depressant intoxication can present as a sedated state, whereas CNS-depressant withdrawal can produce an agitated, anxious state. Untreated CNS-depressant withdrawal can progress to an agitated psychosis, with risk of seizures and death commencing toward the end of the first week after stopping drug use.

Stimulant drug intoxication produces a transient euphoria or agitated state. Depending on degree of intoxication, a paranoid psychotic or organic psychotic state can result. Acute intoxication tends to last hours and clears spontaneously within 24 to 48 hours. Acute stimulant withdrawal produces a dysphoric, depressive state. Suicidal tendencies have been reported during the stimulant crash. Several types of medication are available to help patients deal with the stimulant withdrawal crash, and these will be reviewed later in this chapter. Stimulant withdrawal tends to clear spontaneously within 24 to 72 hours of last use. Chronic stimulant use tends to produce a dysphoric, anhedonic state, with decreased interest in work and in social and sexual relationships [4,5]. A post-cocaine-use panic disorder has recently been identified. In these cases, panic attacks begin during cocaine abuse but continue after cessation of cocaine for months to years. The absence of premorbid panic and of family history of panic attacks characterize these patients. A kindling model has been invoked to explain the postcocaine residual panic. Tegretol (carbamazepine), rather than the classic antipanic agents, is recommended to treat this syndrome [6,7]. Dosage in the 800-mg/day range has been employed.

Phencyclidine (PCP) intoxication produces an emotional lability state of psychotic proportions. Agitation, grandiosity, synthesis, and violent behavior are not uncommon manifestations. Physical signs include increase in heart rate and blood pressure diminished pain response, nystagmus, and ataxia. No withdrawal state is noted.

Hallucinogen intoxication produces mood lability, depersonalization, derealization, and synthesis. Bad trips or panic-type reactions following hallucinogen ingestion, which occur in up to one in ten uses, are frequently associated with the experience of loss of control and are best treated conservatively with support and occasional use of minor tranquilizers. Bad trips tend to disappear within 24 hours. Although no withdrawal state exists, "flashbacks," or the recurrence of the hallucinatory state in the absence of recent drug ingestion, has been reported. A personality alteration as a result of chronic hallucinogen use has been documented and consists of a chronic psychotic condition. The incidence of this disorder is 1/500 [8,9].

Although it remains unclear whether individuals who develop prolonged psychotic symptoms following chronic hallucinogen use have underlying psychopathology that predisposes them to psychosis, there is sufficient evidence that, once present, the psychotic symptoms do not respond well to standard antipsychotic medications [10].

Cannabis intoxication tends to be associated with a calming or tranquilization effect. However, paradoxical anxiety, panic, and paranoid reactions to acute intoxication have been reported. No clear-cut withdrawal reaction has been documented although autonomic arousal beginning 48 hours after heavy use has been reported [11]. Chronic regular use of cannabis can produce a developmental arrestlike syndrome. The cardinal features of this amotivational syndrome appears to be a loss of interest in personal affairs and hygiene [12,13]. Table 1 summarizes the mental changes associated with acute intoxication and withdrawal of the most commonly abused substances [14].

The preceding descriptions clearly underscore that timing is a critical factor in evaluating the interpretation of symptoms in dual-diagnosis patients. Whenever possible, longitudinal assessment over two to three weeks, coupled with comprehensive assessment of premorbid history and family history, should precede medication trials.

The evaluation of substance use and/or abuse in a psychiatric population requires an index of suspicion on the part of the examiner. Table 2 summarizes some of the signs and symptoms that may help alert the physician to an abuse problem. Taken alone, any of these signs can be part of an underlying emotional disorder. Taken as a clustering of behaviors, these clues point in the direction of a substance abuse problem. In addition to data gathered from the patient, outside sources are extremely helpful if a substance abuse problem exists. Family members, as well as other treating physicians, can provide compelling evidence to substantiate drug abuse problems. Naturally, patient cooperation is mandatory before accessing data from any outside source.

One further intervention that can provide data about substance abuse involves urine and blood screening. These methods are routinely employed in hospital settings and are gaining wider use in monitoring substance abuse practices in outpatient settings. Repeated quantitative drug abuse testing provides critical data for both diagnosis and treatment. Chronic use of lipid-soluble substances, such as marijuana or PCP, can provide a false-positive urine test. A patient may not have used these substances for days and may

**Table 1** Drug Effects

| Drug | Acute Intoxication Intoxication | Drug Withdrawal Withdrawal |
|---|---|---|
| Alcohol | Slurred speech; incoordination; unsteady gait; nystagmus; flushed faces; irritability; mood lability; decreased attention | Nausea; vomiting; hand or facial tremors; tachycardia; elevated blood pressure; sweating; anxiety; irritability, seizure |
| Opioids | Miosis, lethargy, sedation, decreased attention span | Lacrimation; rhinorrhea; dilated pupils; piloerection; diarrhea; tachycardia; fever; mild hypertension; insomnia; agitation |
| CNS depressants (other than alcohol, including glutethimide, ethchlorvynol, meprobamate, chloral hydrate, methaqualone, barbiturates, and benzodiazepines) | Slurred speech; incoordination; unsteady gait; impaired attention and memory | Nausea; vomiting; coarse tremors of the hand or face; tachycardia; elevated blood pressure; weakness; anxiety; irritability |
| CNS stimulants including cocaine, amphetamine, and, other sympathomimetic amines | Tachycardia; pupillary dilation; elevated blood pressure and pulse rate; psychomotor agitation; nausea; vomiting; elation; hypervigilance | Irritable or depressed mood; fatigue; disturbed sleep with increased dreaming |
| PCP or Similar Agent | Vertical or horizontal nystagmus; increased blood pressure and heart rate; diminished responsivity to pain; dysarthric; ataxic, psychomotor agitation; emotional lability; grandiosity; synthesis | |
| Cannabis | Tachycardia; injected conjuctivae; dry oral mucosae; euphoria or apathy; sensation of slowed time and increased perception; increased appetite; recent memory failures. A motivational syndrome | Controversial; case reports of anxiety, irritability, sweating, chills, insomnia, anorexia and tremclousness occurring, 48 hours of cessation following regular use of high-potency THC preparations. |

**Table 2** Warning Signs of Substance Abuse

| | |
|---|---|
| Increased isolation from family and friends | Dramatic weight loss or gain |
| Increased irresponsible actions | Decreased physical coordination/increased physical injuries and complaints |
| Increase in lying or blaming others for irresponsible actions | Burns on hand and clothing |
| Suspicion of theft from family members or work place | Mental or physical disorientation |
| Sells possessions for money | Decreased attention to personal hygiene |
| Increased secretiveness about personal problems or activities | Increased anxiety and nervousness (can't sit still) |
| Elusive about friends or whereabouts | Incidents of accidents or reckless driving |
| Violence — verbal or physical abuse | Trouble with the law |
| Erratic eating or sleeping habits | |
| Sudden drop in performance at work | In adolescence: |
| Absenteeism or lateness on the job | |
| Inattentive at work | Sudden drop in grades/academic failure |
| Increased boredom or lethargy/decreased discipline or motivation | Truancy — skipping classes or entire days |
| | Inattentive in class/sleeping in class |
| Increased disregard of rules and the consequences in breaking them | Drops out of sports or other extracurricular activities |
| Lack of response to previously desired rewards | Change in friends or peer group, especially to an older crowd (elusive about new friends) |
| Frequent visits to bathrom | Incidence of fighting with peers |
| Changes in personality/severe mood swings | Increased disrespect toward parents, teachers and authority |

still show trace amounts in the urine. Thus, sequential testing to determine if levels of substance are decreasing or not may be much more meaningful than just one random test.

Table 3 summarizes the laboratory findings in cases of suspected substance abuse problems [15].

It should be noted that EEG testing, as well as drug surveillance, provides valuable data in both CNS-depressant and CNS-stimulant withdrawal cases.

In view of the fact that the most frequently employed specific test to confirm active drug use is urine testing, the currently available methods should be briefly reviewed. Three different types of drug surveillance testing are currently available.

Thin-layer chromatology is a qualitative measure to separate out or screen out a series of drugs. This method requires relatively higher quantities (toxic doses) to be positive. Sensitivity is frequently in low micrograms (one-millionth of a gram). Drugs that can be tested for include opiates, ampheta-

**Table 3**  Test to Confirm Suspected Drug Use by Class of Drugs for States of Drug Withdrawal and Drug Intoxication

Suspected problems

| | | |
|---|---|---|
| Opioids | Intoxification | Blood or urine levels of opioids |
| | Withdrawal | Urine test for opioids or quinine, which may be present for 24–84 hr after the last dose |
| Depressant | Intoxication | Blood or urine levels of depressant; EEG nonspecific depressant effect |
| | Withdrawal | EEG showing bursts of spiked high-amplitude slow waves in nonepileptics |
| Stimulants | Intoxication | Blood or urine levels of amphetamine or cocaine |
| | Withdrawal | Abnormal sleep EEGs; urine screen for amphetamine or cocaine metabolites |
| Hallucinogens | Intoxication | None widely available; some laboratories can assay urine and blood levels |
| | Withdrawal | |
| Phencyclidine | Intoxication | Blood or urine levels of phencyclidine; either EIA or GC apparatus with a nitrogen detector or GC-MS is required for detection in the low nanogram range; otherwise, a false negative may confuse the diagnosis |
| | Withdrawal | The test may be positive up to 7 days after the last dose |
| Cannabis | Intoxication | Blood or urine level of |
| | Withdrawal | This test may be positive for several weeks after last dose |

mines, and barbiturates. Marijuana, PCP, and LSD are not identified at all in most TLC systems although a highly sensitive TLC marijuana assay (20 ng/ml) is now available. Positive results should be confirmed by a more sensitive methodology, such as immunoassay or gas chromatography. It is important to realize that negative results do not mean that levels below the cutoff level are not present in the sample.

Gas chromatography mass spectrometry is the most reliable, most sensitive, and most expensive assay method. It is sufficiently sensitive to produce forensic quality "fingerprinting" of molecules. The sensitivity ranges from monograms to picograms and is thus 100 to 1000 times more sensitive than

TLC. (A nanogram is one-billionth of a gram; one picogram is one-tril-lionth of a gram.)

Radioimmunoassay and enzyme immunoassay techniques show a sensi-tivity between micrograms and picograms. The methodology is easily auto-mated and not very expensive to operate. The basic principle relies on anti-gen antibody florescence.

Figure 1 depicts the heterogeneity of the dual-diagnosis population. Sev-eral studies of substance abuse patients have found that 50% of patients have no psychiatric Axis I diagnosis. This subset of patients frequently have polydrug abuse problems and are frequently diagnosed as antisocial person-ality disorders on Axis II [16,17]. Other studies have looked at the lifetime incidence of psychiatric disorders in a substance abuse population [18]. Rates as high as 80% have been noted [19]. One of the popular relationships between drug and psychiatric problems is the self-medication hypothesis. According to this concept, patients will select certain drugs to "treat" under-lying symptoms and disorders.

It has been previously discussed that drugs cause psychiatric symptoms. A number of researchers have demonstrated a relationship between drug abuse and underlying psychiatric disorders, "selective comorbidity."

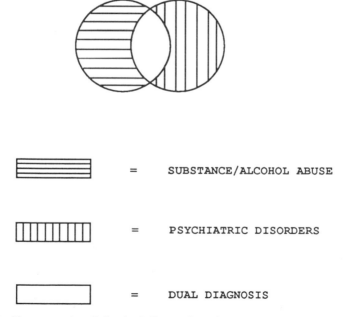

**Figure 1** Heterogeneity of the dual-diagnosis patient.

Four separate studies have shown that cocaine abusers have a fairly high rate of depressive disorders (30–35% for major depression, atypical depression, and dysthymic disorder) and 20–25% for bipolar [4,17,20,21]. In addition, a smaller subset (5–10%) has been noted to have a residual attention deficit disorder (ADD) [4,10,21]. Other literature reviews documented that opiate addicts and sedative/hypnotic abusers have high rates of anxiety disorders as well as affective disorders [18,20,22]. A summary of the data on 160 inpatient substance abusers at McClean Hospital revealed the following: " . . . among opiate or CNS-depressant abusers 51.4% received a nondepression DSM-III Axis I diagnosis, exclusive of substance abuse or alcoholism. Of these, the majority were found to be suffering from either generalized anxiety or panic disorders." [23]

Although alcoholism and depression have been studied for years, the relationship between the two needs careful investigation. It has been proposed by some researchers that most depression in alcoholism is secondary depression, depression beginning after the onset of alcoholism, and that less than 10% of alcoholics have primary depression [24]. Others [25,26] have identified that both phobics and panic attacks precede the self-medication with alcohol in a subset of alcoholics. Thus, the prevalence and incidence of non–substance abuse psychiatric disorders in substance abuse patients warrants careful diagnostic and pharmacotherapeutic investigation.

The first step in pharmacotherapy of dual-diagnosis patients is medical stabilization. Even in a crisis situation, such as an emergency room setting, it is prudent to wait several hours, if possible, to gather lab data and wait for intoxicating drug effects to clear. Addicted dual-diagnosis patients generally require inpatient settings for medical detoxification. This controlled setting is ideal for comprehensive medical stabilization. Medical stabilization includes establishing a protective, drug-free environment, where normal sleep-wake cycles and adequate nutritional needs can be promoted. Also, attention to medical illnesses, medication schedules, and evaluation of medical sequelae of drug abuse can be readily implemented.

Detoxification for addicted patients is the first pharmacologic step in dual-diagnosis medication treatment. For opiate addicts, several options are available. Patients can be stabilized on methadone and then treated for the psychiatric problem. The advantages of methadone maintenance include avoiding hospitalization and defining a treatment course for the drug problem. The liability is that abstinence from abuse of other drugs is not always achieved [27]. Opiate detoxification can be done on either an inpatient or outpatient basis, with the decision being made by a physician on a case-by-case basis.

Patient motivation, as well as medical status, needs to be carefully evaluated to rule out cases with cardiac or blood pressure problems before clonidine detoxification is considered [28].

CNS-depressant addiction, including alcohol addiction, can be treated on either an inpatient or outpatient basis, again, the decision being made on a case-by-case basis. In addition to motivation and severity of psychopathology, medical status and environmental support require careful assessment before deciding on inpatient or outpatient detoxification. Detoxification with benzodiazepines has stood the test of time. Once a patient is stable on a 24-hour total dose of benzodiazepines as reflected by vital signs, detoxification can be safely implemented by reducing the total dose of benzodiazepines 10% a day. Recent reports of the use of Tegretol (carbamazepine) as an effective alternative to benzodiazepines for alcohol detoxification have appeared in the psychiatric literature [29–31].

Sedative/hypnotic detoxification requires inpatient treatment. The risk of seizures in undermedicated cases, as well as the varying half-lives of different sedative/hypnotic preparations, makes initial stabilization more complicated than with CNS-depressant drugs. Once stabilization has occurred, detoxification can be safely implemented by reducing the total dose of benzodiazepines 10% a day.

Stimulants as a class, and cocaine in particular, produce a dysphoric withdrawal state. Several different agents have been tried to treat cocaine cravings. Amino acid supplementation to increase catecholamine precursors has not achieved popular support [32]. Use of antidepressants of the imipramine grouping has been studied by several different research groups. The findings are fairly consistent. In both controlled and open studies of small patient groups, these antidepressants help prevent relapse by decreasing cravings for cocaine [33,35]. It is noteworthy that the jitteriness that can occur with the administration of desipramine has been associated with relapse into cocaine abuse. In these cases, it appears that the autonomic stimulation produced by the medication is similar to the autonomic arousal produced by prior cocaine use [36]. A different strategy employed in treating cocaine cravings has been the use of the dopamine agonist bromocriptine. The rationale for this type of drug relates to the role of dopamine depletion in cocaine cravings [37].

One final area of pharmacotherapy of substance abuse problems in dual-diagnosis patients needs comment. This area involves the use of blocking agents. Antabuse interferes with alcohol metabolism in the liver, resulting in the accumulation of acetaldehyde, which causes the alcohol-Antabuse reaction. Naltrexone binds to the postsynaptic opiate receptor and prevents opiate euphoria and analgesia [38]. Blocking agents are not appropriate for all alcoholics and opiate addicts. Both these agents can cause or aggravate liver problems. Medical limitations, motivation, and compliance with ongoing treatment are all factors that need to be assessed in deciding which patients are appropriate candidates for one or both blocking agents. Block-

ing agents should be prescribed as adjuncts in the treatment of appropriate
addicts.


## DEPRESSION

Although the different pharmacologic strategies for the treatment of affective disorders is fairly straightforward, the dual-diagnostic patient presents a
potential problem. Frequently, a clinician considers utilizing some form of
tranquilization or sedation during the early phase of treatment of agitated
nondelusional depression. The simplest and least complicated approach
avoids the use of any form of addictive drug. Emotional support and nonaddictive sleeping aids, such as tryptophan, antihistamines, or low-dose sedating neuroleptics, can be employed. Agitation and/or anxiety can be treated
with low-dose neuroleptics or antihistamines, such as hydroxyzine and beta-
blocking agents. Both antimonic drugs carbamazepine and lithium carbonate can produce a calming effect in some patients. However, side effects and/
or lack of symptom reduction occurs frequently. For these patients, the
clinician may choose a time-limited course of minor tranquilizers until an
adequate dose of antidepressant agent begins to produce its desired effect.
The symptom relief must be weighed against the potential struggle of having
a patient give up an addictive medication that reduces symptoms. Another
potential problem centers around the use of fluoxetine (Prozac), with which
many patients experience nervousness that is clearly a drug side effect.
Continued treatment for these patients may necessitate some form of tranquilization.


## ANXIETY

Treatment of anxiety disorders presents another challenge for the clinician.
From the discussion of drug withdrawal states presented in Table 1, anxiety
can be triggered by withdrawal from CNS depressants, alcohol, and opiates.
In the case of patients with generalized anxiety disorder (GAD), buspirone
(Buspar) represents a potential successful pharmacologic treatment. Other
agents employed to reduce sympathetic arousal and anxiety include both
alpha- and beta-blockers (propanolol, clonidine) as well as low-dose neuroleptics and antihistamines such as hydroxyzine. The most commonly employed drugs, the benzodiazepines, have no role in the dually diagnosed
patient with GAD. Unlike depression, in which major symptom reduction
will be achieved through use of antidepressants, in GAD the benzodiazepine
is the principal pharmacologic agent. Since tolerance, dependence, and
abuse may occur, it is difficult to rationalize long-term use of benzodiazepine treatment of GAD in a substance abuse problem population. Similarly,

it is not appropriate to consider short-term use of these agents since GAD is a chronic problem.

In addition to the prescription of nonaddictive medications for this population, the physician should consider employing a number of nonpharmacologic interventions that may form the nucleus of treatment for GAD. Among these interventions are relaxation techniques, hypnotherapy, behavioral therapy, acupuncture, exercise programs, and imagery techniques.

## PANIC DISORDERS

Panic attacks are a discrete entity within the anxiety disorder classification. As mentioned earlier in this chapter, panic induced by cocaine kindling may represent a subset of panic disorder patients who respond to carbamazepine. The large majority of panic disorder patients respond to either traditional tricyclic antidepressants, such as imipramine and MAO inhibitor drugs, [39,40] or alprazolam (Xanax) [41]. Of the three different classes of drugs, alprazolam seems to be most effective. Since Xanax is a minor tranquilizer, tolerance, dependence, abuse, and addiction are all potential problems to be anticipated. In addition, withdrawal from Xanax has to be carefully titrated to prevent seizures. Thus, patients who abuse Xanax in the treatment of panic may require inpatient detoxification. Therefore, the most prudent course for treating panic attacks is to begin with a course of either imipramines or MAOI-type antidepressants. Since both of these types of medication take one to two weeks to develop a therapeutic dose, short-term use of low-dose alprazolam may be justified. The argument for use would be similar to that for employment of a sedative/hypnotic or tranquilizer in the beginning phase of treatment of agitated depressive disorders.

The responsibility of the clinician who embarks on such a treatment alternative is to make sure that the following objectives are maintained:

1. Length of time of prescription of potentially addictive drug is realistically set and adhered to.
2. Upper limit of dosage/day is established.
3. Some form of monitoring system is strictly adhered to, such as blood level monitoring and giving only weekly prescriptions.

Finally, if the three objectives cannot be maintained, it is suggested that the clinician consult with a colleague before extending a course of addictive medications. After consultation, if symptom severity and impairment in functioning support continue, use of drugs such as Xanax and a new set of objectives should be established that reflect dose, time frame, and monitoring.

The rule of behavioral techniques to counteract and reduce the agoraphobia that accompanies panic attacks, as well as support groups to reduce isolation, is critical in the treatment of panic disorders. In this regard, the dual-diagnosis patient may be able to derive support from the peer-oriented 12-step meetings that should be a fundamental element of any substance abuse recovery program.

## Obsessive Compulsive Disorder

Patients with COD may have addictive problems with sedative/hypnotic and CNS-depressant drugs. Fortunately, there are many reports that serotonergic agents such as fluoxamine, fluoxetine (Prozac), and clomipramine (Anafranil) may be extremely beneficial in relieving the suffering of the patients' irrational, ritualistic thinking and actions [42–45]. Prozac is currently available with newer similar agents soon to be released. Clonipramine, at the time of publication of the chapter, is available from Ciba Geigy for humanitarian use and has been utilized by psychopharmacologists in the United States for several years now.

## Post-Traumative Stress Disorders

The treatment of patients who have experienced a traumatic, overwhelming stress must be divided into the recent poststress phase (days to weeks) and treatment, once a clear-cut PTSD syndrome develops. Abbreviated use of calming agents and sedating medicines in sufficient doses to provide symptom relief but not stupefation is reasonable during the first month following the traumatic event. However, as noted above in regard to the use of minor tranquilizers and/or hypnotics for GAD, parameters around length of prescription and total dosage need to be carefully monitored. If symptoms of fear, helplessness, and terror persist in terms of (1) reexperiencing the event, (2) avoidance of stimuli associated with the event or numbing of general responsiveness, and (3) symptoms of increased psychologic arousal, a diagnosis of PTSD should be entertained. If a PTSD develops, the pharmacologic picture must reflect the awareness that psychoactive drug abuse is a common complication. The physician must not complicate the situation by maintaining symptomatic treatment with sedative hypnotics and/or minor tranquilizers.

A number of studies have demonstrated a significant role for antidepressants, both tricyclics and MAO-inhibitor drugs, to treat sleep problems, startle reactions, and mood disturbances associated with PTSD [46–49]. These different groups have all demonstrated symptom relief without relying on addictive drugs.

As Figure 1 illustrates, dual-diagnosis patients may initially be more readily perceived as drug abusers. This is certainly the case for Vietnam veterans who may have polydrug abuse problems, including opiates and CNS-depressant abuse. It is the responsibility of the clinician to be alert to the possible PTSD diagnosis and not to misinterpret current symptoms as being exclusively withdrawal phenomena or conscious attempts at manipulation for medication. The role of history and confirming data from family is particularly helpful in substantiating an underlying PTSD.

Given the role that MAO inhibitors and tricyclic antidepressants may play in reducing some of the PTSD symptoms in conjunction with support and behavioral treatments for anxiety, it is imperative that this disorder be accurately diagnosed and aggressively treated [50].

## Eating Disorders

It has been noted that a significant number of eating-disorder patients have substance abuse problems [51]. It is fairly common for patients with anorexia nervosa to abuse laxatives, diuretics, and stimulants. Patients with bulimia have similar concerns about weight loss. In a comprehensive study of 126 bulimic patients, almost one-fifth of the patients met criteria for either alcohol or substance abuse diagnosis [52]. Another 14% had received previous chemical-dependency treatment. Of abusing patients in the bulimic population, 17% abused alcohol, 51% abused stimulants, and 9% abused sedatives. Since bulimia is present in 5–10% of young adult women, this population represents a large subset of dual-diagnosis patients.

Several books have chapters that review the use of pharmacologic treatments in the eating-disorder population [53]. There is fairly clear evidence that antidepressant drugs, both MAO-inhibitor drugs and tricyclic antidepressants, are useful in curbing bingeing in bulimic patients. Newer agents, such as the opiate antagonist Naltrexone and the anticonvulsant drugs such as Tegretol, have been less effective in consistently stabilizing weight or loss of weight. Anticonvulsant drugs have been shown to play a role in eating disorders where EEG abnormalities have been documented.

In patients with anorexia nervosa, a subset with a history of low birth weight gained weight when treated with cyproheptadine [53]. Antidepressant drugs are effective in treating the depressive disorder that frequently develops in anorexia nervosa and some bulimia patients. As will be mentioned again, these agents have no effect on the fundamental problems of body-image distortion or food dyscontrol.

Weight stabilization in anorexia patients should precede vigorous effects at pharmacologic control of symptoms since it has been shown that many of the secondary symptoms of anorexia are due to starvation. With weight stabilization and restoration of weight to a normal range, symptoms of confusion, lethargy, depression, and insomnia improve. Medications, including the neuroleptic agents and tricyclic antidepressants that have been used along with behavioral approaches to stimulate appetite and weight gain, are not specific and do not treat the underlying abnormalities in perception. Detoxification from cathartics is common in severe cases of abuse and frequently requires aggressive involvement by a gastroenterologist to prevent surgical intervention for paralytic ileus.

## Attention Deficit Disorder

A 5–10% prevalence of attention deficit disorders has been reported in a number of different studies of dual-diagnosis patients [20,23]. A self-medication hypothesis would support a comorbidity with stimulant abuse [22]. The cardinal symptoms of adult ADD—hyperactivity, distractibility, impaired concentration, and short attention span—can be very difficult to distinguish from opiate or sedative withdrawal symptoms. However, the history of ADD symptoms that clearly precede the onset of substance abuse should alert the clinician to assess for a possible ADD diagnosis.

Pharmacologic intervention using a variety of nonaddictive agents has been effective for a number of patients. Trials of stimulant molecules [54] and antidepressants [20] have been reported to be quite helpful. Other groups report that magnesium pemoline is also effective in treating ADD [55]. Other agents that treat hyperactive symptoms, such as lithium carbonate, carbamazepine, and neuroleptic medication, are less effective and less well tolerated by the patients.

## Schizophrenia

Treatment of schizophrenia represents a challenge for the clinician. Treatment of psychosis in a schizophrenic with substance abuse problems represents a further complication. Schizophrenics who abuse drugs or who use illicit drugs do not conform to any pattern or grouping. The drug abuse pattern tends to be idiosyncratic and bizarre. While it is possible to invoke self-medication explanations for use of nonprescribed drugs that alter mood and cognitive, careful history, psychological assessment, and laboratory confirmation with drug abuse screening are essential to give the clinician a clear idea of the drugs at play in creating a particular mental status. The pharmacologic intervention needs to be clarified as to interventions during the first 24–72 hours, the first weeks of treatment (stabilization), and thereafter (maintenance of the acute episode). Treatment of exacerbation of psychosis or chronic psychosis in schizophrenia is another area worthy of comment but beyond the scope of this chapter, since there is no role for addictive medications in the long-term treatment of schizophrenia.

During the first 24 hours of treatment, goals include stabilization of agitation through the commencement of some form of tranquilization. Because of the dangers of toxic anticholinergic effects and central autonomic dysregulation, slow, continued buildup of neuroleptics represents a rational approach in the dually diagnosed schizophrenic patient. Employment of minor tranquilizers as an adjunct during this phase, either by mouth or injection, has gained acceptance. This approach comes from an awareness that rapid tranquilization with large doses of neuroleptic drugs creates the circumstances for the development of the neuroleptic malignant syndrome (NMS). This syndrome, which is characterized by the development of fever and muscle stiffness, can be fatal within days if not diagnosed and treated [56–58]. Thus, the risk of anticholinergic toxicity and NMS justify the gradual buildup of neuroleptics, coupled with the use of minor tranquilizers and hypnotics, in the early phase of treatment in these drug-abusing schizophrenics. Over the course of days, antipsychotic drugs should be increased, with reduction in sleep medication and minor tranquilizers. The fundamental decrease in positive symptoms of schizophrenics is a result of judicious use of neuroleptic medications, which begins to occur during the end of the first week of treatment and continues over the next four to six weeks.

It is difficult to justify continued use of minor tranquilizers during the maintenance phase of treatment of schizophrenia in a dual-diagnosed population. There are serious questions around compliance and abuse of these agents. More importantly, the rationale for continued use of these agents is unclear. The argument that tardive dyskinesia (T.D.) risk may be reduced if minor tranquilizers are employed has not yet been adequately documented. The critical element to reduce the risk of T.D. centers around less neuroleptic being employed during maintenance. It would appear that guidelines to reduce the risk of T.D. through the use of minimal effective doses of neuroleptic medication, drug holidays, informed consent, and careful screening for abnormal involuntary movements is more to the point than long-term use of sedatives or minor tranquilizers. However, several authors have noted that the addition of minor tranquilizers to maintenance neuroleptics has resulted both in an improvement in negative symptoms and a reduction in positive symptoms in a small group of cases [59–61]. Thus, more data are necessary to clarify the potential role of minor tranquilizers in maintenance-phase schizophrenia.

## REFERENCES

1. Crowley T, Chesluk D, Dilts S. et al. Drug and alcohol abuse among psychiatric admissions. *Arch Gen Psychiatry* 1974; 30:13–20.
2. Regier D, Boyd J, Burke J. et al. One month prevalence of mental disorders in the United States. *Arch Gen Psychiatry* 1988; 45:977–986.
3. McLellan AT, Druley K, Carson J. Evaluation of substance abuse problems in a psychiatric hospital. *J Clin Psychiatry* 1978; 39:425–430.

4.  Weiss RD, Mirin SM, Michael JL, Sollogub AC. Psychopathology in chronic cocaine abusers. *Am J Drug Alc Abuse* 1986; 12:17–29.
5.  Washton D, Gold M. Chronic cocaine abuse evidence for adverse effects on health and functioning. *Psychiatr Annals* 1989; 14:733–739.
6.  Louie D, Lannon R, Keller T. Treatment of cocaine induced panic disorder. *Am J Psychiatry* 1989; 146:40–44.
7.  Aronson TA, Craig TJ. Cocaine precipitation of panic disorder. *Am J Psychiatry* 1986; 143:643–645.
8.  Rosenthal SH. Persistent hallucinosis following repeated administrations of hallucinogenic drugs. *Am J Psychiatry* 1964; 121:238–244.
9.  Glass GS, Bowers MB. Jr. Chronic psychosis associated with long term psychotomimetic drug abuse. *Arch Gen Psychiatry* 1970; 23:97–103.
10. Tucker GJ, Quinlan D, Harrow M. Chronic hallucinogenic drug use and thought disturbances. *Arch Gen Psychiatry* 1972; 27:443–447.
11. Knight F. Role of cannabis in psychiatric disturbance. *Ann NY Acad Sci* 1976; 282:64–71.
12. Estroff T, Gold M. Psychiatric Presentations of Marijuana Abuse. *Psychiatr Annals* 1986; 16:221–225.
13. Smith DE. Acute and chronic toxicity of marijuana. *J Psychoact Drugs* 1968; 2:37–47.
14. Dimilio L, Gold M, Martin O. *Evaluation of the Substance Abuse in Diagnostic and Laboratory Testing in Psychiatry*. New York: Plenum, 1986; 235–247.
15. Verebey K, Martin D, Gold M. Diagnostic and laboratory testing in psychiatry. In: Gold M, Pottash ALC, eds. *Drug Abuse: Interpretation of Lab Tests*. New York: Plenum, 1986: 155–167.
16. Schnoll SH, Karrigan J, Kitchen SB, Daghestani A, Hansen T. Characteristics of cocaine abusers presenting for treatment. *NIDA Research Monographs* 1985; 61:171–181.
17. Nunes E, Quitkin F, Klein O. Psychiatric Diagnosis in cocaine abusers. *Psychiatr Res* 1989; 28:105–114.
18. Rounsaville BJ, Weissman MM, Kleber HD, Wilbur CH. Heterogeneity of psychiatric diagnosis in treated opiate addicts. *Arch Gen Psychiatry* 1982; 39: 161–166.
19. Ross R, Ball W, Sullivan K, Caroff S. Sleep disturbances as the hallmark of posttraumatic stress disorder. *Am J Psychiatry* 1989; 146:697–706.
20. Sternberg D. Dual diagnosis: Addiction and affective disorders. *Psychiatr Hosp* 1989; 20:71–77.
21. Gawin F, Kleber H. Abstinence symptomatology and psychiatric diagnosis in cocaine abusers: Clinical observations. *Arch Gen Psychiatry* 1986; 43:107–113.
22. Khantzian EJ. The self-medication hypothesis of addictive disorders: Focus on heroin and cocaine dependence. *Am J Psychiatry* 1985; 42:1259–1264.
23. Mirins, Weiss R. Psychopathology in substance abusers: Diagnosis and treatment. *Am J Drug Alc Abuse* 1988; 14(2):139–157.
24. Schukit M. Alcoholic patients with secondary depression. *Am J Psychiatry* 1983; 140:711–714.

25. Kushner M, Sherk, Bertman B. The relationship between alcoholic problems and the anxiety disorders. *Am J Psychiatry* 1990; 147:685-691.
26. Stravynski A, LaMontagne Y, Lavellee YJ. Clinical phobias and avoidant personality disorder among alcoholics admitted to an alcoholism rehabilitation setting. *Can J Psychiatry* 1986; 31:714-719.
27. Dupont R, Saylon K. Marijuana and benzobiazepines in patients receiving methadone treatment. *JAMA* 1989; 261:23 3409.
28. Gold MS, Pottash ALC, Sweeney DR, Kleber HD. Opiate withdrawal using clonidine. Safe, effective, and rapid nonopiate treatment. *JAMA* 1980; 243(4): 343-346.
29. Malcolm R, Ballenger J, Sturgis E, Anton R. Double blind controlled trial of carbamazepine to oraxepam treatment of alcohol withdrawal. *Am J Psychiatry* 1989; 146:617-621.
30. Ritola E, Malinen L. A double-blind comparison of carbamazepine and clomethiazole in the treatment of alcohol withdrawal syndrome. *Acta Psychiatr Scand* 1981; 64:254-259.
31. Poutanen P. Experience with carbamazepine in the treatment of withdrawal symptoms in alcohol abusers. *Br J Addict* 1979; 74:201-204.
32. Gold MS et al. Cocaine Withdrawal: Efficacy of Tyrosine. Presented at the 13th Annual Meeting of the Society for Neuroscience, Boston, Nov 6-11, 1983.
33. Tennant FS, Rawson RA. Cocaine and amphetamine dependence treated with desipramine. *NIDA Research Monographs* 1982; 43:351-355.
34. Rosecan JS. The treatment of cocaine abuse with imipramine, L-tyrosine, and L-tryptophan. Presented at the VII World Congress of Psychiatry, Vienna, July 14-19, 1983.
35. Gawin F, Kleber H, Byck R et al. Desipramine facilitation of initial cocaine abstinence. *Arch Gen Psychiatry* 1989; 46:117-121.
36. Weiss R. Relapse to cocaine abuse after initiating desipramine treatments. *JAMA* 1988; 17(11):2545-2546.
37. Dackis CA, Gold MS. New concepts in cocaine addiction: The dopamine depletion hypothesis. *Neurosci Biobehav Rev* 1985; 9:469-477.
38. Hayman M. Antabuse in the treatment of the alcoholic. *Quart J Stud Alc* 1965; 26:460-467.
39. Gold MS, Pottash ALC, Sweeney DR, Kleber HD. Opiate withdrawal using clonidine. Safe, effective, and rapid nonopiate treatment. *JAMA* 1980; 243(4): 343-346.
40. Ballenger JC, Peterson GA, Laraia M, Hucek A, Lake CR, Jimerson D, Cox D, Trockman C. A study of plasma catecholamines in agoraphobia and the relationship of serum tricyclic levels to treatment response. In: Ballenger JC, ed. *Biology of Agoraphobia*. Washington, DC: American Psychiatric Association Press, 1984: 27-63.
41. Ballenger J, Burrow G, Dupont R et al. Alprazolam in panic disorders and agoraphobia: Results from a multicenter trial. *Arch Gen Psychiatry* 1988; 45: 413-422.
42. Zohar J, Insel TR, Sohar-Kadouch RC et al. Serotonergic responsivity in obsessive-compulsive disorder: effects of chronic clomipramine treatment. *Arch Gen Psychiatry* 1988; 45:167-172.

43. Thoren P, Asberg M, Cronholm B et al. Clomipramine treatment of obsessive-compulsive disorder, I: a controlled clinical trial. *Arch Gen Psychiatry* 1980; 37:1281–1285.

44. Price LH, Goodman WK, Charney DS et al. Treatment of severe obsessive-compulsive disorder with fluvoxamine. *Am J Psychiatry* 1987; 144:1059–1061.

45. Fontaine R, Chouinard G. An open clinical trial of fluoxetine in the treatment of obsessive-compulsive disorder. *J Clin Psychopharmacol* 1986; 6:98–100.

46. Ross R, Ball W, Sullivan K, Caroff S. Sleep disturbances as the hallmark of posttraumatic stress disorder. *Am J Psychiatry* 1989; 146:697–706.

47. Bleich A, Siegel B, Garb R et al. Post-traumatic stress disorder following combat exposure: clinical features and psychopharmacological treatment. *Br J Psychiatry* 1986; 149:365–369.

48. Hogben GL, Cornfield RB. Treatment of traumatic war neurosis with phenelzine. *Arch Gen Psychiatry* 1981; 38:440–445.

49. van der Kolk BA. Psychopharmacological issues in posttraumatic stress disorder. *Hosp Community Psychiatry* 1983; 34:683–691.

50. Friedman MJ. Toward rational pharmacotherapy for posttraumatic stress disorder: an interim report. *Am J Psychiatry* 1988; 145:281–285.

51. Jonas JM, Gold MS, Sweeney D, Pottash ALC. Eating disorders and cocaine abuse: A survey of 259 cocaine abusers. *J Clin Psychiatry* 1987; 48:47–50.

52. Hatuskami D, Owen P, Pyle R, Mitchell J. Similarities and differences on the MMPI between women with bulimia and women with alcohol and drug abuse problems. *Addict Behav* 1982; 7:435–439.

53. Johnson C, Stuckey M, Mitchell J. Psychopharmacology of anorexia nervosa and bulimia. In: Mitchell J, ed. *Anorexia and Bulimia Diagnosis and Treatment*. Minneapolis: University of Minnesota Press, 1983: 134–152.

54. Khantzian EJ. An extreme case of cocaine dependence and marked improvement with methylphenidate treatment. *Am J Psychiatry* 1983; 140:784–785.

55. Weiss RD, Mirin SM, Michael JL, Sollogub AC. Psychopathology in chronic cocaine abusers. *Am J Drug Alc Abuse* 1986; 12:17–29.

56. Levenson JL. Neuroleptic malignant syndrome. *Am J Psychiatry* 1985; 142:1137–1145.

57. Pearlman CA. Neuroleptic malignant syndrome: a review of the literature. *J Clin Psychopharmacol* 1986; 6:257–272.

58. Addonizio G, Susman VL, Roth SD. Neuroleptic malignant syndrome: review and analysis of 115 cases. *Biol Psychiatry* 1987; 22:1004–1020.

59. Wolkowitz OM, Breier A, Doran A et al. Alprazolam augmentation of the antipsychotic effects of fluphenazine in schizophrenic patients. *Arch Gen Psychiatry* 1988; 45:664–671.

60. Csernansky JG, Piney SJ, Lombrozo L et al. Double blind comparison of alprazolam, diazepam and placebo for the treatment of negative schizophrenic symptoms. *Arch Gen Psychiatry* 1988; 45:665–659.

61. Wolkowitz OM, Pickar D, Doran AR et al. Combination alprazolam-neuroleptic treatment of the positive and negative symptoms of schizophrenia. *Am J Psychiatry* 1986; 143:85–87.

# Index

ACCEPT, 3
Adolescent chemical dependency
   syndrome, 255–256
Adolescent drug abuse, 253–288
   assessment, 262–265
   constitutional determinants, 257
   dual diagnosis, 261–262
   extent of problem, 254–255
   family assessment, 270
   family factors in use, 258–261
   family treatment, 278–282
   inpatient treatment, 272–275
   model for understanding, 256–261
   outpatient treatment, 282–283
   psychiatric examination, 269–
     270
   psychological determinants,
     257–258
   psychosocial assessment, 270
   sociocultural determinants, 255–
     259
   therapeutic progression, 277–278

[Adolescent drug abuse]
   twelve steps, 275–280
   treatment, 271–284
Adoption studies
   alcoholism, 37–40
   antisocial personality, 37–40
Affective disorders
   alcoholism, 7–12, 151
   cannabis, 111, 130–131
   drug use, 65–70
   dual diagnosis, 173, 192–195,
     210–213
   opiates, 111
   sedative hypnotics, 110–111
   solvents, 111
   stimulants, 109–110
   substance abuse, 105–116
Alcohol
   abuse, 7–14
   adoption studies, 37–40
   affective disorders, 151
   agoraphobia, 47–49

[Alcohol]
   anorexia nervosa, 117–118
   anxiety, 15
   bulimia nervosa, 118–119
   community surveys, 149–150
   depression, 107–109
   dual diagnosis, 223–226, 228–233
   genetic studies, 31–36
   mania, 109
   panic disorder, 47–49
   seizures, 97–100
Anorexia
   disorder and alcoholism, 152
   nervosa, 117–126
      alcoholism, 117–118
      genetic studies, 121–122
Anticholinergics, 61–62
Antisocial personality
   adoption studies, 37–40
   personality, 36–37
   personality disorder and dual diagnosis, 180–182
Anxiety disorders, 45–56
   dual diagnosis, 173–178, 213–215
   pharmacotherapy with dual diagnosis patient, 328–329
Attention deficit disorder
   benzodiazepine
   cocaine use, 95–96
   controversy, 52–53
   dual diagnosis, 178–179
   psychopharmacotherapy with dual diagnosis patient, 329
   use and dual diagnosis, 20–21

Borderline personality and dual diagnosis, 182–183
Bulimia nervosa, 117–126
   alcoholism, 118–119

Cannabis
   acute abuse, 129
   adulterants, 134–135
   affective disorders, 111, 130–131
   chemistry, 129
   chronic abuse, 129–130
   epidemiology of use, 135–136
   detoxification, 132
   dual diagnosis, 127–138
   history of use, 128
   mode of usage, 129
   physiology, 132
   source, 128
   treatment, 133–134
   withdrawal, 131–132
Cerebrovascular disorders and cocaine, 78–83
Cocaine
   cerebrovascular disorders, 78–83
   dual diagnosis, 17–19
   headache, 83–85
   neurological disorders, 76–85
   panic disorder, 49
   seizures, 76–78
   use and attention deficit disorder, 95–96
Cognitive impairment and substance abuse, 96–97
Conduct disorder and dual diagnosis, 179–180

Depression
   alcoholism, 107–109
   dual diagnosis, 169–173
   genetic studies, 31–36
   pharmacotherapy with dual diagnosis patient, 325
Dissociatives, 59–61
Dual diagnosed thought disorders, 57–73
Dual diagnosis

[Dual diagnosis]
adolescents, 261–262
addiction treatment, 224–237
affective disorders, 166–173,
210–213
alcoholism, 228–233
anorexia nervosa, 117–126
antisocial personality disorder,
180–182
anxiety disorders, 45–56, 173–
178, 213–215
attention deficit disorder, 178–179
bulimia nervosa, 117–126
cannabis, 127–138
clinical history, 160–161
conduct disorder, 179–180
definition, 3–5
diagnosis, 159–186, 205–207
genetics, 29–41
incidence, 4
laboratory studies, 161–162
and medical conditions, 5–7
medical evaluation, 207–208
neurological disorders, 75–104
opiate use, 154–155
personality disorder, 182–183,
217–218
post-traumatic stress disorder,
50–52
precursors, 191–192
prevalence, 139–159
alcoholism treatment units,
150
alcohol detoxification units,
150–151
emergency room, 141–142
inpatient psychiatry, 142–143
private psychiatric hospitals,
146–148
psychiatric practice, 140–141
public psychiatric hospitals,
144–146

[Dual diagnosis]
VA alcohol detoxification
units, 150–151
veterans hospitals, 143–144
psychoactive drug use, 163–166
psychoanalytic theories, 189–191
psychodynamics, 185–204
ego-self deficits, 187–189
deficits in self regulation, 187–
189
psychological testing, 162
psychosis, 215–217
psychotic evaluation, 208–210
self esteem, 195–200
therapy, 22–23
treatment, 152–154
personnel, 246–250
units, 241–246

Eating disorder
psychopharmacotherapy with
dual diagnosis patient, 331–
332
substance abuse, 119–123

Genetics
alcoholism, 31–36
antisocial personality, 36–37
anxiety disorder, 46
depression, 31–36
eating disorders, 119

Headache
cocaine, 83–85
substance abuse, 88–92

Intravenous drug use and neurological disorders, 85–86

Mania
    alcoholism, 109
    dual diagnosis, 167–169
Multiple sclerosis and substance
    abuse, 94–95


Neurological disorders, 75–104
    cocaine, 76–85
    intravenous drug use, 85–86
    solvent use, 86 87
    substance abuse, 87–100
NIDA adolescent assessment-
    referral system, 265–266


Obsessive compulsive disorder,
    pharmacotherapy with dual
    diagnosis patient, 327
Opiates, 62–63
    affective disorders, 110
    use and dual diagnosis, 154–155
Organic mental syndromes and al-
    coholism, 12–14


Pain and substance abuse, 92–94
Panic disorder
    agoraphobia, 47–49
    alcoholism, 47–49
    cocaine, 49
Personality disorders and dual di-
    agnosis, 217–218
    pharmacotherapy with dual di-
    agnosis patient, 329–330
Pharmacotherapy, 319–336
Phencyclidine and affective disor-
    der, 111
Post-traumatic stress disorder, 50–
    52
Psychoactive drug use and dual di-
    agnosis, 163–166

[Psychoactive drug use and dual
    diagnosis]
    psychopharmacotherapy with
    dual diagnosis patients, 327–
    331
Psychosis and dual diagnosis, 215–
    217
Psychostimulants and dual diagno-
    sis, 21
Psychotropie use and dual diagno-
    sis, 21–22


Schizophrenia
    drug use, 16–17
    psychopharmacotherapy with
    dually diagnosed patient, 332–
    333
Sedative-hypnotics and affective
    disorders, 110–111
Seizures
    alcoholism, 97–100
    cocaine, 76–68
Self-medication hypothesis, 107
Sexual dysfunction, 5–6
Solvent use
    dual diagnosis, 19–2
    neurological disorders, 86–87
Steroids, 66
Stimulants and affective disorders,
    109–110
Substance abuse
    affective disorders, 105–116
    chronic pain, 92–94
    cognitive impairment, 96–97
    eating disorders, 119–123
    headache, 88–92
    multiple sclerosis, 54–65
Sympathomimetics, 63–65


Thought disorder, 57–73

[Thought disorder]
  alcohol, 65–70
  anticholinergics, 61–62
  dissociatives, 59–61
  opiates, 62–61
  steroids, 66
  sympathomimetics, 63–65
Treatment
  adult inpatient substance abuse
    units, 242–243
  alcoholism and dual diagnosis,
    223–236
  drug abusers and dual diagnosis,
    237–257
  dual diagnosis treatment units,
    241–246
  dually diagnosed
    anxiety disorder patients, 328–
    329
    attention deficit disorder pa-
    tients, 332
    adolescents, 253–288
    borderline personality disor-
    der patients, 306–308
    depressed patients, 328
    eating disorder patients, 331–
    332

[Treatment]
    elderly patients, 303–306
    impulse control disordered pa-
    tients, 291–303
    obsessive compulsive disorder
    patients, 330
    panic disorder patient, 329–
    330
    post-traumatic stress disorder
    patient, 330–331
    schizophrenics, 332–333
  group therapy, 308–312
  hospitals, 243–244
  inpatient, of patients with pri-
    mary psychiatric diagnoses,
    297–317
  intensive outpatient drug reha-
    bilitation programs, 244–245
  partial psychiatric hospitaliza-
    tion programs, 245–246
  personnel, 246–250
  pharmacologia, 319–336
  problems, 312–315
    with the privileged patient,
    290–296
  psychiatric treatment units, 243
    244